# Dermatology
# for the
# Advanced Practice Nurse

**Faye Lyons, DNP, RN, FNP-C,** is a doctor of nursing practice–prepared family nurse practitioner who has been practicing in family medicine, internal medicine, dermatology, and aesthetic dermatology since 1999. Prior to becoming an NP, Dr. Lyons was a member of the armed services (U.S. Air Force), and an RN in medical, cardiac, and surgical intensive care units and dialysis units. Her experience in dermatology includes working in two large dermatology practices during her NP career and serving rural areas with dermatological services while working in internal medicine. Her responsibilities included skin examinations, biopsies, surgical excisions, and cosmetic procedures that included Botox, cosmetic fillers, and laser therapies. Dr. Lyons is credentialed in dermatology nursing by the Dermatology Nursing Association. Her publications include an award-winning poster presentation on dermatology decision trees at the 2012 Virginia Nurse Practioner Association meeting, dermatological chapters in an upcoming geriatric textbook titled *Healthy Aging: Principles and Clinical Practice for Clinicians* and in *Solving a Skin Rash in Primary Care: Use of a Diagnostic Decision Tree* in the journal *Advance for NPs and PAs*.

**Lisa Ousley, DNP, RN, FNP-C,** is a doctor of nursing practice–prepared family nurse practitioner who has been a primary care provider since 1999. Within primary care, Dr. Ousley has assessed, treated, and referred thousands of skin conditions. Dr. Ousley has been taking photos of skin conditions for many years and has a collection of over 1,000 photos, many of which are used in this book. Dr. Ousley is the director of Eastern Tennessee State University (ETSU) Student/University Health Services. This clinical opportunity supports health promotion and clinical management of acute and episodic illness for a culturally diverse university population. Dr. Ousley's past primary care experiences include Hillsville and Galax Family Care, outpatient hospital-based clinics in Virginia, and she has worked as a hospitalist service provider at Twin County Regional Hospital and in a clinic targeting the public-housing population in Johnson City, Tennessee. Since 2009, Dr. Ousley has been an online graduate instructor at the University of Phoenix, teaching graduate nursing theory.

# Dermatology for the Advanced Practice Nurse

Faye Lyons, DNP, RN, FNP-C
Lisa Ousley, DNP, RN, FNP-C

SPRINGER PUBLISHING COMPANY
NEW YORK

Copyright © 2015 Springer Publishing Company, LLC

All rights reserved.

No part of this publication may be reproduced, stored in a retrieval system, or transmitted in any form or by any means, electronic, mechanical, photocopying, recording, or otherwise, without the prior permission of Springer Publishing Company, LLC, or authorization through payment of the appropriate fees to the Copyright Clearance Center, Inc., 222 Rosewood Drive, Danvers, MA 01923, 978-750-8400, fax 978-646-8600, info@copyright.com or on the Web at www.copyright.com.

Springer Publishing Company, LLC
11 West 42nd Street
New York, NY 10036
www.springerpub.com

*Acquisitions Editor*: Margaret Zuccarini
*Composition*: diacriTech

*ISBN*: 978-0-8261-3643-5
*e-book ISBN*: 978-0-8261-3644-2
*Digital image bank ISBN*: 978-0-8261-2825-6

A digital image bank can be accessed at www.springerpub.com/lyons-image-bank

14 15 16 17 / 5 4 3 2 1

The author and the publisher of this Work have made every effort to use sources believed to be reliable to provide information that is accurate and compatible with the standards generally accepted at the time of publication. Because medical science is continually advancing, our knowledge base continues to expand. Therefore, as new information becomes available, changes in procedures become necessary. We recommend that the reader always consult current research and specific institutional policies before performing any clinical procedure. The author and publisher shall not be liable for any special, consequential, or exemplary damages resulting, in whole or in part, from the readers' use of, or reliance on, the information contained in this book. The publisher has no responsibility for the persistence or accuracy of URLs for external or third-party Internet websites referred to in this publication and does not guarantee that any content on such websites is, or will remain, accurate or appropriate.

**Library of Congress Cataloging-in-Publication Data**
Lyons, Faye, author.
  Dermatology for the advanced practice nurse / authors, Faye Lyons, Lisa Ousley.
       p. ; cm.
  Includes bibliographical references and index.
  ISBN 978-0-8261-3643-5—ISBN 978-0-8261-3644-2 (e-Book)
  I. Ousley, Lisa Ellen, author. II. Title.
  [DNLM: 1. Skin Diseases—nursing. 2. Nursing Diagnosis—methods. 3. Primary Nursing—methods. 4. Skin Care—nursing. WY 154.5]
  RL125
  616.5'0231—dc23
                                                                                            2014008527

Special discounts on bulk quantities of our books are available to corporations, professional associations, pharmaceutical companies, health care organizations, and other qualifying groups. If you are interested in a custom book, including chapters from more than one of our titles, we can provide that service as well.

**For details, please contact:**
Special Sales Department, Springer Publishing Company, LLC
11 West 42nd Street, 15th Floor, New York, NY 10036-8002
Phone: 877-687-7476 or 212-431-4370; Fax: 212-941-7842
E-mail: sales@springerpub.com

Printed in the United States of America by Bang Printing.

# Contents

*Preface    ix*
*Acknowledgments    xi*

## Part I. Overview of Dermatology

### 1. Education: Nurses and Primary Care Providers    3
Epidemiology and Statistics of Skin Disorders    4
Annual Economic Burden    5
Quality-of-Life Implications    5
Evidence-Based Practice and Decision Trees    6
Conceptual Framework for Assessing, Diagnosing, and Treating Skin Rashes    6
Decision Trees and Differential Diagnoses    8

### 2. Basics of Dermatology    15
Skin Anatomy and Physiology    15
Skin Terminology    19
Vascular Lesions    21
Diagnostic Evaluations    21
Distribution, Type, Characteristics, and Pattern of Lesions    22
Special Distribution Category: Patterns of Intentional or Unintentional Injury    22

### 3. Special Considerations for Populations, Culture, and Comorbid Conditions    27
Infants and Children    27
The Elderly    27
Ethnicity    28
Cultural Practices    28
Puberty    29
Pregnancy    29

# Part II. Clinical Management of Dermatology Conditions

### 4. Skin Assessment     35
History     35
Skin Assessment (Physical)     35
Social History     36
Family History     36
Dermatologic Signs     36
Differential Diagnosis     37

### 5. Diagnostics     39
Collecting Specimens     39
Mycology: Microscopic Examination of Scale (Potassium Hydroxide)     40
Use of Mechanical Devices     41

### 6. Treatment Approaches     43
Topical Treatment     43
Systemic Evaluation and Treatment     45
Surgical Treatment     46
Other Treatments     46

### 7. Clinical Management     51
Routine Skin Care     51
Preventive Care     52
Skin Self-Examination     52
Protection From the Sun     53
Moisturizer     54
Nutritional Counseling     55
Appropriate Referrals     56
Genetic Counseling Referrals     58

# Part III. Common Dermatologic Conditions

**Abrasions and Skin Tears**     61
**Acne**     65
**Alopecia**     71
**Aphthous Stomatitis**     79
**Bruise and Contusion**     85
**Burns**     89
**Candidiasis**     95
**Cellulitis/Erysipelas**     109
**Cysts**     115
**Dermatitis**     129
**Erythema Multiforme**     151
**Erythema Nodosum**     157
**Granuloma Annulare**     163
**Herpes Simplex Virus**     169
**Impetigo**     193

Insect Bites     199
Lentigo/Nevi     213
Lichen Planus    223
Molluscum Contagiosum    229
Nail Conditions  235
Pemphigus    249
Perioral Dermatitis    255
Pityriasis Rosea    259
Psoriasis    265
Rosacea    273
Skin Cancer    279
Tinea Infections    303
Urticaria    321
Vasculitis    327
Verruca Vulgaris    337
Vitiligo    345

*Glossary*    351

*Index*    363

# Preface

In primary care, common things occur regularly. This definitely applies to skin conditions. However, each patient and his or her skin is unique. Common dermatological problems seen frequently in primary care practice can be difficult to identify. Becoming educated about the descriptors provides an important foundation for building clinical skills in assessment, differential diagnosis, and preferred management of common skin conditions. Fifteen years ago, when we attended college to become nurse practitioners, there was no formal training in dermatology. Our introduction to dermatology was a 2-hour lecture that covered common rashes and skin cancers. Needless to say, 2 hours is not enough time to cover dermatology.

Dermatology is a complex and challenging field of study. Learning more about the skin reveals that it is one of the most amazing organs in the body. The skin tells us when there are abnormalities or health issues inside the body, it shows us the nutritional status of an individual, and it can also be an indicator of emotional concerns. Knowledge of the most common dermatological presentations elevates the provider's skills and abilities to offer appropriate care to patients.

This book features dermatology diagnostics, treatments, and management strategies. Dermatologic diagnostics include skin assessment, specimen collection, and the use of mechanical devices. Evidence-based topical, systemic, and surgical treatment options for skin conditions are provided. Additionally, wide-ranging management strategies are included.

To facilitate the practitioners' ability to more quickly identify which of the 60 conditions a patient has, the section covering these conditions is organized using a standard format that includes overview, epidemiology, etiology, clinical presentation, histology, differential diagnosis, treatment and management, special considerations and appropriate referrals, patient education, patient follow-up, and clinical pearls. Of utmost importance and to help the clinician in identifying each condition, photos are provided to highlight important visual identifiers for each condition. This collection of photos was taken by Dr. Ousley and her colleagues and captures actual patient presentations observed by them during primary care patient visits. **Additional photos can be found at the Springer Publishing Company website in a digital image bank, which can be accessed through www.springerpub.com/lyons-image-bank.**

An especially unique feature of this book is the dermatological decision trees. These decision trees are clinical tools that were developed by Dr. Lyons. They provide a graphic representation to guide the user from known information at the apex of the tree to a final choice based on observation and logic. Decision trees direct professionals toward diagnoses of common skin conditions.

As APNs, we believe strongly that offering this clinically useful resource captures the most common presentations in primary care that are imperative for all practicing APNs. This book features over 60 dermatological conditions that present and re-present in practice. It provides comprehensive evidence-based information on these common skin diseases and their recommended treatment and management.

**Faye Lyons**
**Lisa Ousley**

# Acknowledgments

Thank you to my husband, Dustin, and my daughter, Kimberly, for being patient and supportive of me while I was writing this book.

This book has been a goal of mine for approximately 15 years and now my goal has been achieved with the help of Springer Publishing Company and my friend Lisa Ousley. I submitted my decision trees and a draft of what I wanted my book to be to Margaret Zuccarini a year ago. She accepted my proposal and asked if I had pictures to submit. When I did not, she told me of a nurse practitioner who had pictures that she wanted to publish. When she gave me Lisa's name and phone number, I laughed because Lisa and I had graduated from school together 14 years before. It seems that this book was meant to be!

—*Faye Lyons*

Since the beginning of my primary care practice I recognized the abundance of presenting skin conditions and this influenced my clinical interest in dermatology. Many generous patients have permitted me to take hundreds of pictures during clinic and the majority of usable photos were taken from my cell or smart phones. I now understand that megapixels do translate to quality photographs.

At a doctor of nursing practice (DNP) conference, I expressed interest in writing my first book about primary care dermatology and including my photographs. The publisher, Margaret Zuccarini, remembered this conversation and a few years later contacted me. A collaborative agreement was arranged with my partner, Dr. Faye Lyons.

This project has been a journey of learning and discovery. Co-authoring a book can be a daunting task and is a learned skill in progress. I have also confirmed that the majority of clinicians lack knowledge and skill in dermatology recognition and treatment. I have discovered generous colleagues who also aspire to increase their skills in dermatology practice. I acknowledge that I continue to have much to learn about the body's largest—and perhaps most complex—organ, the skin.

—*Lisa Ousley*

# PART I
# Overview of Dermatology

1. Education: Nurses and Primary Care Providers   3
2. Basics of Dermatology   15
3. Special Considerations for Populations, Culture, and Comorbid Conditions   27

# 1
# Education: Nurses and Primary Care Providers

Aristotle said, "It is the mark of an educated mind to be able to entertain a thought without accepting it." Aristotle may not have realized how easily this could be applied to a practitioner considering a skin condition. These thoughts, in this case, differential diagnoses, should be based on education, evidence, and experience. However, nurse practitioners, physician assistants, and primary care physicians all too often lack education in basic dermatologic science, dermatopathology, and research.

The need for improving dermatology education has been identified on the basis of the high rates of skin diseases, especially in the elderly population (Shelby, 2008). Realistically, more often than not, it is primary care nurse practitioners and physicians who are the initial providers for patients with a skin condition. All providers are thus challenged to educate themselves to respond competently to common dermatologic conditions in these patients. Although the importance of this education is recognized, the educational needs of practitioners are frequently unmet (Courtenay & Carey, 2006).

The majority of health care professionals agree that rashes are often confusing and can be difficult to diagnose. Studies indicate a knowledge deficit of primary care providers with regard to common dermatoses (Christenson & Sontheimer, 2010). One prospective study of 165 general practitioners found that in 57% of cases, their diagnoses agreed with dermatologists' clinical diagnoses or with histology, but 43% were in disagreement (Moreno, Tran, Chia, Lim, & Shumack, 2007). Inexperience with dermatologic disorders among providers translates into inadequate diagnoses and/or inappropriate treatment of skin conditions, prompting a need for more effective teaching mechanisms in the area of dermatology (Christenson & Sontheimer, 2010).

Inexperience in dermatology for primary care practice providers is related to a lack of dermatology training. Only 10% of nurse practitioners and physician assistants have received formal dermatology training at a teaching institution; however, 53% reported that they had a dermatology rotation in a clinic during their education (Resneck & Kimball, 2008). A systematic review conducted by Loescher, Harris, and Curiel-Lewandrowski (2011) identified the barriers to advanced practice nurses' performance of skin cancer assessment, their ability to recognize and identify suspicious lesions, and their training for skin cancer detection. The research found time constraints and inadequate training to be the prevalent barriers for these providers. Another survey, conducted by the American Academy of Pediatrics, showed that patients younger than age 18 years account for 58% of general dermatology patients. Most dermatologists surveyed had received referrals for common childhood skin conditions, and the vast majority of the children referred were initially diagnosed and treated incorrectly (Dinulos, 2007).

Lack of dermatology education is not exclusive to nurse practitioners. A significant number of U.S. medical school graduates pursue careers in primary care medicine and dedicate 4.1% to 6.2% of their appointment times to dermatologic diseases (Fleischer, Herbert, Feldman, & O'Brien, 2000). Ninety-two primary care physicians and 252 primary care residents were surveyed regarding the training received while in medical school (Hansra, O'Sullivan, Chen, & Berger, 2008). According to the primary care residents, dermatology was not as adequately taught compared with other curricular areas. Less than 40% believed that their medical school adequately prepared them to diagnose and treat common skin diseases. The American Academy of Dermatology surveyed 120 medical school deans to determine the amount of dermatologic training medical students received. According to survey results, the average medical student received fewer than 18 hours of dermatologic didactics and training (Shelby, 2008).

There are two major reasons why primary care physicians, nurse practitioners, and physician assistants have difficulty diagnosing rashes. First, different conditions can produce similar rashes (Ely & Stone, 2010b). For example, both psoriasis and fungal rashes can appear scaled. Second, a single skin condition can result in different presentations. One example is contact dermatitis, which may present with a vesicular, scaled, papular, or macular rash.

Furthermore, primary care providers frequently have appointments scheduled every 10 to 15 minutes. Consequently, when a patient presents with a rash, clinicians do not have time to search databases, Internet resources, textbooks, and articles to assist in diagnosis (Awadalla, Rosenbaum, Camacho, Fleischer, & Feldman, 2008).

Nurse practitioners, physicians, and physician assistants in primary care need accurate, effective, and efficient tools to guide them in diagnosing rashes. Clinical dermatology education requires clinical exposure and experience; interaction with and feedback from instructors; and quality, focused knowledge acquisition. Unfortunately, there is minimal commitment toward dermatology training with respect to clinical requirements of advanced practice, medical, or general nursing programs.

## EPIDEMIOLOGY AND STATISTICS OF SKIN DISORDERS

At any given time, there are more than 3,000 skin conditions affecting one in two Americans (Jones & Kalabokes, 2010). In the United States, the health care system relies heavily on primary care clinics to manage a variety of conditions, including dermatologic conditions. In fact, dermatologists treat only 30% to 40% of patients with skin disease, which leaves the majority of skin disorders to be treated by other specialties, 22% of whom are family medicine providers (Awadalla et al., 2008). As advancements in medical knowledge develop, family medicine providers face the continually rising challenge of diagnosing and applying evidence-based treatments for skin disorders. Providers must maintain competence in disease identification and management, as well as an understanding of when it is appropriate to refer a patient to a dermatologist (Awadalla et al., 2008).

When considering the leading dermatologic disorders for each major racial and ethnic group in the United States, providers should be aware that some dermatologic disorders are known to be much more common in patients of color (Davis et al., 2012). According to Davis et al. (2012), the top five diagnoses for African American patients in dermatology clinics were acne, unspecified dermatitis or eczema, seborrheic dermatitis, atopic dermatitis, and dyschromia. For Asian or Pacific Islander patients, the top five were acne, unspecified dermatitis or eczema, benign neoplasm of the skin, psoriasis, and seborrheic keratosis. By contrast, in Caucasian patients, the top five were actinic keratosis, acne, benign neoplasm of the skin, unspecified dermatitis or eczema, and nonmelanoma skin cancer. In Hispanic patients of any race, the leading diagnoses were acne, unspecified dermatitis or eczema, psoriasis, benign neoplasm of the skin, and viral warts.

The identification of cutaneous diseases affecting the increasing ethnic populations serves to focus research and clinical resources (Taylor, 2003). Undoubtedly, dermatology health care needs to respond to all skin types and colors. Traditional use of Eurocentric tools and scales has little to no relevance to skin of color. The impetus to gain cultural competence is certainly related to population shifts (Czerkasij, 2013). In our current reality, Whites are the majority population in the United States. However, within the next 30 years, the current minority populations (Asians, Hispanics, Blacks, and American Indians) will shift into the majority. Culturally competent health care, both within primary care and dermatology, mandates providers understanding and acquiring skills in treating skin of color.

## ANNUAL ECONOMIC BURDEN

Skin disorders affect 20% to 30% of the U.S. population (Williams et al., 2008). In 2004, the estimated total economic burden of skin diseases in this country was $96 billion (Khatami & Sebastian, 2009). The number of skin problems that present to primary care practices is 15.1 per 100 patient encounters, making dermatologic complaints the third most common reason for primary care appointments. Only respiratory (21.4 per 100 patients) and musculoskeletal (16.3 per 100 patients) complaints are more numerous (Moreno et al., 2007). Because managed care has promoted primary care practitioners to be caretakers for cost-effectiveness and a shortage of dermatologists exists, primary care providers are challenged with diagnosing and treating many skin lesions and conditions (Bruner & Schaffer, 2012). Up to 79% of the U.S. population visit a primary care provider annually, and the majority of these visit are skin related (Shelby, 2008).

## QUALITY-OF-LIFE IMPLICATIONS

The burden of skin disease extends beyond the financial cost and generates intangible costs associated with decreased quality of life (Lewin Group, 2005). It is most often in primary care that the clinician encounters a patient with a skin problem. Primary care is defined as comprehensive care, and providers consider a major advantage of this specialty to be the delivery of general counseling and preventative care of their patients (Feldman & Fleischer, 2000). However, it appears that simple skin disease is not so simple for primary care providers to diagnose and manage. Roughly 20% to 25% of patients encountered in primary care experience a skin disorder at some point in their lives (Bruner & Schaffer, 2012). This was confirmed by Feldman, Fleischer, and Chen (1999) in a study that looked at the prospect of referral of patients from primary care providers to other specialists. Referral of the patient from the primary care provider is more common for skin problems than for other, nonskin medical problems.

The most common reasons for referral of patients with skin disease were not complex or rare disorders but rather common, simple skin problems such as dermatitis, warts, cysts, cellulitis, acne, and other rashes (Feldman et al., 1999). With nearly 2,200 diseases and disorders affecting the skin, accurate dermatologic diagnosis can be difficult (Czerkasij, 2010). Misdiagnosis of skin rashes can result in unnecessary office visits, prescriptions, costs, patient suffering, disfigurement, and even fatality.

## EVIDENCE-BASED PRACTICE AND DECISION TREES

Evidence-based practice (EBP) is the foundation for clinical practice guidelines, and an understanding of EBP is needed to comprehend the basis for these guidelines. EBP uses critical thinking, evaluation, and the application of research data for making clinical decisions to improve the delivery of treatment interventions and to promote the best patient care outcomes (Adamson, 2009). The search for the best evidence starts with systematic reviews and evidence-based clinical practice guidelines (Figure 1.1).

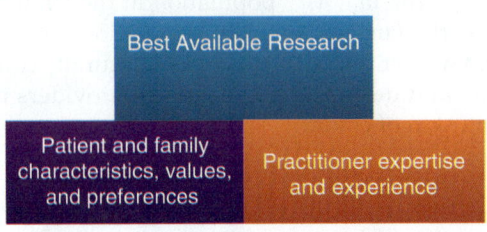

FIGURE 1.1  Evidence-based practice.

A systematic review is a summary of evidence on a specific topic, typically by an expert or experts who uses an arduous process for identifying, appraising, and combining studies to answer a specific question (Vickers, 2009). The large number of clinical studies in dermatology and the lack of agreement on the management of many skin disorders suggest that systemic reviews are a way of improving the evidence and guiding clinical decisions. However, systemic reviews alone cannot be expected to overcome the methodological limitations in dermatologic research. Inversely, it seems that systemic reviews, if not properly guided by important clinical questions, may intensify the unimportant issues and result in a misleading scale of evidence to guide clinical decisions (Williams et al., 2008).

The Agency for Healthcare Research and Quality (AHRQ) provides free online EBP guidelines through the National Guideline Clearinghouse. However, health care providers need to know what to look for when researching this site to access the proper treatment guidelines.

## CONCEPTUAL FRAMEWORK FOR ASSESSING, DIAGNOSING, AND TREATING SKIN RASHES

The concept of assessing, diagnosing, and treating skin disease can be broadly defined yet requires systematic organization. A conceptual framework provides focus and directs rationale for the complex diagnoses of thousands of skin disorders that a provider may encounter in practice. The framework is a tool for integration and interpretation of information provided by the patient during the primary care office visit. Using a conceptual framework (Figure 1.2) to direct the assessment, diagnosis, and treatment of a patient during a primary care office visit, the provider would do the following:

1. Observe the patient who presents with a rash of unknown origin or cause to the primary care office.
2. Obtain a thorough history of the rash and associated symptoms that the patient may have experienced or may currently be experiencing.
3. Perform a complete review of symptoms.

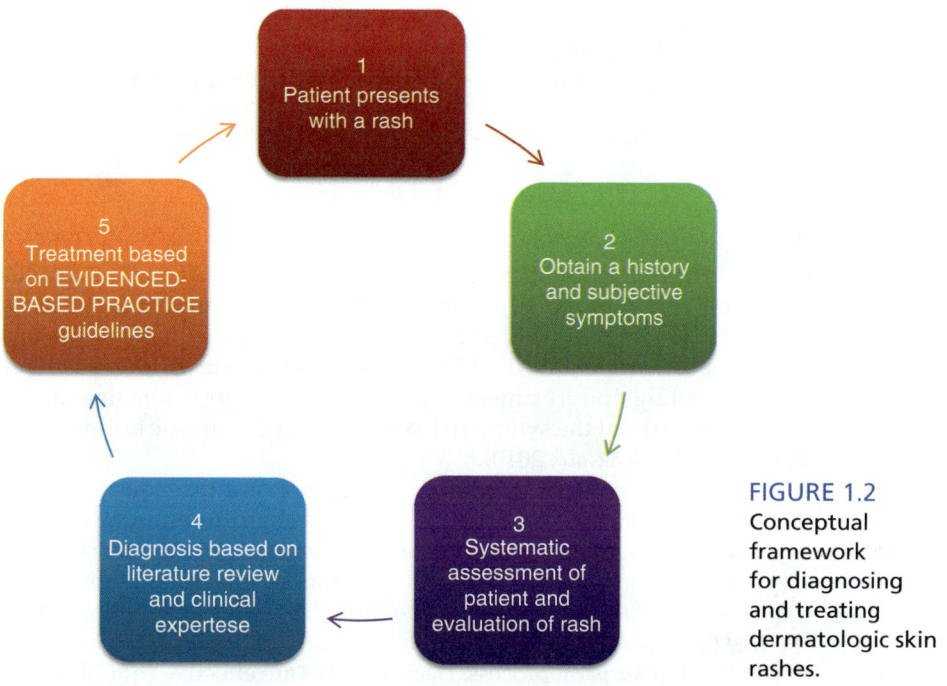

FIGURE 1.2 Conceptual framework for diagnosing and treating dermatologic skin rashes.

First, ask a well-constructed clinical question that includes an accurate description of the patient or problem. The clinical question has four elements: a patient or problem, an intervention, a comparison intervention, and an outcome (referred to with the acronym PICO). A well-informed clinical question offers two benefits: It supports an efficient search for evidence, and it enhances the critical appraisal of the evidence identified through the search (Williams et al., 2008).

Second, ask the patient about recent travel; hobbies; contact with people who are ill, pets, or insects; drug exposure, including over-the-counter, herbal medications, and illicit drugs; relevant sexual history; and whether he or she has had occupational exposures, chemical exposures, chronic illness, and recent symptoms, especially fever. Evaluate for pruritus and painful lesions, and examine the initial site of involvement.

Finally, ask about personal or family history of asthma, eczema, or allergies (Ely & Stone, 2010b).

4. Perform a head-to-toe physical examination after having the patient remove street clothing and shoes and don a hospital gown. Examination of the genital area may be eliminated unless there is a specific complaint or symptom involving this area. Palpate lymph nodes, evaluate neurologic status, assess body temperature, and evaluate general appearance.
5. Evaluate the rash closely. Several signs can help narrow the diagnosis. Ascertain whether the rash is papular, vesicular, scaly, or macular. Identify where the rash is located on the body. Determine any unique association of locations or patterns for the rash. For example, is the rash on one side of the body, not crossing the midline of the body? Is the rash on the feet and hands only? Is there involvement near a site of trauma? Does the rash bleed easily if scale is removed? Does the rash blanch when pressure is applied?
6. Consult a clinical reference. There are many great references for rashes, but sometimes it is not feasible to conduct a thorough literature review within a limited time frame. Located in this chapter are decision trees that will aid the provider

in diagnosing the rash. If the diagnosis remains elusive, refer the patient for a dermatology consultation.
7. After a diagnosis has been established, treatment can be introduced.

## DECISION TREES AND DIFFERENTIAL DIAGNOSES

Because of the large number of skin conditions that present as a rash in primary care, it can be difficult for providers to generate a complete differential diagnosis at the initial office visit (Ely & Stone, 2010a). In a clinical situation in which significant morbidity or mortality can occur, a rapid and accurate skin diagnosis is critical to making treatment decisions. It is imperative that the provider formulate inclusive differential diagnoses to direct testing and treatment strategies. If a diagnosis remains unclear, the clinician may decide to treat the symptoms, order further diagnostic testing, or consult a dermatologist (Kelly & Stone, 2010).

An accurate description of skin lesions allows the clinician to formulate a series of differential diagnoses (Corvette, 2011). Decision trees, originally developed in the 1940s for financial and governmental use, employ a progressive succession of possible choices (O'Brien, 2008). When skin descriptors are placed on decision trees, they supply a graphic representation to guide the provider from known information at the apex of the tree to a final choice based on observation and logic. In this way, they simplify and streamline the decision process. Decision trees are effective clinical tools to aid in obtaining a correct differential diagnosis for the skin rashes commonly seen in primary care. This chapter supplies four original anatomically directed and designed decision trees for assisting a clinician in diagnosing common skin rashes and diseases most often seen in primary care: face, torso, extremities, and genitals.

# FACE

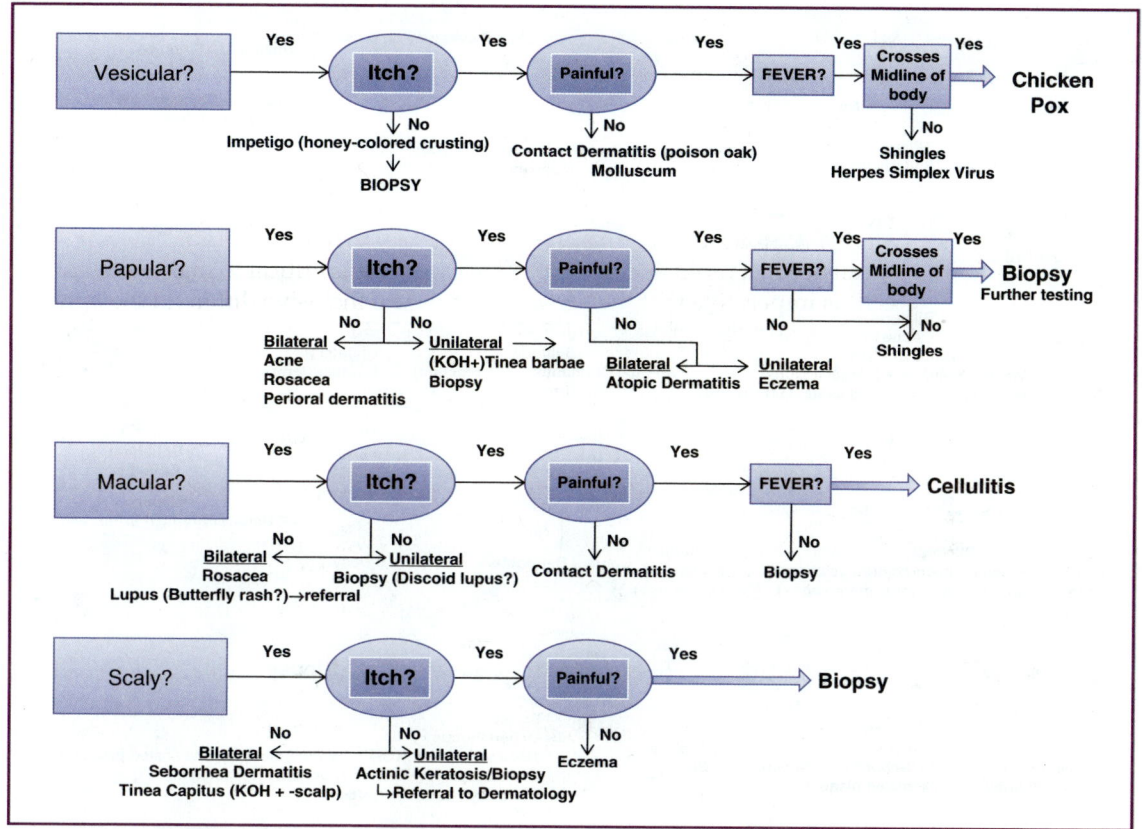

## TORSO

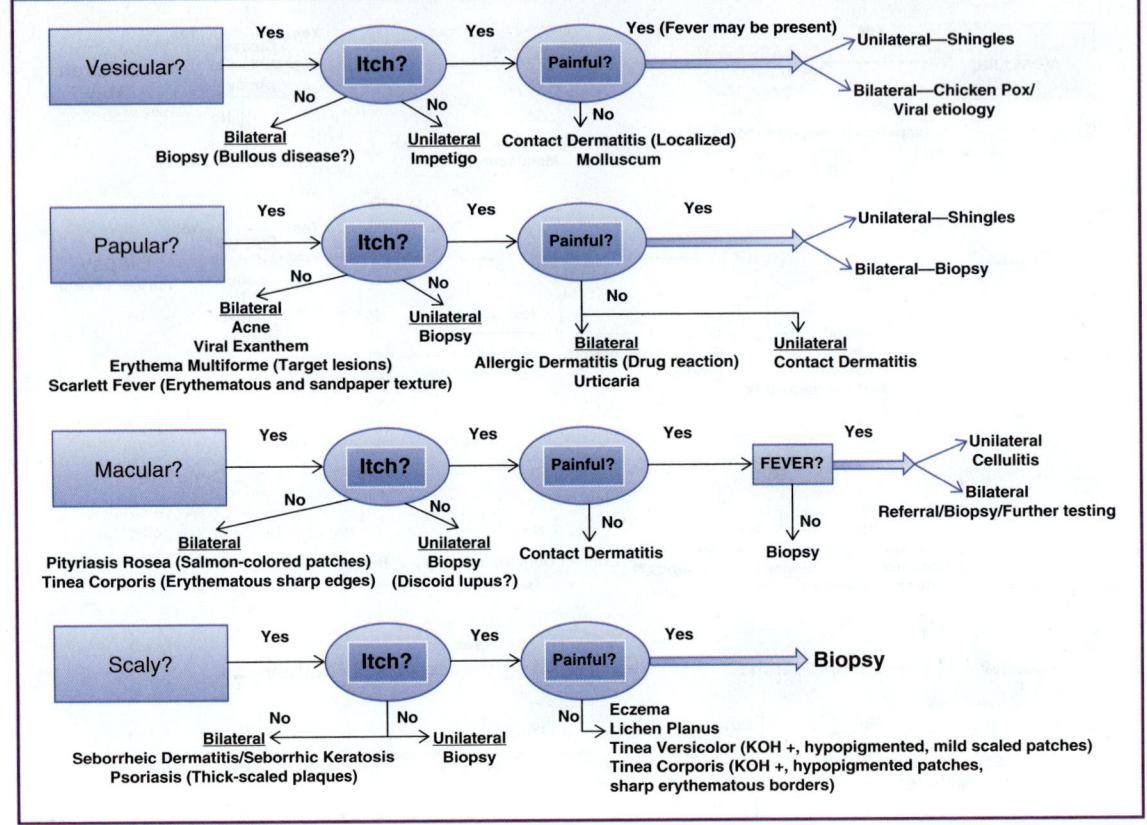

# EXTREMITIES

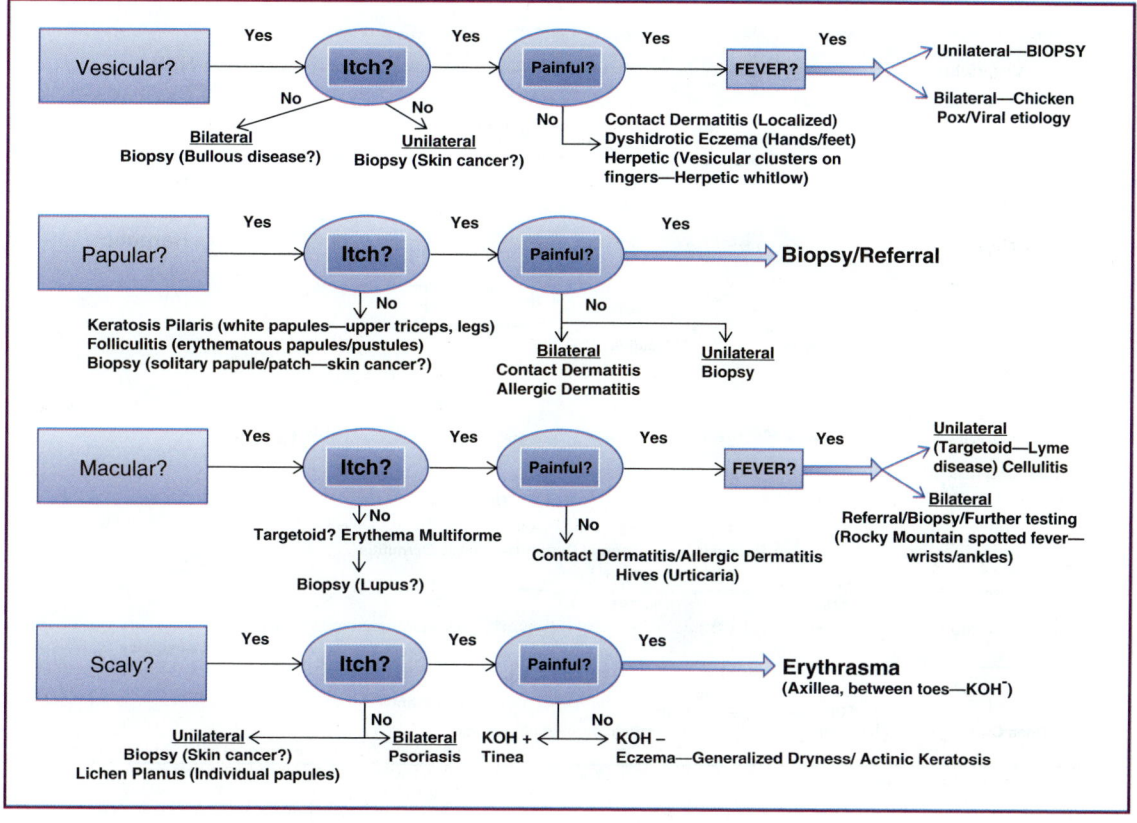

# GENITALS

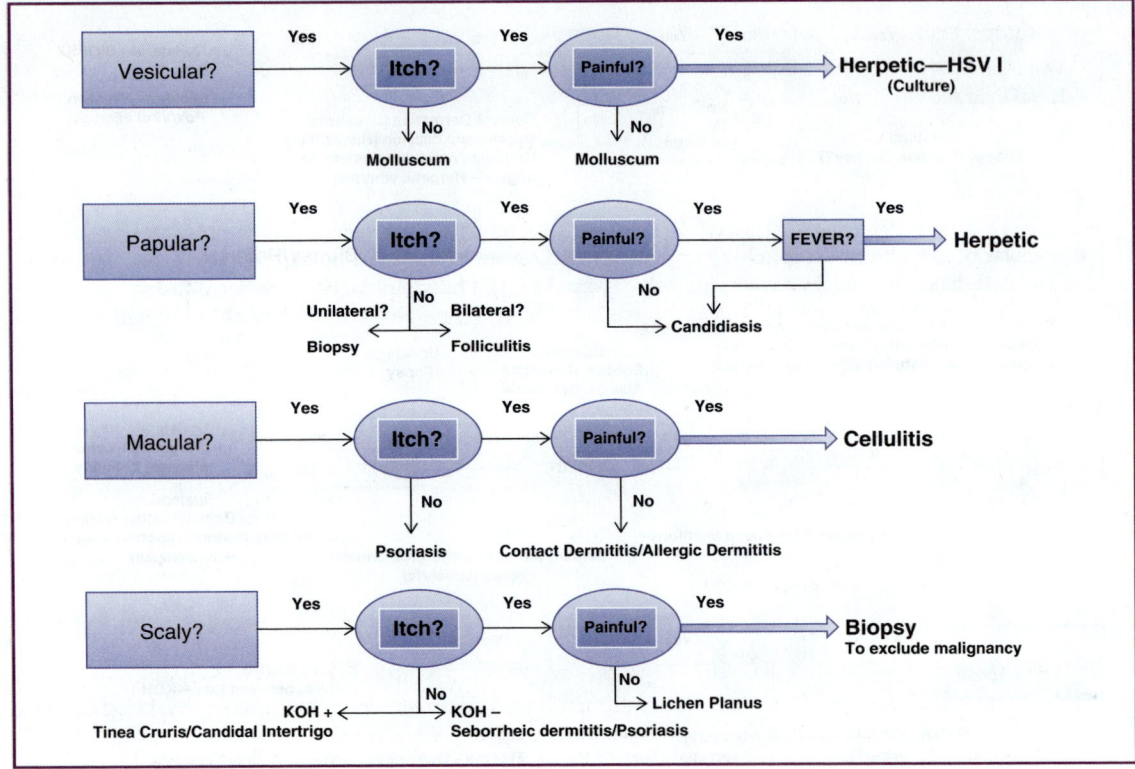

# REFERENCES

Adamson, T. (2009). Dermatology nursing excellence: The impact of professional knowledge on environment. *Journal of the Dermatology Nurses' Association, 1*(1), 48–52.

Awadalla, F., Rosenbaum, D. A., Camacho, F., Fleischer, A., & Feldman, S. R. (2008). Dermatologic disease in family medicine. *Family Medicine, 40*(7), 507–511.

Bruner, A., & Schaffer, S. D. (2012). Diagnosing skin lesions: Clinical considerations for primary care practitioners. *Journal for Nurse Practitioners, 8*(8), 600–604.

Christenson, D., & Sontheimer, L. (2010). Epidemiology and outcomes of dermatology inpatient consultations in a Midwestern U.S. university hospital. *Dermatology Online Journal, 16*(2), 12.

Corvette, D. (2011). Morphology of primary and secondary lesions. In J. E. Fitzpatrick & J. G. Morelli (Eds.), *Dermatology secrets plus* (4th ed., pp. 14–21). Philadelphia, PA: Elsevier/Mosby.

Courtenay, M., & Carey, N. (2006). Nurse-led care in dermatology: A review of the literature. *British Journal of Dermatology, 154*(1), 1–6.

Czerkasij, V. A. (2010). A strategy for learning dermatology. *Journal of Nursing Practice, 67*(7), 555–556.

Davis, S. A., Narahari, S., Feldman, S. R., Huang, W., Pichardo-Geisinger, R. O., & McMichael, A. J. (2012). Top dermatologic conditions in patients of color: An analysis of nationally representative data. *Journal of Drugs in Dermatology, 11*(4), 466–473.

Dinulos, J. (2007). Pediatric dermatology: Past, present and future. *Current Opinion in Pediatrics, 19*, 417–419.

Ely, J. W., & Stone, M. (2010a). The generalized rash: Part 1. Differential diagnosis. *American Family Physician, 81*(6), 726–734.

Ely, J. W., & Stone, M. S. (2010b). The generalized rash: Part 2. Differential diagnosis. *American Family Physician, 81*(6), 735–739.

Feldman, S. R., & Fleischer, A. B., Jr. (2000). Role of the dermatologist in the delivery of dermatologic care. *Dermatologic Clinics, 18*(2), 223–227.

Feldman, S. R., Fleischer, A. B., Jr., & Chen, J. G. (1999). Patients seen by primary care providers for dermatologic problems are frequently referred to dermatologist: Inefficiency of the gatekeeper system. *Journal of the American Academy of Dermatology, 40*, 426–432.

Fleischer, A., Herbert, C., Feldman, S., & O'Brien, F. (2000). Diagnosis of skin disease by nondermatologist. *American Journal of Managed Care, 6*, 1149–1156.

Hansra, N. K., O'Sullivan, P., Chen, C. L., & Berger, T. G. (2008). Medical school dermatology curriculum: Are we adequately preparing primary care physicians? *Journal of the American Academy of Dermatology, 61*(1), 23–29.

Jones, J., & Kalabokes, V. (2010). Coalition of skin diseases. *Journal of the Dermatology Nurses' Association, 2*(5), 214–217.

Khatami, A., & Sebastian, M. S. (2009). Skin disease: A neglected public health problem. *Dermatology Clinics, 27*(2), 99–101.

The Lewin Group. (2005). *The burden of skin diseases.* Retrieved from http://www.lewin.com/~/media/lewin/site_sections/publications/april2005skindisease

Loescher, L. J., Harris, J. M., & Curiel-Lewandrowski, C. (2011). A systematic review of advanced practice nurses' skin cancer assessment barriers, skin lesion recognition skills, and skin cancer training activities. *Journal of the American Academy of Nurse Practitioners, 23*, 667–672.

Moreno, G., Tran, J., Chia, A., Lim, A., & Shumack, S. (2007). Prospective study to assess general practitioners' dermatological diagnostic skills in a referral setting. *Australasian Journal of Dermatology, 48*(2), 77–82.

O'Brien, S. H. (2008). Decision analysis in pediatric hematology. *Pediatric Clinics of North America, 55*(2), 287–304.

Resneck, J. S., & Kimball, A. B. (2008). Who else is providing care in dermatology practices? Trends in the use of nonphysician clinicians. *Journal of the American Academy of Dermatology, 58*(2), 211–216.

Shelby, D. (2008). The development of a standardized dermatology residency program for the clinical doctorate in advanced nursing practice. *Dermatology Nursing, 20*(6), 437–447.

Taylor, S. C. (2003). Epidemiology of skin diseases in ethnic populations. *Dermatologic Clinics, 21*(4), 601–607.

Vickers, A. (2009). Evidence-based practice guidelines for skin cancer screening. *Dermatology Nursing, 21*(1), 15–18.

Williams, H., Bigby, M., Diepgen, T., Herxheimer, A., Naldi, L., & Rzany, B. (2008) *Evidence-based dermatology* (2nd ed.). Maiden, MA: Blackwell Publishing.

# 2
# Basics of Dermatology

## SKIN ANATOMY AND PHYSIOLOGY

The skin, as the largest organ of the body, accounts for approximately 15% of the total adult body weight. It performs many vital functions, including protection against external physical, chemical, and biological aggressors, as well as prevention of excess water loss from the body and thermoregulation (Kolarsick, Kolarsick, & Goodwin, 2011).

The skin is a protective barrier. Specifically, the stratum corneum, the outmost layer of the epidermis, provides protection. The barrier is impermeable. It is made of fatty acids, cholesterol, and ceramides. Keratinocytes are part of the physical barrier as well. The skin assists in fluid balance and protects against infections, toxins, and harmful ultraviolet (UV) radiation (Habif, 2004). Maintaining or restoring the functions of the skin's barrier is an important goal of therapy.

## The Parts of the Skin

The *epidermis* (Figure 2.1) is a continually renewing layer and gives rise to derived structures, such as pilosebaceous apparatuses, nails, and sweat glands (Kolarsick et al., 2011). The epidermis, the outermost portion of the skin, consists of two major layers: the stratum corneum and the cellular stratum. The basement membrane that lies beneath the cellular stratum connects the epidermis to the dermis. Because the epidermis is avascular, it depends on the underlying dermis for nutrition (Jarvis, 2012). The other layers of the skin are as follows:

- The *stratum corneum*, the outermost layer of the epidermis, protects the body against harmful environmental substances and restricts water loss. It has waterproof keratin that lets water out but not in and protects the body from bacteria.
- The *stratum germinativum* is the innermost layer of the epidermis. It is here that mitosis (growth of new cells) takes place, and new cells push old cells to the surface. Merkel cells, the receptors responsible for the sense of touch, are located in this layer.
- *Cellular stratum* is the layer in which keratin cells are synthesized.

The *dermis* (Figure 2.1) is connected to underlying organs by the *hypodermis*, a subcutaneous layer that consists of loose connective tissue filled with fatty cells. This adipose layer generates heat and provides insulation, shock absorption, and a reserve of calories (Jarvis, 2012; Kolarsick et al., 2011; Scanlon & Saunders, 1999).

A number of glands and cell types contribute to the multiple functions of the skin. *Eccrine glands* open directly to the skin and regulate body temperature through water secretion. These glands are all over the body except the lip margins, eardrums, nail beds, inner surface of the prepuce, and the glans penis (Jarvis, 2012; Scanlon & Saunders, 1999).

The *apocrine glands* are specialized structures found only in the axillae, nipples, areolae, anogenital area, eyelids, and external ears. These glands are larger and located more deeply than the eccrine glands. In response to stimuli, these glands secrete a white fluid containing protein, carbohydrate, and other substances. Secretions from these glands are odorless; body odor is produced by bacterial decomposition of apocrine sweat (Jarvis, 2012; Kolarsick et al., 2011; Scanlon & Saunders, 1999).

The *sebaceous glands* secrete *sebum*, a lipid-rich substance that keeps the skin and hair from drying out. Secretory activity, which is stimulated by sex hormones (testosterone mostly), varies according to hormonal levels throughout the life span.

The *Langerhans cells* originate in the bone marrow. These cells break down foreign material, such as bacteria, that enters our bodies through breaks in the skin and travels to the lymph nodes, which triggers an immune response.

*Melanocytes* are found in the lower epidermis where they produce a protein, a pigment called melanin. Melanin gives skin its color. Both heredity and exposure to UV light contribute to melanin production. Additionally, hair color and eye color are derived from melanin.

*Fibroblasts* are cells in connective tissue that produce the skin's collagen and elastin fibers. Their primary function is to maintain the structural integrity of connective tissues. Fibroblasts play a vital role in wound healing.

*Hair follicles* are made up of the hair root, the hair shaft, and the pilomotor or arrector pili muscles. Hair goes through cyclic changes: anagen (growth), catagen (atrophy), and telogen (rest), after which the hair is shed. Males and females have the same number of hair follicles, which are stimulated to differential growth by hormones.

The *nails* are epidermal cells converted to hard plates of keratin. The nail bed is highly vascular and lies beneath the plate, giving the nail its pink color. The white crescent-shaped area extending beyond the proximal nail fold marks the end of the nail matrix, the site of nail growth. The stratum corneum layer of the skin covering the nail root is the cuticle, which pushes up and over the lower part of the nail body. The paronychium is the soft tissue surrounding the nail border. Overall, the skin has multiple functions. These include protection, barrier, perception, temperature regulation, identification, communication, wound repair, absorption and excretion, and vitamin production.

Blood vessels also help maintain body temperature. When arterial constriction decreases blood flow, heat stays in the body. Conversely, dilation increases blood flow, so heat is brought to the surface of the body—the skin—and released. Subcutaneous tissue contains superficial fascia that connects the dermis to underlying muscle. Areolar connective tissue connects the dermis to the muscles and contains white blood cells. Adipose tissue contains stored energy in the form of true fats, cushions the body, and provides insulation from the cold.

Secretion and excretion are significant functions of the skin. Sweat is produced by the eccrine/apocrine glands. Small amounts of urea and sodium chloride are excreted in sweat.

A form of cholesterol exists in the skin that, upon exposure to the sun's UV light, is changed to vitamin D. This vitamin allows calcium to be absorbed into the bones.

2. Basics of Dermatology  17

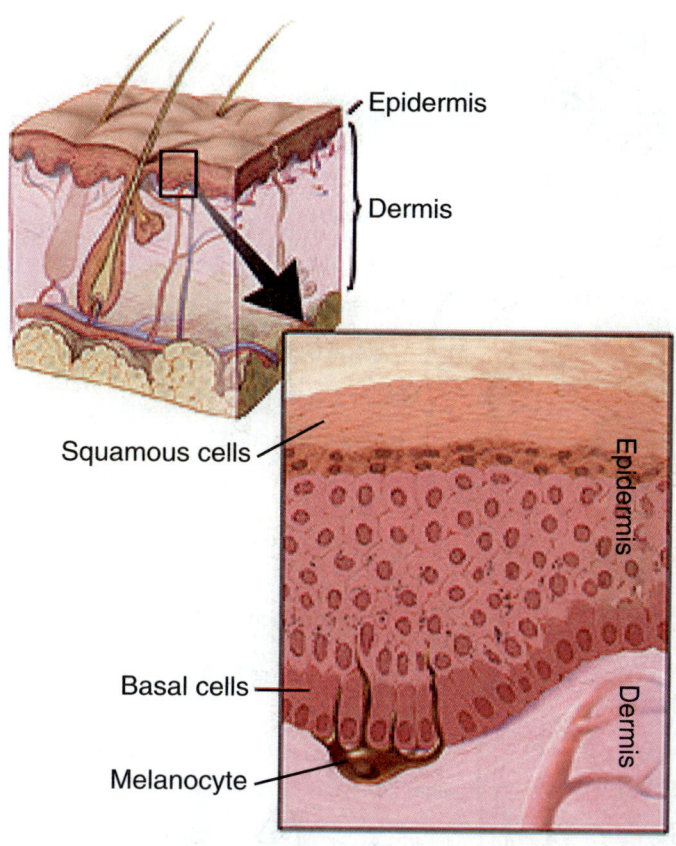

FIGURE 2.1  Skin anatomy
Source: National Cancer Institute

## Dermatomes

The surface of the skin is divided into specific areas. The areas, called *dermatomes*, originate from somite cells, and the somite cells differentiate into three regions. The second region, also called the dermatome, forms connective tissues, including the dermis.

Dermatomes are predominantly supplied by a single spinal nerve root (Apok, Gurusinghe, Mitchell, & Emsley, 2011). There are 31 segments of the spinal cord that comprise the 8 cervical nerves, 12 thoracic nerves, 5 lumbar nerves, 5 sacral nerves, and 1 coccygeal nerve. Each spinal nerve provides sensation to a predictable area of skin and that region of skin relays a message to the brain.

Understanding the nerve distribution along the dermatomes helps determine how certain diseases, such as herpes zoster (shingles) and varicella (chicken pox), target one area of the body. Dermatomes stack like discs along the thorax and abdomen but run longitudinally along the limbs (Figure 2.2). Although dermatomes' patterns are similar in all individuals, the exact areas of innervation are distinctive for each person.

**18** ■ I. Overview of Dermatology

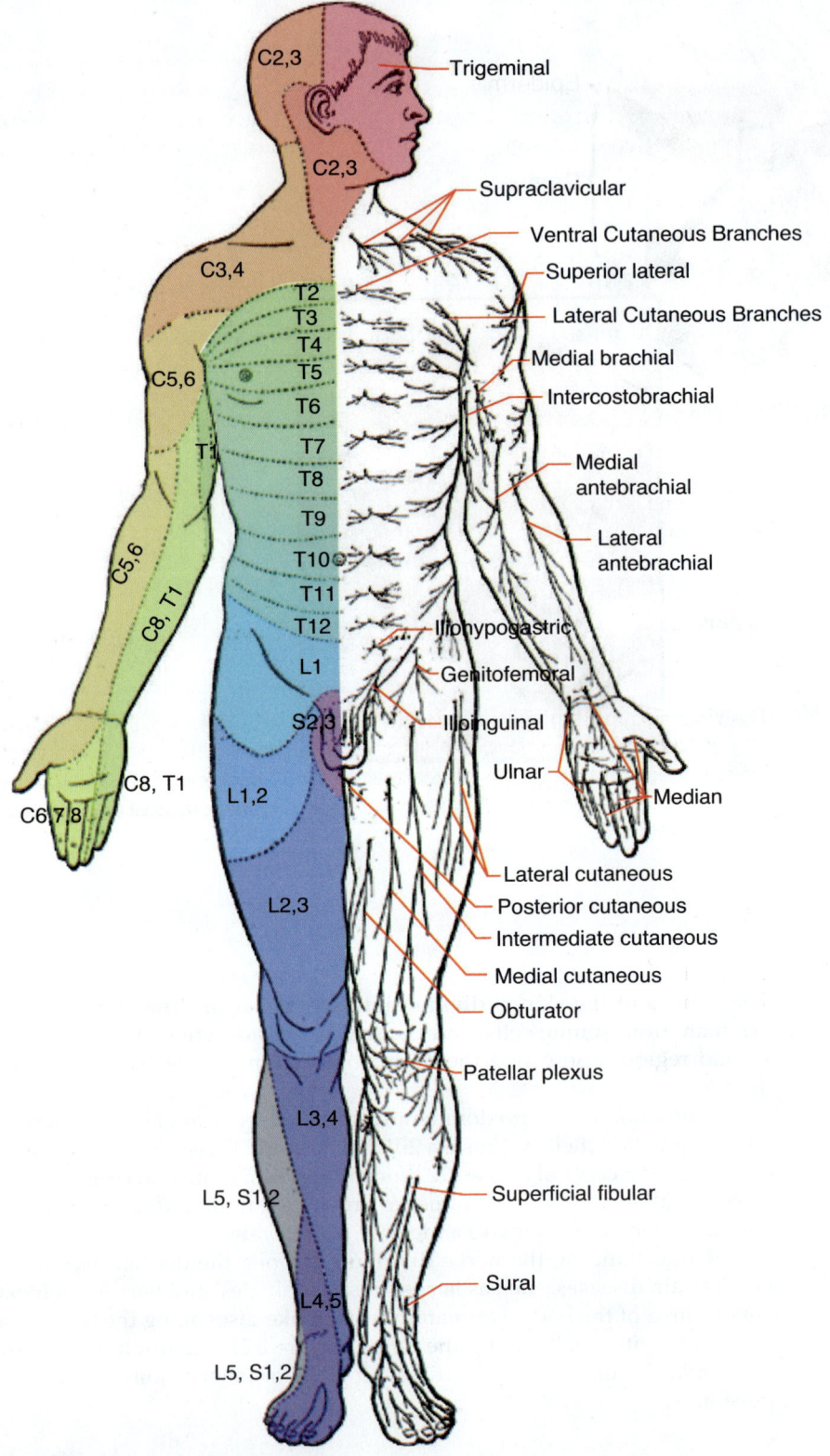

**FIGURE 2.2** Dermatomes

# SKIN TERMINOLOGY

Extensive terminology has been developed to standardize the description of skin lesions, including lesion type (primary morphology), lesion arrangement (secondary morphology), distribution, texture, and color. A *lesion*, for example, is an area of skin that has suffered damage through injury or disease; this can include wounds, bruises, abscesses, or tumors, among other things. A *rash* is a widespread eruption of lesions, and *dermatosis* is another name for skin disease.

## Documentation of Rashes and Lesions

The body of dermatology language is distinctive, and recognizing common skin conditions in the primary care setting requires knowledge of skin terminology. Providers are encouraged to develop a glossary of skin terminology to describe conditions and demonstrate competence in documentation of these skin rashes and lesions.

Documentation of skin rashes and lesions includes diagnostic evaluations made considering arrangement, distribution, type and characteristics, patterns of lesions, and specific lesion sites. Understanding dermatologic terminology facilitates accurate diagnoses (Draper, 2011). Skin lesions are referred to as either primary or secondary lesions.

## Primary Skin Lesion Terminology

The majority of skin diseases begin with a basic lesion, called a *primary skin lesion* (Habif, 2004). Primary skin lesions initially appear in reaction to external or internal environment and are physical changes in the skin caused by a disease process. However, types of primary lesions are rarely specific to a single disease entity. The shape, size, and colors of a primary lesion as well as the symptoms associated are important in describing skin lesions. A primary lesion is described with established dermatologic terminology. Identifying the primary lesion(s), when possible, is the first step toward identification of the disease or cutaneous process. Thus, it is important for a clinician to have the skill to identify a primary skin lesion. Habif (2004) confirmed that it was often at the initial office examination that the primary lesion was identified and a diagnosis was confirmed. Identifying these basic lesions in primary care is vital to making an accurate diagnosis—or at least to forming differential diagnoses—and to initiating appropriate treatment of the identified cutaneous disease.

The following are examples of primary skin lesion terminology.

- *Abscess* or boil (also called a furuncle): A deep infection of the hair follicles
- *Bulla* or blister: A raised fluid-filled or pus-filled lesion 0.5 cm or larger
- *Macule*: A circumscribed change in skin color without elevation or depression that may be brown, blue, red, or hypopigmented
- *Nodule*: A palpable solid lesion of varying size that is greater than 0.5 cm and less than 2 cm in diameter and which may be present in the epidermis, dermis, or subcutis; a large nodule is called a tumor (Habif, 2004)
- *Papule*: A solid raised lesion usually 0.5 cm or less in diameter that varies in color and may become confluent or form plaques
- *Plaque*: A raised superficial solid lesion more than 0.5 cm in diameter that can be formed by the confluence of papules (Habif, 2004)
- *Pustule*: A circumscribed elevated lesion that contains pus; a pustule is usually in the dermis or subcutis, and it varies in size

- *Vesicle*: A circumscribed elevated lesion that contains free fluid and is 0.5 cm or less in diameter
- *Wheal* (or hive): A rounded or flat-topped elevated firm plaque formed by local dermal edema that is generally transient and may last only a few hours

## Secondary Skin Lesion Terminology

Secondary lesions result from changes over time caused by disease progression, manipulation (scratching, picking, rubbing), trauma, infection, the healing process, or treatment. Secondary lesions may evolve from primary lesions. The distinction between a primary and secondary lesion is not always clear. Secondary skin lesion terminology is made up of the following.

- *Atrophy*: A thinning of epidermis, dermis, or subcutaneous fat, creating a depression in the skin
- *Crust*: An accumulation of serum, blood, or purulent exudate that results from the drying of plasma or exudate on the skin; it is also called a scab
- *Desquamation* (scaling, exfoliation, peeling): The shedding of stratum corneum or keratin
- *Erosion*: A loss of epidermis above the basal layer, leaving a denuded surface; because of location, erosions do not leave a scar
- *Eschar*: A hard, usually darkened, plaque covering an ulcer implying extensive tissue necrosis, infarct, or gangrene
- *Fissure*: A linear crack in the skin with sharply defined walls; it is created by a loss of the dermis and epidermis (e.g., cracked lips or a fungal infection such as athlete's foot)
- *Keloid*: An exaggerated connective tissue response of injured skin that extends beyond the edges of the original wound
- *Scale*: Flakes or plates that represent compacted desquamated layers of stratum corneum; desquamation occurs when there are peeling sheets of scale following acute injury to the skin
- *Scar*: A dermal and epidermal change associated with wound healing; scars are permanent fibrotic changes that occur on the skin after damage to the dermis. They can have secondary pigment characteristics. They may be hypertrophic (raised), atrophic (depressed), or icepick-like (Glickman & Shalita, 1990).
- *Ulcer*: A loss of epidermis through necrosis of the epidermis and part or all of the dermis, which leaves a depressed moist lesion
- *Special skin lesions*: Those that are produced by special circumstances within a body system—some special skin lesions—are as follows:
  - *Burrow*: A narrow, raised, twisting canal formed by a parasite
  - *Comedo*: A hair follicle opening plugged by sebaceous and keratinous material; it can be a dilated blackhead or a narrowed whitehead
  - *Cyst*: A sac containing liquid or semisolid material usually in the dermis
  - *Excoriation*: Linear crusts and erosions or traumatized or abraded skin caused by scratching or rubbing.
  - *Lichenification*: An accentuation of skin markings commonly associated with thickening epidermis usually caused by scratching or rubbing; it is marked by the presence of fine papules
  - *Milia*: A small superficial keratin cyst that has no evident opening
  - *Petechiae*: A confined deposit of blood less than 0.5 cm in diameter (Habif, 2004)
  - *Purpura*: A confined deposit of blood greater than 0.5 cm in diameter
  - *Telangiectasia*: Superficial dilated blood vessels

## VASCULAR LESIONS

### Petechiae, Purpura, and Ecchymosis

Bleeding that occurs in the skin can be categorized as petechiae, purpura, and ecchymosis. Generally, the term *petechiae* refers to smaller lesions. *Purpura* and *ecchymosis* are terms that refer to larger lesions. In certain situations, purpura may be palpable. In all situations, petechiae, ecchymoses, and purpura do not blanch when pressed.

## DIAGNOSTIC EVALUATIONS

### Arrangement

The arrangement of lesions in relation to one another as well as their distribution are also important in fully describing dermatosis. Arrangement or configuration refers to the shape or outline of a single lesion or a cluster of skin lesions because skin lesions are often grouped together. The pattern or shape may help in diagnosis because many skin conditions have a characteristic configuration or arrangement. The following terms may apply to the shape or the arrangement:

- *Acneiform*: Follicular eruptions that consist of papules and pustules that appear to be similar to acne; the dermatoses include acne vulgaris, rosacea, folliculitis, and perioral dermatitis
- *Annular*: Lesions seen in a ring shape with central clearing; examples include tinea corporis, granuloma annulare, erythema migrans (the lesion associated with lyme disease), some dermatophyte infections (ringworm), drug eruptions, and secondary syphilis
- *Clustered*: Lesions that are grouped together; seen in herpes simplex or with insect bites
- *Confluent*: Lesions that run together
- *Dermatomal*: Zosteriform lesions follow a dermatome; lesions of herpes zoster (also known as shingles) are the classic example, but there are other lesions that assume the same pattern
- *Discrete*: Lesions that tend to remain separate
- *Grouped*: Lesions that group together (e.g., herpetic, zosteriform, agminate, reticular)
- *Herpetiform*: Grouped umbilicated vesicles, as arise in herpes simplex and herpes zoster infections
- *Iris-target*: Lesions that form a series of concentric rings that have a dark or blistered center; frequently seen with erythema multiforme
- *Linear*: Lesions that occur in a straight line or band-like configuration; this descriptive term may apply to a wide variety of disorders and can be suggestive of some forms of contact dermatitis, linear epidermal nevi, and lichen striatus
- *Morbilliform*: A rash consisting of macular lesions that are red and are usually 2 to 10 mm in diameter but may be confluent in places; patients with the measles, Kawasaki disease, drug reactions, or other conditions may have a morbilliform rash
- *Multiform*: Lesions with a variety of shapes
- *Nummular*: Round or coin-shaped lesions also known as *discoid*; an example is nummular eczema
- *Polycystic*: Lesions having or containing many cysts
- *Serpiginous*: Lesions that appear wavy or serpentlike
- *Target* (or bull's eye or iris): Lesions that appear as rings with central duskiness; this is a classic arrangement for erythema multiforme

## DISTRIBUTION, TYPE, CHARACTERISTICS, AND PATTERN OF LESIONS

Not only is the appearance of lesions important, but their pattern and distribution on the skin is as well. *Distribution* refers to how the skin lesions are scattered or spread out. Skin lesions may be isolated (solitary or single) or multiple. The localization of multiple lesions in certain regions helps diagnosis because skin diseases tend to have characteristic distributions. A practitioner should ask, "What is the extent of the eruption and its pattern?" The following terms are helpful in describing the distribution of skin lesions.

- *Asymmetrical*: Lesions that fail to correspond to one another in shape, size, or arrangement
- *Bilateral*: Lesions that are two-sided in context of the body
- *Generalized or universal*: Lesions that may be mild or severe, scattered, or diffuse
- *Intertriginous*: Lesions that appear in a region of the skin where two areas rub or touch (*Candida* [perleche], tinea, or erythrasma)
- *Localized*: Lesions that are confined to a definite skin location
- *Sunlight exposed*: Lesions involving light eruption, drugs, seborrheic dermatitis, acne rosacea, acne vulgaris, and acute contact dermatitis, and lesions located on the arms and legs
- *Palms and soles*: The areas of lesions in syphilis (palms), Rocky Mountain spotted fever, and erythema multiforme
- *Symmetrical*: Lesions that are in the same region; the left side is affected in a similar way to the right side
- *Unilateral*: Lesions that appear on one side of the affected skin region

## SPECIAL DISTRIBUTION CATEGORY: PATTERNS OF INTENTIONAL OR UNINTENTIONAL INJURY

One important category of skin lesions involves a form of skin lesion that may present in primary care in cases of child abuse and other intentional injury (bite marks, slap marks, strap marks, burns) or in cases of unintentional injury. Additionally, abrasions are considered traumatically caused erosions. Specific skin sites that could indicate trauma and require examination include:

- Face
- Eyes
- Ears
- Mouth
- Nose
- Genital area

Six sections in the genital area that require assessment for trauma and injury include the following:

- Pubis
- Upper thighs next to the groin
- Creases between the groin and thigh
- Genitals (vulva, penis, scrotum)
- Skin between anus and vulva, around anus, and between anus and scrotum
- Creases between the buttocks

## Risk Factors

Risk factors for the skin include anything that affects the chance of a person getting a skin disease (American Cancer Society, 2013). Some of the risk factors surrounding skin diseases, such as amount of sun exposure, can be changed, and some, like age and genetics, cannot. Undoubtedly, different skin diseases have diverse risk factors and having one or more risk factors does not mean the patient will develop a skin disease. However, the absence of risk factors does not exclude skin disease.

## Congenital/Genetic Diseases

The formation of almost all components of the skin (e.g., hair texture and color and skin pigmentation and thickness) is under genetic control. A large number of common skin diseases also are directly or indirectly determined by a person's genotype (genetic constitution), but their expression may require an external influence or an altered hormonal milieu. The hereditary diseases psoriasis and atopic eczema are examples of skin disorders in which sunlight (as an extrinsic factor) or stress (as an intrinsic factor) activate the condition. Even when heredity has a determining role, other factors also influence the skin disease. Some of the complex hereditary disorders that primarily affect the skin require special diagnostic and management expertise. These skin disorders include (Genetic Skin Disorders, 2013) the following:

- Ectodermal dysplasias
- Ehlers–Danlos syndrome
- Ichthyoses
- Incontinentia pigmenti

A genetic disease is any disease that is caused by an abnormality in an individual's genome. The abnormality can range from minuscule to major—from a discrete mutation in a single base in the DNA of a single gene to a gross chromosome abnormality involving the addition or subtraction of an entire chromosome or set of chromosomes. Some genetic disorders are inherited from the parents; other genetic diseases are caused by acquired changes or mutations in a preexisting gene or group of genes. Mutations occur either randomly or because of some environmental exposure.

Congenital skin disorders cover an extensive range of different diseases. Some of the diseases include acrodermatitis enteropathica, congenital ichthyosis, xeroderma pigmentosum (XP), epidermolysis bullosa, hereditary hyperbilirubinemia, keratosis follicularis, pseudoxanthoma elasticum, and urticaria pigmentosa. Syndromes also exist, such as Ehlers–Danlos syndrome and Wiskott–Aldrich syndrome.

## Congenital Ichthyosis

Congenital ichthyosis is a rare genodermatosis that belongs to a group of heterogeneous cornification disorders. Ichthyosis results from the abnormal function of proteins required for epidermal development. The disease has been linked to eight distinct genes (Goldsmith et al., 2013). When the disease is limited to the skin, it has a significant impact on the quality of the patient's life. Autosomal recessive congenital ichthyosis can present with numerous phenotypes, including the most severe form, harlequin ichthyosis.

## Harlequin Ichthyosis

One of the most severe congenital skin disorders is harlequin ichthyosis. The cause of this usually fatal disorder is still unknown, but the symptoms are unmistakable. The baby is often born premature and covered with a thick, armorlike covering that makes it difficult, if not impossible, for the baby to move. The skin can further dry out, flake, and form into what looks like scales. Most affected are the lips, eyelids, ears, and nose area, which are covered in the plating. Although babies have been able to survive longer than they used to with this disorder thanks to advanced neonatal intensive care, anyone with this disorder is most likely going to face a life of disfigurement and constant infection.

## Xeroderma Pigmentosum

Xeroderma pigmentosum (XP) is a rare, genetic condition resulting from a defect in an enzyme that normally repairs damage to DNA. Young patients with XP have a high risk for developing melanoma and other skin cancers. Because people with XP are less able to repair DNA damage caused by sunlight, they can develop many cancers on sun-exposed areas of their skin (American Cancer Society, 2013).

## Epidermolysis Bullosa

Epidermolysis bullosa is a group of skin conditions, with the majority being inherited. Four major types have been identified: epidermolysis bullosa simplex, junctional epidermolysis bullosa, dystrophic epidermolysis bullosa, and epidermolysis bullosa acquisita. The disease initially affects infants and young children. It presents as blisters in response to minor trauma, heat, friction from rubbing, scratching, or adhesive tape (Mayo Clinic, 2011). Mild forms may improve with age; however, severe forms have significant complications and can be fatal.

Epidermolysis bullosa has no known cure. Treatment of the disorder focuses on symptom management, which includes pain control, wound prevention and disinfection, and control of pruritus related to continuous wound healing (Mayo Clinic, 2011).

## Acquired Diseases

Several risk factors can make a person more likely to develop melanoma. For example, UV radiation, either from the sun or tanning beds and lamps, is a major risk factor for most melanomas. People who get a lot of exposure to light from these sources are at greater risk for skin cancer, including melanoma. Nevi (moles), which are pigmented tumors, are usually benign and typically not present at birth but begin to appear in childhood and young adulthood. Unfortunately, persons with multiple nevi are more likely to develop melanoma. Conversely, moles present at birth—congenital melanocytic nevi—increase the lifetime risk of getting melanoma by between 0% and 10%, depending on the size of the nevus (American Cancer Society, 2013).

For individuals with fair skin, freckling, and light hair, the risk of melanoma is more than 10 times higher compared with African Americans. Whites with red or blond hair, blue or green eyes, or fair skin that freckles or burns easily are at increased risk. Risk increases for people with a first-degree relative who has a history of melanoma. Approximately 10% of all people diagnosed with melanoma have a family history of this disease. Familial risk factors can be linked to shared lifestyles, such as frequent sun exposure and also fair skin coloring and gene mutations. From 10% to 40% of families with a high rate of melanoma have gene mutation (American Cancer Society, 2013). Five percent of people with a history of melanoma will have a reoccurrence. Immune suppression increases the risk of melanoma as well.

Melanoma risk increases as people age. Unfortunately, melanoma is found in patients of any age with a family history of the disease. It is one of the most common cancers in people younger than age 30. At this age, the risk is higher in women. However, after age 40, the risk of melanoma is higher in men. In the United States, men have a higher overall risk of melanoma.

## REFERENCES

American Cancer Society. (2013). *Melanoma skin cancer*. Retrieved from http://www.cancer.org/acs/groups/cid/documents/webcontent/003120-pdf.pdf

Apok, V., Gurusinghe, N., Mitchell, J., & Emsley, H. (2011). Neurological signs: Dermatomes and dogma. *Practical Neurology, 11*(2), 100–105.

Draper, R. (2011). *Dermatological descriptive terms*. Retrieved from http://medical.cdn.patient.co.uk/pdf/1033.pdf

Glickman, F., & Shalita, A. (1990). *Fundamentals of dermatology*. New York, NY: Marcel Dekker.

Goldsmith, T., Fuchs-Telem, D., Israeli, S., Sarig, O., Padalon-Brauch, G., Bergman, R., ... Nousbeck, J. (2013). The sound of silence: Autosomal recessive congenital ichthyosis caused by a synonymous mutation in *ABCA12*. *Experimental Dermatology, 22*(4), 251–254. doi:10.1111/exd.12110

Habif, T. (2004). *A color guide to diagnosis and therapy: Clinical dermatology*. Philadelphia, PA: Mosby.

Jarvis, C. (2012). *Physical examination & health assessment* (6th ed., rev.). St. Louis, MO: Elsevier/Saunders.

Karlene, S., & Gaffney, K. *Genetic Skin Disorders*. (2013). Retrieved from http://www.karlenedermatology.com/offered-services/conditions/genetic-disorders.html

Kolarsick, P. A., Kolarsick, M. A., & Goodwin, C. (2011). Anatomy and physiology of the skin. *Dermatology Nurses' Association, 3*(4), 203–212.

Mayo Clinic. (2011). *Epidermolysis bullosa*. Retrieved from http://www.mayoclinic.com/health/epidermolysis-bullosa/DS01015/DSECTION=treatments-and-drugs

Scanlon, V. C., & Saunders, T. (1999). *Essentials of anatomy and physiology* (4th ed., rev.). Philadelphia, PA: F.A. Davis.

# 3

# Special Considerations for Populations, Culture, and Comorbid Conditions

## INFANTS AND CHILDREN

The newborn's skin is similar in structure to the adult's, but many functions of the skin are not fully developed. Infants' skin has a thinner stratum corneum and papillary dermis. The newborn's skin is smooth and elastic and is relatively more permeable than that of the adult, so the infant is at greater risk for fluid loss. Infant skin has higher water content and is able to absorb more water and lose excess water more quickly compared with adult skin (Lio, 2011). Sebum, which holds water in the skin, is present during the first few weeks of life, producing milia and cradle cap in some infants.

There are significant structural and functional differences that make infant skin more susceptible to certain skin conditions. For example, there is little temperature regulation. Eccrine sweat glands do not secrete in response to heat until 2 to 3 months of age and then only marginally throughout childhood. As the child grows, the epidermis thickens, toughens, and darkens; the skin becomes better lubricated; and hair growth quickens. Also during infancy, there are significant developments of the skin and subcutaneous fat that warrant handling infants carefully (Lio, 2011).

## THE ELDERLY

When people age, their skin atrophies. Aging skin has decreased elasticity, skin folds develop, and sagging occurs. Wrinkles appear on the face. By age 70, the skin will appear thin and paperlike. Senile purpura occurs because of decreased vascularity and increased vascular fragility. A loss of elastin, collagen, and subcutaneous fat occurs, as well as a reduction in muscle tone. Sweat glands and sebaceous glands decrease in number, which predisposes elderly people to heat stroke and dry skin. Sun exposure and cigarette smoking will increase the aging of the skin: coarse wrinkling, decreased elasticity, atrophy, speckled and uneven coloring, more pigment changes, and a yellow, leathery texture occurs.

All of these factors place the elderly person at risk for skin disease and skin breakdown because the skin is thin and has less vascularity and protein, which aids in healing. Skin ulcerations and skin cancers are prominent in the elderly.

## ETHNICITY

Blacks, Hispanics, and American Indians have a lower incidence of skin cancers because of a greater amount of melanin in their skin. Melanoma is 20 times higher among Whites than Blacks and four times higher among Caucasians than Hispanics.

The apocrine and eccrine glands are also different among cultures. Most Asians and American Indians have a mild body odor or none at all, whereas Whites and Blacks tend to have a strong body odor. In Artic regions, Inuits have adapted to their environment: They sweat less than Whites on the extremities and more on the face.

Blacks are prone to having keloids, increased postinflammatory hyperpigmentation after skin trauma, pseudofolliculitis, and melasma. Blacks may develop linear hyperpigmented vertical bands under the nails, which may be a normal variation, whereas a linear hyperpigmented vertical band under the nail of a White person might indicate melanoma. The incidence of childhood eczema in the United States is approximately 10.7% and Black and Asian children are diagnosed with atopic dermatitis more often than White children are (Buster, Stevens, & Elmets, 2012).

## CULTURAL PRACTICES

Approximately 30% of the U.S. population is comprised of people of races other than White (Ravanfar & Dinulos, 2010). Providers often encounter unusual skin findings that are the result of cultural practices. Frequently, patients and families do not reveal information about their cultural practices, which can lead to misdiagnosis and improper treatments. The following are some examples of different cultural practices (Ravanfar & Dinulos, 2010).

Coin rubbing and spooning is repeated pressured strokes over lubricated skin and moving down the muscles with a smooth edge such as a worn coin, a metal cap with a rounded edge, a ceramic Chinese soup spoon, rounded animal bone, a piece of jade, or a piece of ginger root. The skin manifestation that result from these cultural practices cause petechial and ecchymosis in linear streaks along the back in a Christmas tree pattern, which is referred to in Chinese medicine as the *Sha* rash. These practices are used to treat fever and colds.

Gridding is a folk remedy that is most commonly practiced in Russian cultures as well as the Ukraine. Gridding is the practice of painting the back with iodine in a crisscross pattern. This results in a hyperpigmented gridlike pattern on the back. This practice is often used to treat respiratory illness.

Cupping is a cultural practice that dates back to 3,000 BCE and is practiced in a variety of cultures, including Egyptian, Chinese, Greek, European, and Middle Eastern. Cupping is the practice of creating a small area of low pressure next to the skin with a cup, leading to suction. This practice leads to annular ecchymosis and annular hyperpigmentation across the skin. The use of oils and lubricants can cause blistering and contact dermatitis.

Moxibustion is a traditional Chinese therapy that is also used in other Asian cultures. The procedure involves using moxa, a mugwort herb, either by placing it on an acupuncture point, with or without the needle in place, and directly burning it on the skin or indirectly burning by lighting one end of the moxa stick and holding it near the skin or placing it on the inserted acupuncture needle. The results are often a burn to the skin that can resemble a cigarette burn and results in scarring to the skin.

Herbal applications can cause contact dermatitis and photodermatitis. One such herbal application is black henna, most commonly known for its use as a temporary ornamental tattoo applied traditionally in Indian, Middle Eastern, and Mediterranean cultures. Turkish populations often apply ash, olive oil, tar, or coffee to the infant's umbilical stump. Salting of the infant skin for an hour is a cultural practice that is another practice unique to Turkey, which can lead to severe, life-threatening hypernatremia and dehydrated, scalded skin. Hispanic populations may use heated aloe vera, capsaicin, and gentian violet on the skin.

## PUBERTY

Puberty is the time of sexual maturation (Stoppler, 2012). Secretion from apocrine sweat glands increases in response to heat and emotional stimuli, which produces body odor. Sebaceous glands become more active, the skin becomes oily, and acne develops. Subcutaneous fat deposits increase, especially in females. Coarse pubic hair, axillary hair, and in males facial hair develops.

## PREGNANCY

Several common physiologic changes occur during pregnancy, including some that affect the skin. Often hyperpigmentation of the skin (*melasma*) after sun exposure appears on the face in response to estrogen and progesterone. The only symptom of melasma is a darkening of skin color. The following are other changes that may occur during pregnancy.

### Striae Distensae

Striae distensae (commonly referred to as "stretch marks") represent linear dermal scars accompanied by epidermal atrophy (Samer, 2012). Striae form in up to 90% of American women during pregnancy because the skin is often exposed to continuous and progressive stretching (especially on the breasts and abdomen). The increased stress is placed on the connective tissue as a result of increased size of the various parts of the body (Samer, 2012).

### Palmar Erythema

Palmar erythema (superficial reddening of the skin) in pregnancy usually appears within the first trimester. It is most prevalent in Whites. Palmar erythema during pregnancy is attributed to venous capillary engorgement (Soutou et al., 2009). The erythema generally fades within 1 week postpartum.

### Areolas

The areolas darken as a result of increased estrogen and progesterone during pregnancy. This skin around the nipples continues to darken as the pregnancy progresses. The color can begin changing in the first or second week of pregnancy, and some women will also develop Montgomery tubercles (tiny bumps on the areolas). Genetics determines whether the patient has brown- or red-pigmented areolas. The areolar color can range from pale yellow to black but usually stays paler among light-skinned people and darker among dark-skinned people (Pregnancy Corner, 2013).

## Hair

During pregnancy, women's hair loss slows. Normally, 85% to 95% of the scalp hair is growing, and the other 5% to 15% of hair is in a resting stage. After the resting period, this hair naturally sheds at about 100 hairs a day. This shedding often occurs during brushing or shampooing the hair and is replaced by new growth (Baby Center, 2013).

## Diabetes

Diabetes can affect every organ of the body, including the skin. Up to a third of all diabetic individuals will develop a skin disorder at some point. In fact, skin problems can often be the first indication of diabetes. Diabetic persons are more likely than the general population to develop bacterial and fungal infections and itching. Furthermore, those with diabetes are more prone to several of the following skin conditions.

### Acanthosis Nigricans
Acanthosis nigricans is a skin condition that causes darkening and thickening of skin mainly in the skinfolds of the neck, axillae, under breasts, and groin. This disorder is typically seen in obese patients, and although not curable, it may improve with weight loss. In most people, acanthosis nigricans precedes diabetes and is a skin manifestation of insulin resistance. Acromegaly and Cushing syndrome are also known to cause acanthosis nigricans.

### Bullosis Diabeticorum
Bullosis diabeticorum, or diabetic blisters, resemble burn blisters. The blisters occur in diabetic patients with severe disease who have diabetic neuropathy. They occur on the fingers, hands, toes, feet, legs, or forearms. These painless blisters typically heal without treatment.

### Diabetic Dermopathy
Diabetic dermopathy develops from changes to the small blood vessels that supply the skin. The lesions appear light brown or red, round or oval, are shiny and often form on the front of the lower legs. The lesions (patches) are painless but can itch and burn in some patients. Generally no treatment is required.

### Digital Sclerosis
Digital sclerosis causes the skin on the toes, fingers, and hands to become thick, waxy, and tight. Stiffness of the finger joints can also occur. Lotions and moisturizers can be helpful in softening the skin.

### Disseminated Granuloma Annulare
Disseminated granuloma annulare causes sharply defined, ring- or arc-shaped areas on the skin. These lesions occur most often on the fingers and ears, but they can occur on the chest and abdomen. The rash can be red, red-brown, or skin colored. Treatment is typically not required, but a topical hydrocortisone may be beneficial.

### Eruptive Xanthomatosis
Eruptive xanthomatosis is a skin lesion that occurs in diabetic individuals with uncontrolled blood glucose and extremely elevated serum triglycerides. The lesions form as firm, yellow, pea-like papules on the skin of the feet, arms, legs, buttocks, and backs of the hands. The lesions are surrounded by red halos and can cause pruritus.

### Fungal Infections
Fungi, particularly *Candida albicans*, cause a large amount of fungal infections in people with diabetes. *Candida* creates a pruritic red rash that is often surrounded by small blisters and scales. The fungus frequently occurs in warm, moist skinfolds. Treatment involves a combination of topical steroids and antifungals.

Itching skin, or pruritus, can be caused by infections, xerosis, and altered circulation. The lower legs and feet are most often affected by altered circulation. Using lotions or creams, avoiding hot showers, and using gentle soaps are strategies to keep skin soft and moist. Moisturizers reduce itching caused by dry skin.

### Necrobiosis Lipoidica Diabeticorum
Necrobiosis lipoidica diabeticorum (NLD) is caused by changes in the blood vessels and the collagen and fat content underneath the skin. The overlaying skin area becomes thinned, raised, waxy in appearance, and reddened. Most lesions are found on the lower parts of the legs and have fairly well defined borders between normal skin. These lesions can ulcerate if subjected to trauma. NLD can be itchy and painful. If the lesions do not break open, treatment is not necessary.

### Scleredema Diabeticorum
Scleredema diabeticorum causes a thickening of the skin on the back of the neck and upper back. This rare condition most often affects people with type 2 diabetes. The treatment is to improve blood glucose levels. Lotions and moisturizers may help soften the skin.

### Vitiligo
Vitiligo is a skin condition that affects the skin's color. In vitiligo, melanin, which controls skin color, is destroyed, and the results are patches of discolored skin. Vitiligo affects the chest, abdomen, and the face around the mouth, nostrils, and eyes. The condition often occurs with type 1 diabetes.

## REFERENCES

Baby Center. (2013). *Hair and nail changes during pregnancy*. Retrieved from http://www.babycenter.com/0_hair-and-nail-changes-during-pregnancy_1456563.bc

Buster, K. J., Stevens, E. I., & Elmets, C. A. (2012). Dermatologic health disparities. *Dermatology Clinics, 30*, 53–59.

Lio, P. (2011). *How does infant skin differ from adult skin?* Retrieved from http://www.medscape.org/viewarticle/743529

Pregnancy Corner. (2013). *Darkened areolas*. Retrieved from http://www.pregnancycorner.com/pregnant/pregnancy-symptoms/darkened-areolas.html

Ravanfar, P., & Dinulos, J. G. (2010). Cultural practices affecting the skin of children. *Current Opinion in Pediatrics, 22*, 423–431.

Samer, A. (2012). *Striae distensae*. Retrieved from http://emedicine.medscape.com/article/1074868-overview

Soutou, B., Régnier, S., Nassar, D., Parant, O., Khosrotehrani, K., & Aractingi, S. (2009). *Dermatological manifestations associated with pregnancy: Pigmentary changes*. Retrieved from http://www.medscape.org/viewarticle/706769_3

Stoppler, M. (2012). *Puberty*. Retrieved from http://www.medicinenet.com/puberty/article.htm

# PART II
# Clinical Management of Dermatology Conditions

| | |
|---|---|
| 4. *Skin Assessment* | *35* |
| 5. *Diagnostics* | *39* |
| 6. *Treatment Approaches* | *43* |
| 7. *Clinical Management* | *51* |

# 4
# Skin Assessment

## HISTORY

When a patient presents with a rash or skin lesion, obtaining a medical history is important. The skill of interpreting what is seen is even more significant (Habif, 2011). An organized approach should be used for all patients presenting with a skin disease. First, obtain a thorough history; this includes the natural history of the disease, duration of the skin condition, rate of onset, and the rash or lesion location. Include any symptoms, allergies, family and occupational histories, and previous treatment, prescribed or over the counter.

Marks (2001) suggested three basic questions that should always be asked on a dermatologic history.

1. "Where did the rash start?"
2. "How long have you had the rash?"
   *Acute rashes* (hours or days) are often associated with a diagnosis of urticarial and allergic reaction, insect bites, drug reaction, herpes simplex/zoster, and viral exanthema. Acute chronic rashes (days or weeks) are linked with eczema, impetigo, scabies, drugs, pityriasis rosea, psoriasis, tinea, and *Candida*. *Chronic rashes* (weeks or months) are often associated with psoriasis, eczema, tinea, pityriasis versicolor, warts, or cancers.
3. "Does the rash itch?"
   Warts, tinea, pityriasis versicolor, impetigo, psoriasis, skin cancers, and viral exanthema may cause mild itching. Urticaria, eczema, scabies, insect bites, or drug reactions may cause moderate to severe itching.

## SKIN ASSESSMENT (PHYSICAL)

The skin examination should be methodical. When assessing the distribution (extent of eruption) of the rash, have patients remove their clothes and dress in an examination gown to enable complete examination of the skin. Thorough visualization of the skin surfaces is imperative for accurate diagnosis, any necessary testing, and determination of treatment strategies.

According to Marks (2001), there are two important features to look for:
1. The characteristics of individual lesions
2. The overall distribution of the lesions

It is important to evaluate whether the eruption affects the epidermis (Marks, 2001). Nearly every disease affecting the skin has a dermal component to it, so the area in question is the epidermis. Epidermal changes include scaling, crusting, fissures, vesicles, and weeping or oozing.

Examination for the overall distribution is linked to the history of the rash location. There are specific areas that, when affected, give insight to the diagnosis. Examples of epidermal lesions include eczema, psoriasis, tinea, pityriasis rosea, impetigo, herpes, warts, skin cancers, and scabies. Dermal lesions include urticaria, insect bites, drugs, skin infiltrations, and viral exanthema. The practitioner should examine the skin to determine the primary lesion, also known as the basic lesion. Magnification with a hand lens affords careful lesion examination. The diagnosis can often be determined if the primary lesion is identified. If the diagnosis is not evident, recognition of the primary lesion assists the provider in forming relevant differential diagnoses. Next assess for evidence of secondary skin lesions or special lesions (Habif, 2011).

Secondary lesions form as skin diseases evolve. These lesions may be created from a secondary infection or from a patient's scratching. Secondary lesions may be the only evident lesions on examination; in this situation, the primary cutaneous disease would be presumed.

Testing may be required after the skin is examined to confirm a diagnosis or exclude a differential diagnosis. Tests that can be ordered or performed by all skilled providers include skin biopsies and lab tests; serology; bacterial, viral, or fungal cultures; cytology; Wood's light examination; and patch tests.

## SOCIAL HISTORY

Social history can supply the information a provider requires to create appropriate differential diagnoses. Consideration of work, home, play, travel, and contacts is significant. Contact with an occupational substance is often a frequent source of dermatitis. Workplace irritants can cause allergic reactions. Furthermore, determine whether there are pets in the patient's home. Does the patient live or work with a pregnant person or immunocompromised individual? Has the patient traveled to other countries where a parasite may be the cause of a rash? Does the patient use herbal products or illicit drugs? The patient's responses will often direct the provider to the next line of questioning.

## FAMILY HISTORY

Establishing a family history of any disease that could be related to the skin disease is important. This is particularly relevant if immediate family members have a history of eczema, hay fever, asthma, psoriasis, allergies, urticaria, or skin cancers.

## DERMATOLOGIC SIGNS

Several dermatologic signs may help in the diagnosis of a rash (Ely & Stone, 2010b). For example, *Koebner phenomenon* is the development of typical lesions at the site of a trauma and is characteristic of psoriasis and lichen planus. *Nikolsky sign* is the easy separation of the epidermis from the dermis with lateral pressure and is associated with staphylococcal scalded skin syndrome and toxic epidermal necrolysis. *Auspitz sign* is the appearance of bleeding points when scale from a rash is removed from psoriatic lesions (Figure 4.1). *Blanching* of erythematous lesions with a small amount of downward pressure indicates that the erythema is the result of vasodilation rather than dermal bleeding. Blanching is often seen with drug eruptions, viral exanthems (Figure 4.2), Kawasaki disease, roseola, and scarlet fever, whereas meningococcemia and the late stage of Rocky Mountain spotted fever do not blanch.

## DIFFERENTIAL DIAGNOSIS

Because of the large number of skin conditions that present as a rash in primary care, it can be difficult for providers to generate a complete differential diagnosis at the initial office visit (Ely & Stone, 2010a). In a clinical situation in which significant morbidity or mortality can occur, a rapid and accurate skin diagnosis is critical to make treatment decisions. It is imperative for the provider to formulate inclusive differential diagnoses to direct testing and treatment strategies. If a diagnosis remains unclear, the clinician may decide to treat the symptoms, order further diagnostic testing, or consult a dermatologist (Ely & Stone, 2010a).

An accurate description of skin lesions allows the clinician to formulate a series of differential diagnoses (Corvette, 2011). More significant, when descriptors are placed on decision trees, they supply a graphic representation to guide the provider from known information at the apex of the tree to a final choice based on observation and logic; this simplifies and streamlines the decision-making process. Decision trees are thus useful clinical tools that can aid in obtaining a correct differential diagnosis for the skin rashes commonly seen in primary care. Chapter 1 in this book contains four original decision tree charts that can guide any provider in correctly diagnosing common rashes and lesions.

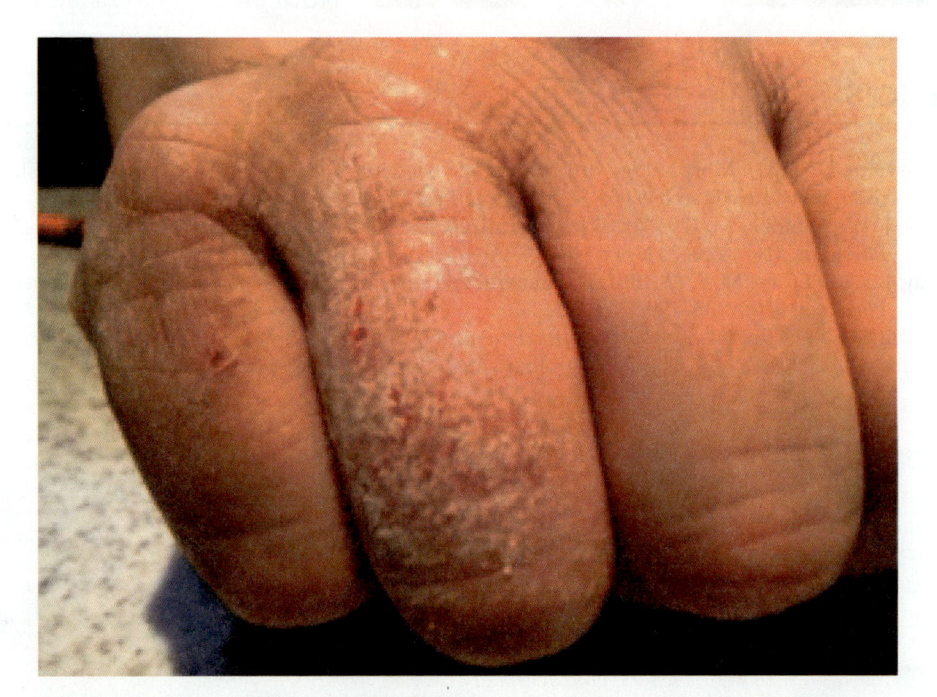

FIGURE 4.1   Auspitz sign is the appearance of bleeding points when scale from the rash is removed from psoriatic lesions.

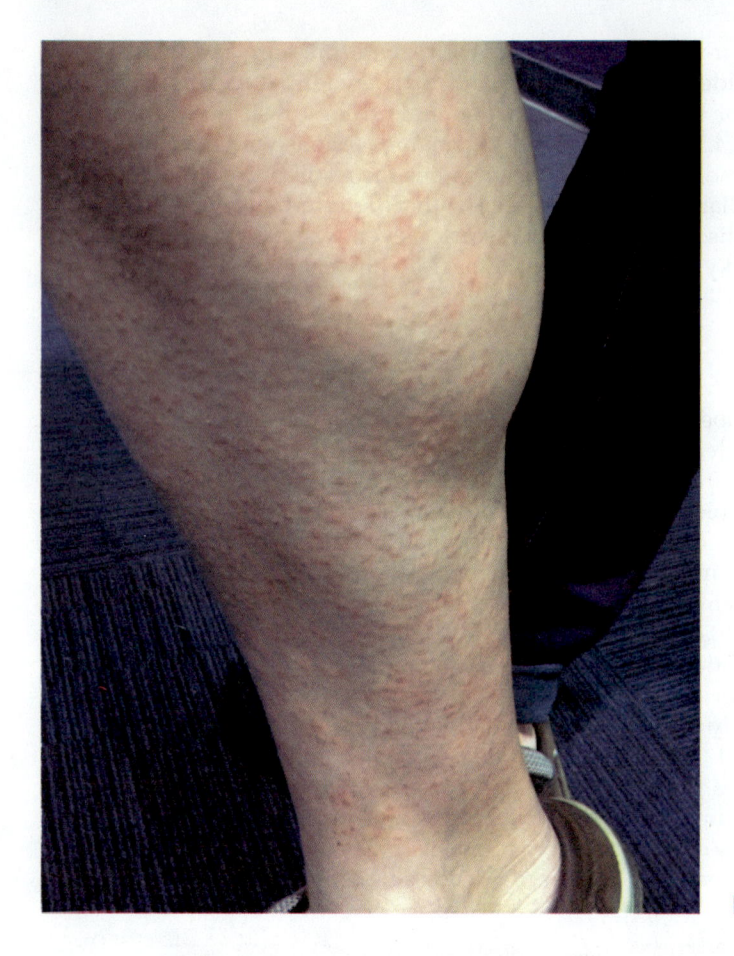

FIGURE 4.2  Viral exanthem of the leg

# REFERENCES

Corvette, D. (2011). Morphology of primary and secondary lesions. In J. E. Fitzpatrick & J. G. Morelli (Eds), *Dermatology secrets plus* (4th ed., pp. 14–21). Philadelphia, PA: Elsevier/Mosby.

Ely, J. W., & Stone, M. (2010a). The generalized rash: Part 1. Differential diagnosis. *American Family Physician, 81*(6), 726–734.

Ely, J. W., & Stone, M. S. (2010b). The generalized rash: Part 11. Diagnostic approach. *American Family Physician, 81*(6), 735–739.

Habif, T. (2011). *Skin disease diagnosis and treatment* (3rd ed.). Edinburgh, Scotland: Elsevier.

Marks, R. (2001). Diagnosis in dermatology. *Australian Family Physician, 30*(11), 1028–1032.

# 5
# Diagnostics

## COLLECTING SPECIMENS

### Biopsy (Shave, Punch, Excisional)

A skin biopsy is used to remove the skin cells or obtain skin samples. The sample taken from the biopsy is given further microscopic examination to diagnose or rule out skin disease. Skin biopsies are performed to diagnose a number of cutaneous conditions, most frequently to diagnose moles, rashes, or skin cancer. A biopsy may be indicated when a mole or other marking on the skin has changed in its shape, color, or size. Skin biopsies are also sometimes used to diagnose infections of the skin.

The three main types of skin biopsies are:

1. *Shave biopsy*: The provider uses a scalpel to remove a small section of the epidermis and a portion of the dermis.
2. *Punch biopsy*: The provider uses a circular punch tool to remove a small section of skin, including the epidermis, dermis, and superficial fat.
3. *Excisional biopsy*: The provider must use a scalpel to remove an entire area or mass of abnormal skin (generally larger and deeper than the other types of biopsies), including a portion of normal skin down to or through the fatty layer of skin.

A skin or wound culture is used to diagnose the etiology of an infection in a sore, burn, surgical wound, or injury. Wounds that are more likely to become infected include injuries, animal bites, human bites, marine stings, and/or scrapes, cuts, and puncture wounds (Figure 5.1). A skin culture directs the best treatment for an infection. This is called *sensitivity testing*.

### Bacterial: Aerobic and Anaerobic

Bacterial cultures are used to diagnose skin infections. Before the culture is taken, the wound should be cleaned with an alcohol pad and carefully swabbed. Attention should be given to the maximum point of inflammation when collecting the culture. Cellulitis can be cultured by injecting the leading edge with saline with a 20-gauge needle on a tuberculin syringe. The specimen can be kept in the syringe and taken immediately to the laboratory for culture, or the aspirate can be transported in a bacterial Culturette. Cultures have higher yields in superficial infections such as impetigo, ecthyma, and ulcers and lower yields in cellulitis.

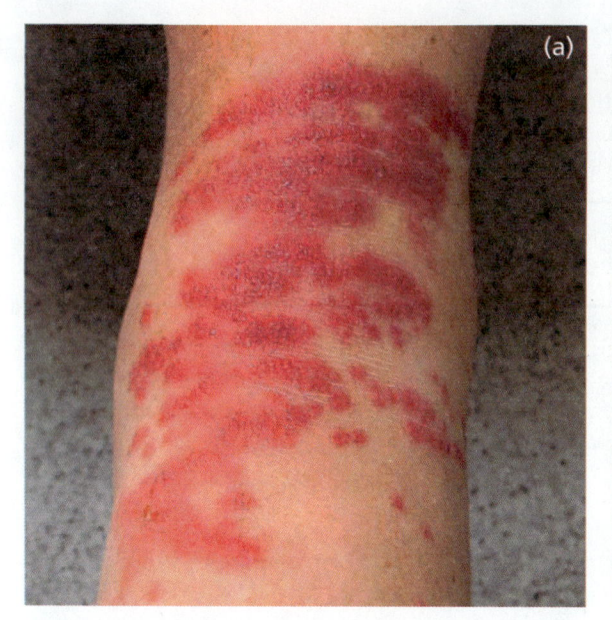

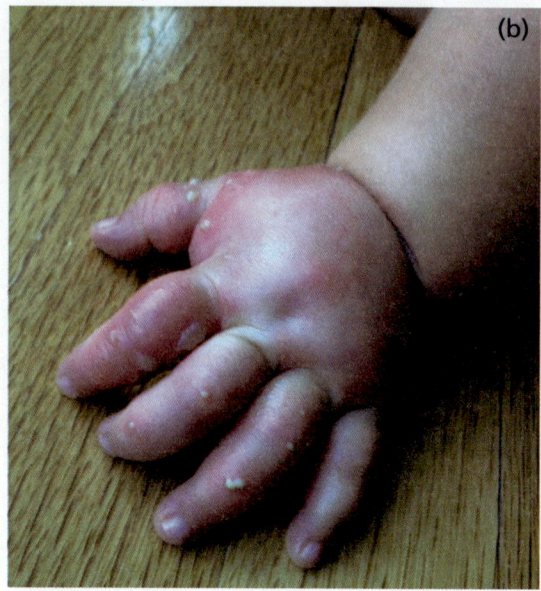

FIGURE 5.1: **(a)** A jellyfish sting and **(b)** fire ant stings. Marine and insect stings are examples of wounds that may become infected. A wound culture may be beneficial in these instances.
Courtesy of Jeri Brehm, FNP, APRN-BC, and Elizabeth A. Lineberry, RN, BSN

## Viral: Tzanck Smear

*A Tzanck smear* is used to assist in the rapid diagnosis of herpes simplex virus (HSV) and herpes zoster virus (VZV; Goodheart, 2011), although the smear cannot distinguish between the two. The base of the blister is scraped with a scalpel blade, and then the adhering cells and material are spread onto a microscope slide. After the specimen air dries, the glass slide is then stained with Giemsa, Wright, or Sedi stain (Spates, 2011). Examination under oil immersion (×100; Goodheart, 2011) assists in identifying a multinucleated giant cell or atypical large nuclei keratinocytes that are visible in the presence of HSV or VZV.

## MYCOLOGY: MICROSCOPIC EXAMINATION OF SCALE (POTASSIUM HYDROXIDE)

### Scraping

Another basic, common technique is the microscopic evaluation of skin scrapings. To evaluate a scaly lesion of suspected fungal etiology, a scalpel with a number 15 blade can be used to gently scrape the superficial surface or active border of the lesion edge (Goodheart, 2011). The scrapings can be collected onto a microscope slide; a couple of drops of potassium hydroxide solution are added to the slide and then it is placed under the microscope for viewing. The presence of hyphae or spores confirms the presence of dermatophytes. To assess for the presence of scabies within a lesion, scrap the lesion more vigorously to remove the entire top surface and add a drop of mineral oil to the scrapings on the slide. When viewed under the microscope, the examiner looks for an eight-legged mite, oval-shaped ova, or feces in the form of red-brown asymmetrical clusters (Bruner & Schaffer, 2012).

## USE OF MECHANICAL DEVICES

### Wood's Light

A *Wood's light* is a handheld black light that produces invisible long-wave (360 nm) ultraviolet radiation. The black light is held over the skin in a darkened room; when the black light strikes the skin, it produces fluorescence. Hypopigmented skin appears lighter, and depigmented skin areas appear milk white. Several skin conditions can be assessed and diagnosed with the use of the Wood's light. Under the black light, tinea capitis and tinea versicolor appear dull yellow, erythrasma appears coral red, and *Pseudomonas* infection of the skin appears green. The black light is useful in screening for porphyria cutanea as well by revealing that the urine fluoresces a coral color (Fitzpatrick & Morrelli, 2011). The Wood's light can also be applied to certain pigmentation disorders, accentuating superficial epidermal pigment and exposing complete depigmentation, as in vitiligo (Spates, 2011).

### Magnification

*Dermatoscopy*, also known as surface and epiluminescence microscopy or dermoscopy, is a noninvasive diagnostic technique used to evaluate skin lesions (Rosendahl et al., 2010). Either a nonpolarized light source using a transparent plate and a liquid medium or the newer option of a polarized light that cancels the skin surface reflection is used. The images or videos can also be digitally produced.

## REFERENCES

Bruner, A., & Schaffer, S. D. (2012). Diagnosing skin lesions: Clinical considerations for primary care practitioners. *Journal for Nurse Practitioners, 8*(8), 600–604.
Fitzpatrick, J., & Morelli, J. (2011). *Dermatology secrets plus* (4th ed.). Philadelphia, PA: Elsevier/Mosby.
Goodheart, H. (2011). *Goodheart's same-site differential diagnosis: A rapid method of diagnosing and treating common skin disorders*. Philadelphia, PA: Lippincott Williams & Wilkins.
Rosendahl, C., Kittler, H., Cameron, A., Balinska, A., McColl, I., & Plaine, H. (2010). *Introduction to dermatoscopy*. Retrieved from http://basicdermatoscopy.blogspot.com
Spates, S. (2011). Diagnostic techniques. In J. E. Fitzpatrick & J. G. Morelli (Eds.), *Dermatology secrets plus* (4th ed., pp. 14–21). Philadelphia, PA: Elsevier/Mosby.

# 6

# Treatment Approaches

## TOPICAL TREATMENT

A *topical medication* is applied directly to the surface of the skin. The advantages of topical application include the ability to apply the dose of medication where it is needed and reduced possibility of systemic side effects and toxicity. Some disadvantages of topical formulations include the time required for application and that they can be messy to apply and uncomfortable; some formulas also make usage complex (Oakley, 2012).

Topical medications contain an active ingredient, a drug or botanical, and a base or vehicle. The vehicle contains water, oil, alcohol, or propylene glycol mixed with preservatives, emulsifiers, absorption promoters, and fragrances. This base may be directed to a specific body location or category of skin disorder. The formula may be moisturizing, or it may penetrate into or through the skin. Other ingredients in the formula may interact to increase or reduce potency or absorption rates (Oakley, 2012).

The amount of the active ingredient that is absorbed through the skin depends on certain factors: skin's thickness (this varies by body location, age, and skin disorder), barrier function, and hydration (up to 10 times more absorption if the skin is occluded). The molecular size, lipophilic properties, and concentration of the chemical all influence absorption as well.

Topical medications are applied to the skin in a thin layer. One gram of cream covers a 10 cm$^2$ area of skin; ointments cover a slightly larger area. It takes 20 to 30 grams of cream or ointment to cover an adult once (Oakley, 2012).

Oakley (2012) lists the following classes of topical formulations.

- Solutions are water or alcoholic lotions containing a dissolved powder.
- Lotions are typically thicker than a solution and contain oil and water or alcohol.
- Creams are thicker than lotions and maintain their shape. They consist of a 50/50 emulsion of oil and water. Creams require preservatives and tend to be moisturizing.
- Ointments are semisolid, generally water free, and contain approximately 80% oil. They are greasy, sticky, emollient, protective, and can be occlusive. Contact allergy is

rare because of the absence of preservatives. Ointments may contain paraffin; wax; or vegetable, coconut, or olive oil.
- Gels are aqueous or alcoholic monophasic semisolid emulsions. Gels are frequently based on cellulose and liquefy on contact with skin. Gels can and often do include preservatives and fragrances.
- Pastes are a concentrated suspension of oil, water, and powder.
- Aerosol foams or sprays are solutions with a pressurized propellant.
- Powders are made from minerals such as talc, or vegetables such as cornstarch.
- Solids melt at body temperature. Two examples are antiperspirant sticks and suppositories.
- Transdermal patches are adhesives placed on the skin; this medication delivery method affords defined dosing and ensures correct skin placement.

When dermatosis is wet or oozing, creams, lotions, and drying pastes are used; if the skin is dry and scaly, ointments or oils are used; for inflamed skin, wet compresses or soaks, followed by creams or ointments, are used; and for cracks and sores, bland applications are used, avoiding alcohol and acidic formulations (Oakley, 2012).

The selection of topical preparations is also directed by the body location of the lesion. For the palms and soles, select ointment or cream; for skin folds, select cream or lotion; for hairy areas, select lotion, solution, gel, or foam; and for mucosal surfaces, select nonirritating formulations.

## Steroids

Prescribing topical corticosteroids is an effective strategy for treating the multiple skin conditions that providers encounter. Knowing how to prescribe the correct dose and the appropriate use of topical steroids significantly affects the success of patient outcomes when treating skin problems. Several steroid formulations are available. Topical corticosteroids work by causing vasoconstriction of the small vessels in the upper dermis. Generally, all corticosteroid preparations have the same basic anti-inflammatory properties; the differences are found in their potency, base, and cost (Habif, 2004).

The seven groups of topical corticosteroids are divided by strength. Group I is the most potent, and group VII is the least potent. All the drugs in a particular group are essentially equivalent in strength. When choosing the dosage of the topical steroid, the provider should consider the skin diagnosis, the potency needed, and any limitations of using that medication. For the best response from the drug, it is vital to prescribe an adequate strength and appropriate time frame for treatment.

The concentration of the corticosteroid must be understood and not compared with strengths of other formulations. Some steroids are much stronger than others, and the amount used must be adjusted accordingly. Most steroids have added fluorination to increase potency.

The base, also called the vehicle, is the substance in which the active ingredient is mixed. The base determines the rate of absorbency (Habif, 2004). Some patients are allergic or sensitive to the bases. The following are types of bases: creams, ointments, gels, solutions, lotions, and foams.

It is important to dispense the appropriate amount of medication for the skin's surface area. Using the fingertip unit (0.5 g) and the rule of hand (which represents 1% of the body surface area) can assist the practitioner in calculating the treatment amount. When considering the entire skin surface, consider that 20 to 30 grams of cream cover an average-sized adult.

Generic topical steroids are readily available and cost much less. This may come at the price of inferior products and inconsistencies, however. Generic steroids are different from brand names.

## Antibacterial

Topical antibiotics are prescribed to treat bacterial skin infections; they are ineffective for fungal or viral infections. They are used directly on the skin's surface to treat or prevent superficial infections. Topical antibiotic use can accelerate healing and prevent complications. These medications are available by prescription and over the counter depending on the type and strength of the medication within the base. Topical antibiotics are available in powders, creams, ointments, and sprays and allow the patient to self-treat. Typical skin conditions that warrant topical antibiotic use include impetigo, folliculitis, pseudofolliculitis barbae, and mild acne.

## Antifungals

The majority of antifungals are commercially available over the counter. Most of these topical antifungal medications are available in the form of creams or lotions, and some are available as powders and aerosols. Antifungal preparations are effective for the majority of dermatophyte infections, with the exception of deep inflammatory lesions of the body and scalp (Habif, 2004). Antifungal creams and lotions should be applied topically twice daily until the infection has resolved and for a minimum of 2 weeks. Habif (2004) suggested discontinuing topical medication after inflammation has resolved and also endorsed avoiding mixing topical preparations for convenience because it dilutes the treatments' potencies and decreases effectiveness. Topical medications do not work for nail fungus and should not be prescribed for this condition. Some of the commonly prescribed antifungal creams available include ketoconazole 2% cream (Nizoral), clotrimazole 1% cream or lotion (Lotrimin, Mycelex), econazole 1% cream or lotion (Spectazole), miconazole 2% cream (Monistat), terbinafine (Lamisil), and butenafine hydrochloride (Mentax Cream 1%, Lotrimin Ultra).

## Topical Chemotherapeutics

5-Fluorouracil is commonly prescribed for superficial actinic keratosis. It is an effective topical chemotherapy used to disrupt rapidly dividing abnormal superficial cells and destroy them. Normal cells appear to be unaffected by this drug (Habif, 2004). The treatment provokes inflammation and thus can be painful in the first week or two of therapy. Treating small areas decreases the pain experienced. Drug companies supply educational material to inform and prepare the patient about the inflammation that will occur. Treatment strategies should consider the extent of disease, the patient's occupation, and natural ultraviolet exposure.

Imiquimod (Aldara) 5%, an immune response modifier cream, can be used to treat a variety of skin diseases, including genital warts, actinic keratosis, and superficial basal cell cancers. Patients with actinic keratosis apply imiquimod three times weekly for 6 to 8 weeks. Diclofenac sodium and acid peels are additional topical chemotherapy agents prescribed to clear superficial skin lesions.

## SYSTEMIC EVALUATION AND TREATMENT

Individual providers are mandated to consider the possible connections between the presenting rash or lesions and a variety of systemic illnesses. Certain systemic diseases have long been known to cause mild and at times severe cutaneous symptomology. Being alert to the "great mimickers"—amelanotic melanoma, lupus erythematosus, sarcoid, mycobacteria, and cutaneous T-cell lymphoma—is imperative (Borton, 2011).

# SURGICAL TREATMENT
## Cauterization of Lesions

### Acid
*Chemical cautery*, also called chemotherapy or chemosurgery, is the selective destruction of skin tissues using chemical agents. Chemical cautery is generally used on chronic skin ulcers with poor granulation, flat warts, chloasma, syringoma, angiokeratoma, and other common skin lesions. Commonly used chemicals include strong acids and alkali, trichloroacetic acid, and carbolic acids.

During application of the cauterizing agents, the practitioner must use caution to avoid contact with surrounding normal skin surfaces. The greatest challenge of using chemical cautery is precisely controlling the amount of chemical applied to the lesion. The practitioner should also exercise caution to avoid the self-exposure of clothes or skin during treatment. When applied correctly, treatment outcomes are excellent. Temporary postinflammatory hyperpigmentation can occur after treatment with chemical cautery.

### Electrocautery
*Electrocautery* uses a low-voltage, high-amperage electric current that heats a filament tip. The tip transfers the heat to the patient's superficial tissue, inducing coagulation (Fitzpatrick& Morelli, 2006). No electrical current is transferred to the deep tissue or the patient, making this a good choice of treatment for patients with implanted electrical devices such as pacemakers.

### Electrodessication and Curettage
*Electrodessication* and *curettage* are treatment methods used to remove or destroy benign superficial skin lesions (Goodheart, 2011). Some of the lesions commonly treated include warts, seborrheic keratosis, skin tags, molluscum contagiosum, and condylomata acuminatum. Electrodessication and curettage can also be used to treat both basal and squamous cell skin cancers. Electrodessication uses high-voltage, low-amperage electric current, and there is contact between the electrode tip and the patient (Fitzpatrick& Morelli, 2006). Desiccation results when the heat is transferred to the tissue. Curettage involves scraping or scooping techniques performed with a dermal curette (Goodheart, 2011).

Treatment of the skin lesion usually includes both electrodessication and curettage, but at times electrodessication is used as the sole treatment for lesions without curettage. Conversely, curettage can be used independent of electrodessication for the treatment of epidermal lesions.

# OTHER TREATMENTS
## Cryotherapy

Cryotherapy is the controlled application of a cold substance, usually liquid nitrogen, used with the intent of causing tissue damage to treat a skin lesion. The intracellular and extracellular ice formation dehydrates and destroys the targeted tissue. Freezing the tissue denatures the protein liquid complexes and creates vascular stasis that causes tissue anoxia and necrosis (Fitzpatrick & Morelli, 2006; Goodheart, 2011). With this treatment the practitioner controls the freezing to direct the tissue damage to the abnormal lesion, avoiding the normal surrounding skin. The most effective technique is rapid freezing with slow thawing. This creates greater tissue damage, increasing the chance of lesion destruction. Melanocytes have a greater affinity for freezing and thus can be damaged at higher temperatures. Knowing this should guide treatment choices for melanocytic lesions and patients with darkly pigmented skin.

Cryotherapy is an appropriate treatment for both benign and malignant lesions. Liquid nitrogen is most commonly used because it is readily available, easy to use and store, and works quickly (Fitzpatrick & Morelli, 2006). Cryotherapy is most commonly used in primary care for the treatment of common dermatologic conditions such as warts, actinic keratosis, seborrheic keratosis, and molluscum contagiosum. Contraindications to cryotherapy are any cold-related conditions, such as Raynaud phenomenon or cold hypersensitivity. Patients with these conditions should not be treated with cryotherapy.

## Excision of Skin Lesions

*Mohs micrographic surgery* is a precise microscopically controlled serial method of skin cancer removal. The goal of the surgery is to completely excise the tumor and maximize tissue conservation (Brown & Mellette, 2011). The cure rate is the highest of any treatment option for basal and squamous cell carcinomas; lesions larger than 2 cm; and cancers located on lips, ears, nose, or nasolabial folds (Goodheart, 2011).

Mohs surgery is ideal for the excision of recurrent skin tumors. Often cancer cells reside in the scar tissue of these recurrent tumors, and their clinical margins are not clear (Brown & Mellette, 2011). Cure rates of up to 95% are achieved for recurrent skin cancers treated by Mohs surgery.

## Interlesional Injection of Corticosteroids

Interlesional injections of corticosteroids are often an effective treatment for various skin lesions, such as acne cysts, hypertrophic scars, keloids, localized psoriatic plaques, lichens planus, and prurigo nodularis (Goodheart, 2011). Using a 30-gauge needle, the practitioner injects triamcinolone acetonide (Kenalog, 2.5, 5, 10, 40 mg/mL) intralesionally. The treatment can be repeated at 4- to 6-week intervals.

## Incision and Drainage

Incision and drainage (I&D) is the primary management for cutaneous abscess formation (Fitch, Manthey, McGinnis, Nicks, & Pariyadath, 2007). Most localized abscesses, without evidence of cellulitis, do not require antibiotic therapy and can be treated with simple I&D. Although an abscess can form in any body location, undoubtedly the axillae, buttocks, and extremities are the most common sites. I&D is a common outpatient procedure performed in most primary care practices.

Diagnosing an abscess is vital for the provider to make the appropriate treatment choice. Abscesses are generally tender, fluctuant, and/or erythematous. After diagnosing the abscess, the provider needs to determine whether I&D is needed. It is imperative that the abscess is in an accessible location. Generally the provider considers abscesses 5 mm or larger in size as appropriate for I&D.

Referrals to a specialist for treatment of an abscess are necessary in several clinical scenarios. The potential bacteremia associated with I&D should be considered in patients with artificial or abnormal heart valves (Fitch et al., 2007). A very large or deep abscess mandates surgical intervention. Abscesses on the face or breasts often generate cosmetic concerns and should dictate referral. Problematic skin areas such as palms, soles, and nasolabial folds prompt specialist care.

## Treatment of Ingrown Toenails

In the early stage of ingrown toenail inflammation, nonsurgical management is appropriate (Goldstein & Goldstein, 2012; Tolen, 2013). Ingrown toenails (Figure 6.1) can be treated by gently dislodging the lateral edge of the nail plate from the inflamed nail fold where it is embedded. The next step is to place a sterile nonabsorbent gauze or cotton under the corner of the nail. The gauze or cotton should be replaced each day, and the toe should be soaked in warm water several times daily. The patient should also be prescribed a cutout shoe and activity should be modified to minimize pressure. The patient should be educated on proper nail care, which includes trimming the nail with squared corners that extend distally to the hyponychium.

The provider should suspect an abscess has formed when the ingrown toenail fold extends over the nail plate and erythema and edema has developed. Nonsurgical management may be an option at this stage if cautious care is provided. At this point, the toenail requires absolutely no pressure, including shoes and socks. In addition to the previously described care, warm-water soaks several times a day are needed. Antibiotic use is generally not indicated unless there is evidence of cellulitis or the patient is diabetic or immunocompromised.

A wound culture should be performed if antibiotics are needed. There are several alternative choices for conservative management, including splints or shape memory alloys (Goldstein & Goldstein, 2012; Tolen, 2013).

Advanced disease is evidenced by heavy granulation tissue formation accompanied by pain with walking. This is indicative of the need for surgery and it is highly unlikely nonsurgical treatment would be successful. An abscess forms when the drainage is obstructed, and this occurs when the epithelium grows over the granulation tissue. The excess tissue cannot be lifted off the nail edge.

Ingrown toenail removal begins with a digital block using 1% lidocaine. The two dorsal and two volar nerves must be blocked to achieve successful anesthesia. Injection is made with a 27-gauge needle and 5-mL syringe at 2, 4, 8, and 10 o'clock positions

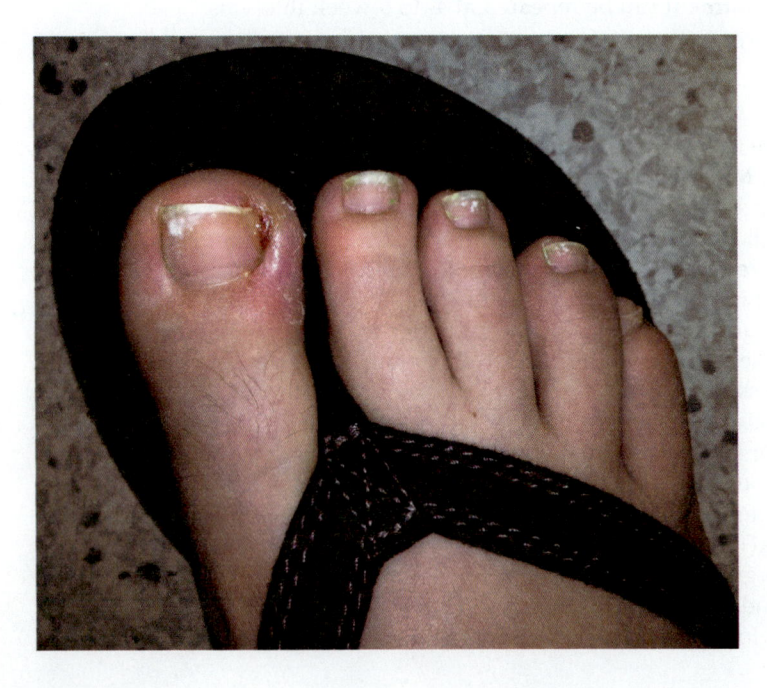

FIGURE 6.1  An ingrown toenail

(Goldstein & Goldstein, 2012; Tolen, 2013). A superficial wheal is created at the dorsal nerve. The needle is advanced, and 1 mL lidocaine is injected to the side of the bone with an additional 0.5 mL as the needle is withdrawn. The procedure is then repeated on the other side.

# REFERENCES

Borton, C. (2011). *Dermatological history and exam*. Retrieved from http://www.patient.co.uk/doctor/dermatological-history-and-examination

Brown, M., & Mellette, J. R. (2011). Mohs surgery. In J. E. Fitzpatrick & J. G. Morelli (Eds.), *Dermatology secrets plus* (4th ed., pp. 374–377). Philadelphia, PA: Elsevier/Saunders.

Fitch, M., Manthey, D., McGinnis, H., Nicks, B., & Pariyadath, M. (2007). Abscess incision and drainage [video]. *New England Journal of Medicine, 357*, e20. doi:10.1056/NEJMvcm071319

Fitzpatrick, J. E., & Morelli, J. G. (2006). *Dermatology secrets in color* (3rd ed.). Philadelphia, PA: Elsevier/Mosby.

Goldstein, B. G., & Goldstein, A. O. (2012). *Paronychia and ingrown toenails*. Retrieved from http://uptodate.com/contents/paronychia-and-ingrown-toenails

Goodheart, H. (2011). *Goodheart's same-site differential diagnosis: A rapid method of diagnosing and treating common skin disorders*. Philadelphia, PA: Lippincott Williams & Wilkins.

Habif, T. (2004). *Clinical dermatology: A color guide to diagnosis and therapy* (4th ed.). Philadelphia, PA: Elsevier/Mosby.

Oakley, A. (2012). *Topical formulations*. Retrieved from http://dermnetnz.org/treatments/topical-formulations.html

Tolen, R. W. (2013). *Ingrown nails*. Retrieved from http://emedicine.medscape.com/article/909807-overview

# 7

# Clinical Management

## ROUTINE SKIN CARE

Routine skin care requires consistent skin hygiene, skin protection, and a lifetime of healthy habits. The strategies that should be employed for routine skin care include diet, exercise, stress management, smoking avoidance, and limited sun exposure.

Daily skin hygiene requires patients to treat their skin carefully during cleaning. Bathing once daily is generally adequate using gentle soaps and warm, not hot, water. Limiting time in the shower and bath helps reduce oils that can be lost during bathing and promotes moisture. Shaving in the direction of hair growth and using shaving cream, lotion, foam, or gel helps protect and lubricate the skin. Providers should educate the patient to pat or blot the skin dry after bathing to allow retention of oils and moisture. Also, patients should be instructed to moisturize the skin's surface after bathing with a product that meets the needs of their skin type. Additionally, applying moisturizer within 3 minutes of bathing helps maintain the skin's hydration.

Protection from the sun is one of the most important strategies to protect the skin. Sun exposure over a person's lifetime causes wrinkles, age spots and benign lesions (Figure 7.1), and disfiguring and deadly skin cancers. For the most complete sun protection and skin cancer prevention, patients should avoid the sun; if they are unable or unwilling to stay out of the sun, encourage the use of broad-spectrum sunscreen with a sun protective factor (SPF) of at least 15. Sunscreen should be reapplied to the skin's surface every 2 hours or more often when swimming or perspiring. Instruct patients to avoid the sun between 10 a.m. and 4 p.m. and wear protective clothing to block the sun's ultraviolet (UV) rays. Long sleeves and pants, wide-brimmed hats, sun-protective laundry additives, and special protective clothing offer protection from exposure. It is the weave of clothing that promotes sun protection, not necessarily the type of cloth—the tighter the weave the more sun protection.

Routine skin care includes not smoking. Educate patients that smoking ages the skin and creates wrinkles. Smoking constricts small blood vessels in the epidermis and decreases blood supply, depleting the skin of oxygen and nutrients. It also damages collagen and elastin, decreasing elasticity. The repetitive facial expressions made during smoking (pursing of lips and squinting of the eyes) can also contribute to increased wrinkling.

Inform patients that eating a healthy diet promotes skin health and should be included as a strategy of routine skin care. A diet high in vegetables, fruits, and lean protein is understood to promote skin health and help the skin look healthier. Research indicates a diet high in vitamin C improves the skin's appearance as well.

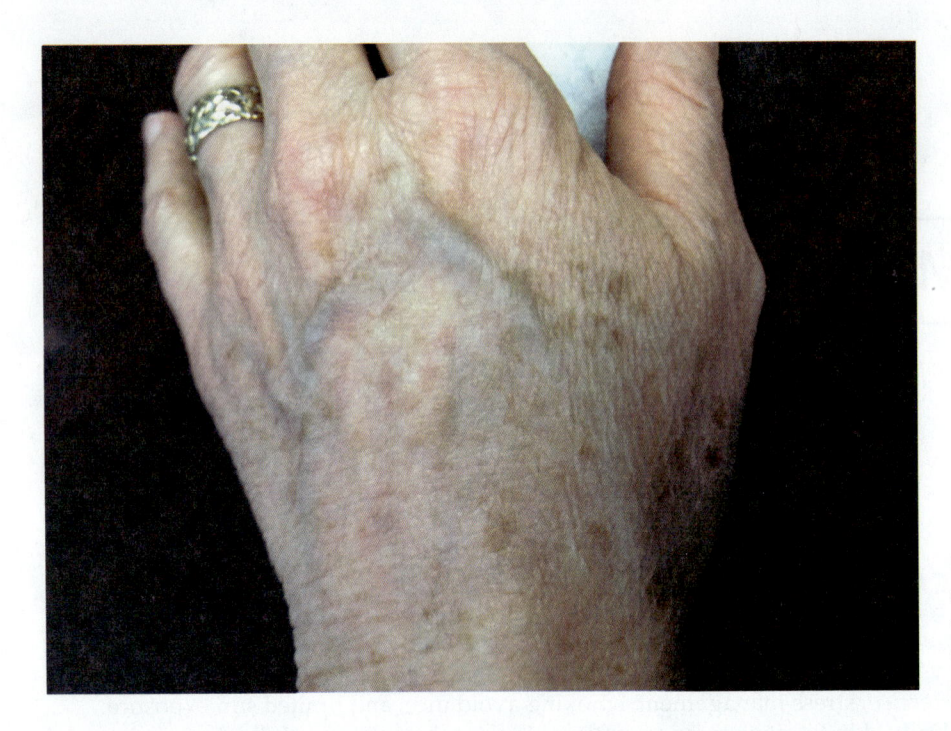

FIGURE 7.1 Age spots are among the benign lesions caused by sun exposure.

Having patients manage and reduce stress promotes healthy skin and is equally important in maintaining skin health. Increased stress can trigger acne and provoke other skin problems such as psoriasis, eczema, and urticaria. Other skin diseases have been related to increased stress and are thus an insult to the patient's immune system. Examples of stress-induced skin disorders include rosacea, stys, herpes zoster, genital herpes, vitiligo, alopecia, and aphthous ulcers. Helping patients reduce stress can be imperative to reducing skin condition occurrences.

## PREVENTIVE CARE

There are essentially two things a clinician should teach patients about skin cancer prevention: sun protection from either sun avoidance or sunscreen use and skin self-examination. A self-examination of the skin is an essential part of skin cancer prevention (Yohn, 2011a, 2011b). Research has revealed that most patients discover their own abnormal skin lesions. Equally important is teaching patients the proper methods of self-examination of the skin and that skin cancer treated early is curable. Patients should be taught to examine their entire skin surface monthly (both sun-exposed and non-sun-exposed areas), including the scalp, buttocks, genitalia, and feet. The next sections discuss preventive measures in more detail.

## SKIN SELF-EXAMINATION

The National Cancer Institute and the American Academy of Dermatology recommend that people perform a skin self-examination once a month. Berman and Zieve (2012) suggested instructing patients that, ideally, the room in which they do the self-examination should have a full-length mirror and bright lights so that the entire body can be well visualized. Furthermore, they noted that when performing a skin self-examination, patients should be instructed to look for:

- New skin markings (moles, blemishes, changes in color, bumps)
- Moles that have changed in size, texture, color, or shape
- Moles or lesions that continue to bleed or will not heal
- Moles with uneven edges, differences in color, or lack of even sides (symmetry)
- Any mole or growth that looks different from other skin growths

Recommend that patients examine their skin in the following ways:

- Look closely at the entire body, both front and back, in the mirror
- Check under the arms and on both sides of each arm
- Examine the forearms after bending the arms at the elbows, and then look at the palms of the hands and underneath the upper arms
- Look at the front and back of both legs
- Look at the buttocks and between the buttocks
- Examine the genital area
- Look at the face, neck, back of the neck, and scalp. It is best to use both a hand mirror and full-length mirror, along with a comb, to see areas of the scalp
- Look at the feet, including the soles and the space between the toes
- Have another person help by examining hard-to-see areas

Always instruct patients to report the following:

- Any new or unusual lesions on the skin
- A mole or skin lesion that changes in size, color, or texture
- A sore that does not heal

## PROTECTION FROM THE SUN

As discussed earlier, the leading skin disease prevention strategy is sun protection through sun avoidance, wearing protective clothing, or the use of sunscreens (Levy, 2012). Although sun avoidance is the most effective protection against skin damage, many people work, walk, or play outside. Clothing is the next best protection. Tight cloth weaves and darker colors offer the greatest protection. Nalory and Farmer (as cited in Levy, 2012) found that using sunscreen is also a practical strategy for all patients. In humans, consistent use of sunscreens reduces the occurrence of actinic keratosis, solar keratosis, and squamous cell carcinoma. Additionally, the photosensitivity created by medication use and sun-induced dermatoses can be prevented by the regular use of sunscreens. Consistent use of SPF 15 sunscreen in a child's first 18 years of life reduces the incidence of basal and squamous cell carcinomas by 78% (Truhan, 1991). The following paragraphs will talk about some of these sun protection techniques in more detail.

As discussed earlier, clothing can provide protection from UV radiation. Clothes that are bright or dark colored (red or black) absorb more UV radiation than white or pastel shades. Also, synthetic fibers (polyester) can offer more protection than materials such as refined cottons or crepe. Still, the weave density is more important for protection than the type of cloth. On cooler days, tightly woven or closely knitted fabrics such as denim and denser fabrics, such as heavyweight flannel, will absorb less UV light than thinner materials (Skin Cancer Foundation, 2011).

Sun-protective garments should have an ultraviolent protection factor (UPF) label. This indicates what fraction of the sun's UV rays can penetrate the fabric.

For example, a shirt with a UPF of 50 will let 1/50 of the sun's UV radiation reach the skin. The Skin Cancer Foundation recommends clothing with a UPF of 30+ (2011).

A broad-spectrum sunscreen provides protection through the entire spectrum of both UVB (ultraviolet B, short-wave) and UVA (ultraviolet A, long-wave) radiation, and water-resistant sunscreens maintain an SPF level after 40 to 80 minutes of water immersion. The SPF is defined as the dose of UV radiation required to produce one minimal erythema dose (MED) on protected skin after the application of 2 mg/cm$^2$ of product divided by the UV radiation required to produce 1 MED on unprotected skin (Levy, 2012).

Sunscreens are categorized by their ability to absorb or block UV radiation. Chemical sunscreens absorb high-intensity radiation. Physical sunscreen blockers reflect and scatter radiation. It has been suggested that microsized physical blockers or nonchemical sunscreens may also work in part by absorption (as cited in Levy, 2012). Levy (1995) noted that sunscreens with an SPF of at least 15 provide approximately 93% of UVB protection, and an SPF of 30 protects up to 97%. Unfortunately, sunscreens do not adequately protect patients from UVA radiation, especially UVA I (Levy, 2012). In addition to the SPF, the thickness of sunscreen application affects the skin's protection from UVA. SPF of 30 provides better protection than SPF of 15 and sunscreens do not provide adequate UVB protection. It is imperative that patients who spend time in the sun and expect sunscreens to protect their skin understand that they are still at risk for sun damage, especially UVA radiation damage.

Recommendations for extra precautions are:

- Avoid reflective surfaces such as water, sand, concrete, and white-painted surfaces.
- Remember that cloudy, hazy days can intensify UVB exposure.
- Keep in mind that UV intensity depends on the angle of the sun, not the heat or brightness, so dangers are greater closer to the start of summer.
- Be aware that skin burns faster at higher altitudes. One study suggested that a person of average complexion burns in 6 minutes at 11,000 feet at noon compared with 25 minutes at sea level.
- Avoid sun lamps, tanning beds, and tanning salons; the machines use mostly high-output UVA rays.

## MOISTURIZER

According to Habif (2011, p. 2), "a moisturizer is a compound that serves four principal functions: (1) repairs the skin barrier, (2) maintains skin integrity and appearance, (3) reduces transepidermal water loss, and (4) restores the lipid barrier's ability to hold and redistribute water." To minimize the drying effects of bathing, patients should be taught to pat the skin dry and apply moisturizer within 3 minutes.

Occlusive moisturizers work by preventing water loss from the skin's surface. Petroleum, lanolin, mineral oil, and silicones are all occlusive moisturizers. Petroleum feels greasy and can block follicular and eccrine openings but is felt to be the least irritating. Humectant moisturizers, such as glycerin, increase the absorption of water from the air to the skin. Lotions spread more easily on the skin, and they soften and smooth the skin's surface. Some lotions decrease itching and contain camphor and menthol. Lactic acid, salicylic acid, and glycolic acid are keratolytic emollients; these gently exfoliate the skin.

Moisturizers can include various additives, such as fragrances, preservatives, sunscreens, and vitamins. People with sensitive skin should use fragrance-free products. Preservatives added in moisturizing products can cause dermatitis and allergies.

Sunscreens are added to some moisturizers to reduce sun damage and aging effects. Vitamins A, E, and C are added to some products for antiaging.

## NUTRITIONAL COUNSELING

There are numerous cutaneous signs of nutritional disturbances (Demidovich, 2011). Abnormal skin conditions occur when a deficiency or excess of a particular nutrient exist. Nutritional disorders are not exclusive to the skin but involve multiple body systems, and thus obtaining a clinical history, review of systems, and physical examination are imperative to determining the cause of a skin condition suggestive of nutritional disorder (Demidovich, 2011).

The effects of protein and caloric deprivation on the skin include rough, inelastic, pallid, gray skin. Additionally, hair appears thin, and nails grow slowly and can exhibit fissuring. Fat malabsorption syndromes can create generalized dermatitis caused by transepidermal water loss, which results from the loss of the skin's barrier function; dietary or intravenous linoleic acid supplementation can be curative in these cases (Demidovich, 2011). Conversely, cutaneous findings associated with obesity include plantar keratosis (thickened soles), acanthosis nigricans (Figure 7.2), striae, and skin tags (Yosipovitch, Devore, & Dawn, 2007).

Most water-soluble vitamin deficiencies exhibit skin findings (Demidovich, 2011). Skin manifestations of deficiencies in the B-complex vitamins—riboflavin ($B_2$), pyridoxine ($B_6$), and cobalamin ($B_{12}$)—and in biotin include angular cheilitis, periorificial dermatitis, and glossitis (Barthelemy, Chouvet, & Chambazard, 1986). Severe vitamin $B_1$ (thiamine) deficiency, called beriberi, occurs as a result of alcoholism, imbalanced diet, gastrointestinal disease, after some surgeries (gastric bypass), and in pregnancy. Mucocutaneous indicators include limb edema and glossitis (Towbin et al., 2004). Dermatitis is one of the four manifestations (diarrhea,

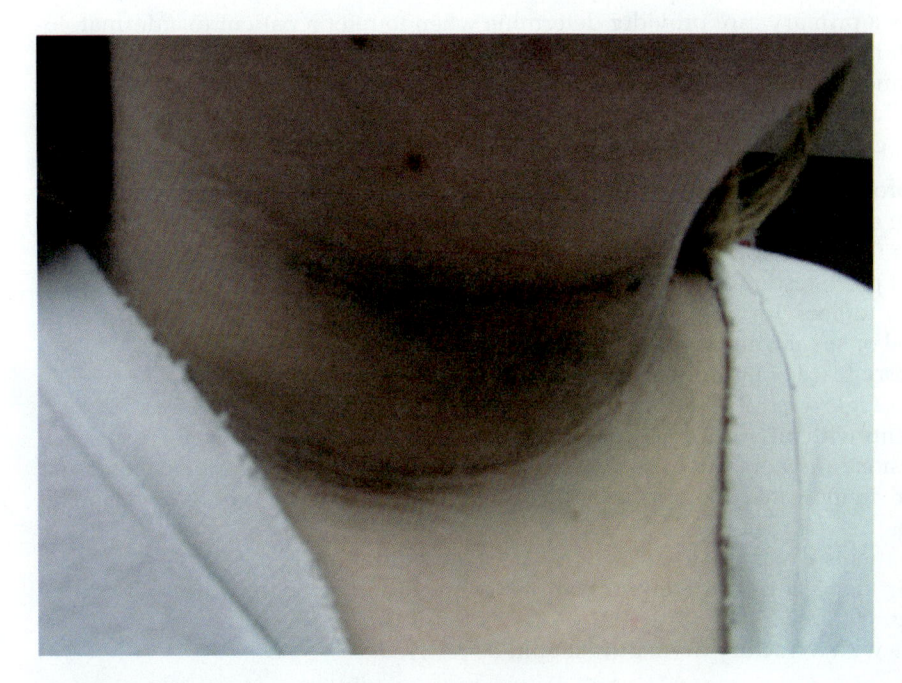

FIGURE 7.2
Acanthosis nigricans is a dark, velvety, hyperpigmentation of the skin, often found at the skin folds.

dermatitis, dementia, and death) of pellagra (niacin deficiency), most commonly seen in alcoholics and patients on isoniazid therapy (Hegyi, Schwartz, & Hegyi, 2004). The dermatitis tends to be photodistributed and turns dry, scaly, and thickened. *Casal necklace* is a term coined to describe the demarcated lesions that develop around the neck. Lesions can also develop on the genital and perineal skin areas, over bony prominences, and on the face. Niacin supplementation allows rapid improvement.

Deficiencies in fat-soluble vitamins can occur but are much less common because these vitamins have substantial storage depots (Fitzpatrick & Morelli, 2011). Vitamin K deficiency occurs during the newborn period before intestinal bacteria forms and also because of malabsorption conditions; skin lesions range from petechiae to mass hemorrhages (Fitzpatrick & Morelli, 2011).

Vitamin A deficiency, most commonly caused by malabsorption disorders, creates cutaneous keratotic follicular lesions appearing first on the extremities. The lesions then erupt on the trunk, back, abdomen, buttocks, and neck. Also called phrynoderma, facial lesions look like large comedones, and eye symptoms can include nyctalopia, night blindness, and xerophthalmia (Maronn, Allen, & Esterly, 2005). A clinical finding for vitamin A deficiency is Bitot spots, areas of shed corneal epithelium (Sommer, 2008).

Vitamin A excess can be acute or chronic. Acute toxicity is generally caused by overdose. A cutaneous sign of hypervitaminosis A is large areas of desquamation. Chronic toxicity creates similar symptoms to retinoid use—alopecia, dryness, and exfoliation. Symptoms resolve in days to weeks once excessive vitamin A is removed (Fitzpatrick & Morelli, 2011).

Acral dermatitis and alopecia are the cutaneous symptoms of the deficiency of the trace element zinc. Oral or intravenous supplementation of zinc rapidly reverses symptoms.

## APPROPRIATE REFERRALS

How does a primary care provider determine when to refer a patient to a dermatologist? Certain cutaneous diagnoses and conditions that fail to respond to conventional skin treatments should alert the clinician that an appropriate dermatologic referral is needed. The following are common cutaneous disorders and conditions that warrant dermatologic referral.

- If the provider suspects a patient with acne may have an endocrine abnormality or scarring acne, referral is in order.
- Eczema that does not improve after a trial of sensitive skin care and treatment may warrant patch testing by a dermatologist.
- Vascular tumors during infancy need to be referred.
- Atypical or suspicious nevi need referral for biopsy.
- Refractory cases of nummular eczema (Figure 7.3) need referral.
- Dermatologic referral is recommended for all bullous diseases (Figure 7.4).
- In patients with pityriasis rosea, a referral is in order when lesion morphology is variable, lesions are more extensive than expected, or lesions last longer than expected.
- Referral is indicated for severe recalcitrant seborrheic dermatitis or widespread disease.
- Refer patients when leg ulcers are large or of long duration.
- Scarring alopecia or erosive mucosal involvement and refractory cases should be referred.
- Patients with refractory dermatitis should be referred.

7. Clinical Management ■ 57

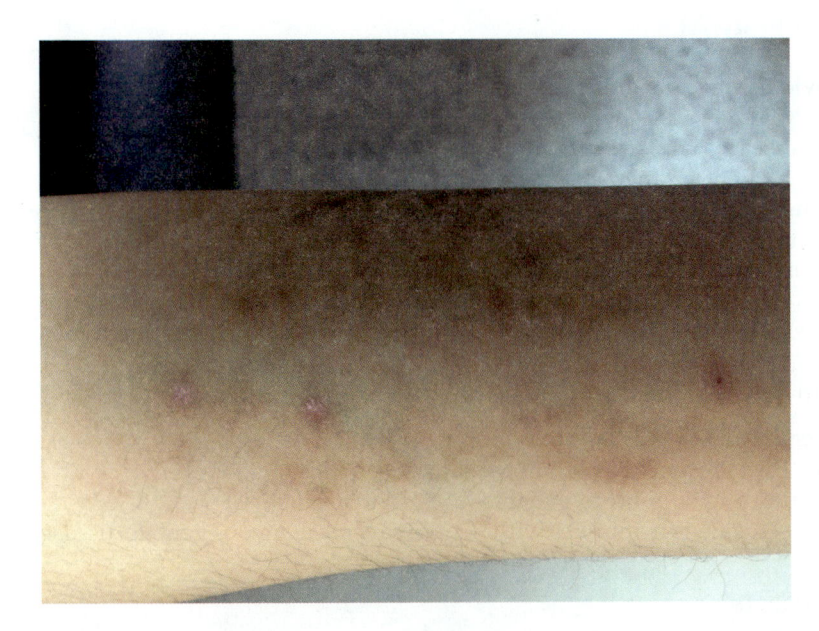

FIGURE 7.3　Nummular eczema

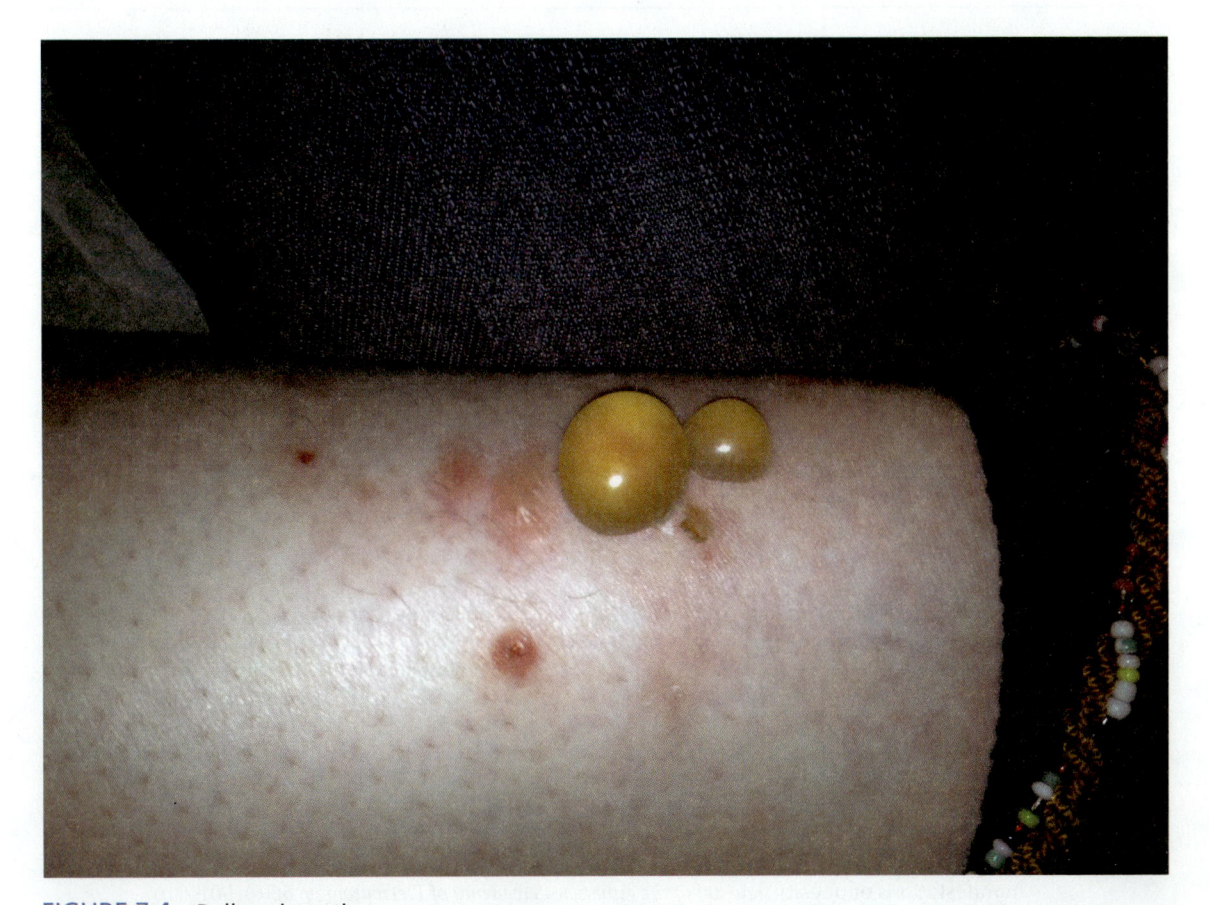

FIGURE 7.4　Bullous impetigo

## GENETIC COUNSELING REFERRALS

Primary care providers have a significant role in making appropriate genetic referrals for their patients. Providers are generally the first-line professionals whom patients ask about genetic skin disease risks, in particularly the individual's or his or her children's risk of inheriting a familial cutaneous disease (Tidy, 2012).

Genetic counseling is an integral part of the genetic testing process. It should be offered in the majority of genetic testing circumstances, and it is the responsibility of the provider ordering the genetic testing to fully inform the patient of the medical facts and consequences. It is also important for any clinician to recognize that genetic counseling requires special skill and education, and clinicians should know their limitations in genetic care.

According to Tidy (2012), primary care providers need to be able to:

- Explain the mechanism of inheritance of disease
- Educate patients on a lifestyle that promotes skin health
- Provide information and support to patients referred to a geneticist
- Advise antenatal screenings in families with known severe cutaneous genetic disease

## REFERENCES

Barthelemy, H., Chouvet, B., & Chambazard, F. (1986). Skin and mucosal manifestations in vitamin deficiency. *Journal of the American Academy of Dermatology, 15*(6), 1263–1274.

Berman, K., & Zieve, D. (2012). *Skin self-exam*. Retrieved from http://www.nlm.nih.gov/medlineplus/ency/article/007086.htm

Demidovich, C. (2011). Cutaneous signs of nutritional disturbances. In J. E. Fitzpatrick & J. G. Morelli (Eds.), *Dermatology secrets plus* (4th ed., pp. 287–291). Philadelphia, PA: Elsevier/Mosby.

Fitzpatrick, J. E., & Morelli, J. G. (2011). *Dermatology secrets plus* (4th ed.). Philadelphia, PA: Elsevier/Mosby.

Habif, T. (2004). *Clinical dermatology: A color guide to diagnosis and therapy* (4th ed.). Philadelphia, PA: Elsevier/Mosby.

Habif, T. (2011). *Skin disease: Diagnosis and treatment* (3rd ed.). New York, NY: Elsevier.

Hegyi, J., Schwartz, R., & Hegyi, V. (2004). Pellagra: Dermatitis, dementia, and diarrhea. *International Journal of Dermatology, 43*(1), 1–5.

Levy, S. (1995). How high the SPF? *Archives of Dermatology, 131*(12), 1463–1464.

Levy, S. (2012). *Sunscreen and photoprotection*. Retrieved from http://emedicine.medscape.com/article/1119992-overview#aw2aab6b3

Skin Cancer Foundation. (2011). *Give up tanning in 2011*. Retrieved from http://www.skincancer.org/prevention/tanning/give-up-tanning-in-the-new-year

Sommer, A. (2008). Vitamin A deficiency and clinical disease: A historical overview. *Journal of Nutrition, 138*, 1835–1839.

Tidy, C. (2012). *Genetic counseling—A guide for GPs*. Retrieved from www.patient.co.uk/doctor/genetic-counselling-a-guide-for-gps

Towbin, A., Inge, T. H., Garcia, V. F., Roehrig, H. R., Clements, R. H., Harmon, C. M., & Daniels, S. (2004). Beriberi after gastric bypass surgery in adolescence. *Journal of Pediatrics, 145*(2), 263–267.

Truhan, A. (1991). Sun protection in childhood. *Clinical Pediatrics, 30*(12), 676–681.

Yohn, J. (2011a). Disorders of pigmentation. In J. E. Fitzpatrick & J. G. Morelli (Eds.), *Dermatology secrets plus* (4th ed.). Philadelphia, PA: Elsevier/Mosby.

Yohn, J. (2011b). Disorders of pigmentation. In T. Habif (Ed.), *Skin disease: Diagnosis and treatment* (pp. 126–134). New York, NY: Elsevier.

Yosipovitch, G., Devore, A., & Dawn, A. (2007). Obesity and the skin: Skin physiology and skin manifestations of obesity. *Journal of the American Academy of Dermatology, 56*(6), 901–916.

# PART III

# Common Dermatologic Conditions

| | |
|---|---|
| *Abrasions and Skin Tears* | *61* |
| *Acne* | *65* |
| *Alopecia* | *71* |
| *Aphthous Stomatitis* | *79* |
| *Bruise and Contusion* | *85* |
| *Burns* | *89* |
| *Candidiasis* | *95* |
| *Cellulitis/Erysipelas* | *109* |
| *Cysts* | *115* |
| *Dermatitis* | *129* |
| *Erythema Multiforme* | *151* |
| *Erythema Nodosum* | *157* |
| *Granuloma Annulare* | *163* |
| *Herpes Simplex Virus* | *169* |
| *Impetigo* | *193* |
| *Insect Bites* | *199* |
| *Lentigo/Nevi* | *213* |
| *Lichen Planus* | *223* |
| *Molluscum Contagiosum* | *229* |
| *Nail Conditions* | *235* |
| *Pemphigus* | *249* |
| *Perioral Dermatitis* | *255* |
| *Pityriasis Rosea* | *259* |
| *Psoriasis* | *265* |
| *Rosacea* | *273* |
| *Skin Cancer* | *279* |
| *Tinea Infections* | *303* |

| | |
|---|---|
| *Urticaria* | *321* |
| *Vasculitis* | *327* |
| *Verruca Vulgaris* | *337* |
| *Vitiligo* | *345* |

# Abrasions and Skin Tears

## OVERVIEW

*Abrasions* and *skin tears* are breakages in the upper layers of the skin caused by trauma from friction. Abrasions and skin tears may ooze blood from injured capillaries (LeBlanc & Baranoski, 2011). Abrasions typically occur to the epidermal layer of the skin, whereas skin tears separate the epidermis from the dermis (*partial-thickness wound*) or separate both the epidermis and the dermis from underlying structures (*full-thickness wound*; Chardon, 2011; LeBlanc & Baranoski, 2011).

## CLINICAL PRESENTATION

When assessing a patient, evaluate for a potential serious injury that may have caused the abrasion or skin tear. Include these questions in your assessment.

- When did you injure yourself (date and time)?
- Describe your pain level on a scale of 0 (*no pain*) to 10 (*worst pain imaginable*).
- Do you have any allergies to medication, tape, latex, or any over-the-counter product?
- Have you had a previous injury in the same area?
- Were you wearing a helmet or other protective gear at the time of the injury?
- Have you had a tetanus vaccine? If so, when?
- What have you done to treat the wound? (Chardon, 2011)

The Payne–Martin Classification System was the only method for classifying a skin tear documented in the literature until 2006, when the Skin Tear Audit Research (STAR) classification system was introduced. In their article, LeBlanc and Baranoski (2011) described the STAR classification system, which organizes skin tears into five categories:

- Category 1a: A skin tear in which the edges can be reapproximated to the normal anatomic position and the skin color is not pale, dusky, or darkened
- Category 1b: A skin tear in which the edges can be reapproximated to the normal anatomic position and the skin flap is pale, dusky, or darkened
- Category 2a: A skin tear in which the edges cannot be reapproximated to the normal anatomic position and the skin flap is not pale, dusky, or darkened

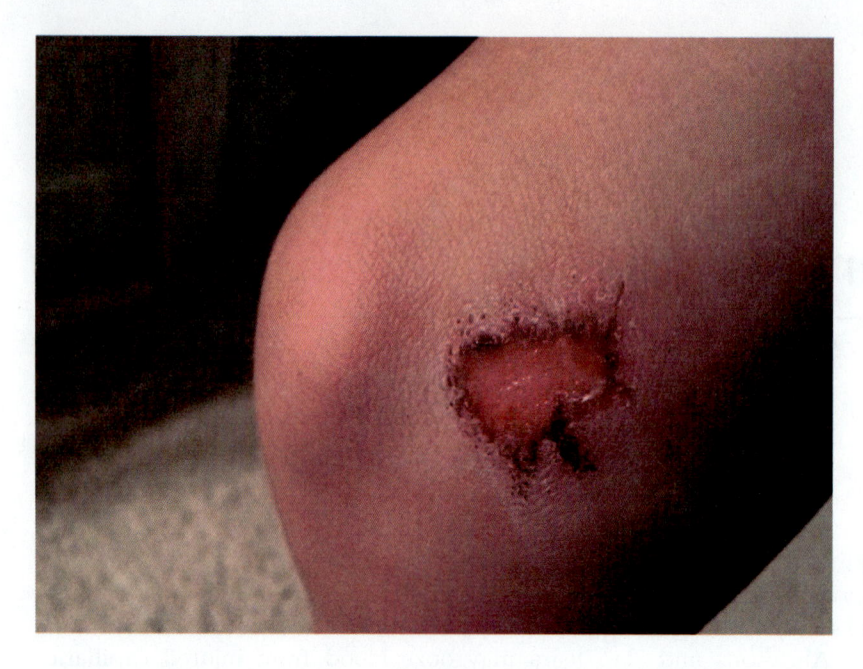

FIGURE III.1 An abrasion on the medial knee
Courtesy of Michael Lineberry

- Category 2b: A skin tear in which the edges cannot be reapproximated to the normal anatomical position and the skin flap is pale, dusky, or darkened
- Category 3: A skin tear in which the skin flap is completely removed

## TREATMENT/MANAGEMENT

Immediately clean the abrasion or skin tear with clear water and soap (Ivory dish soap is preferable) while wearing gloves. Try to remove any foreign material, if present, without scrubbing the area, which could result in additional damage. Keep abrasion and tear areas moist. Instruct the patient to change the dressing several times per day. Keep the areas around or over a joint or moving body part moist until the wound is healed. Use of newer dressings, such as Tegaderm or Bioclusive, will help maintain a moist environment, although covering the wound with an antibacterial ointment, such as bacitracin, Polysporin, or Neosporin, and a nonstick dressing is also acceptable.

## SPECIAL CONSIDERATIONS

### Older Adult or Geriatric Patients

With increasing age, individuals have decreased moisture in the skin as a result of thinning and serum composition changes, which causes decreased skin elasticity. The risk of abrasions and skin tears is greatly increased in older adults who are dehydrated, are poorly nourished, have cognitive impairment or altered mobility, or report decreased sensation. These factors are common in the older patients in all care settings and increase the skin's susceptibility to trauma (LeBlanc & Baranoski, 2011).

## Neonates and Infants

Neonates and infants are also prone to abrasions and skin tears because their skin is underdeveloped and the epidermis is thinner compared with that of older children and adults. Neonates also have less epidermal–dermal cohesion; deficient stratum corneum; limited thermoregulation; and immature immune, hepatic, and renal systems (LeBlanc & Baranoski, 2011).

## When to Refer

The following types of wounds should be referred for additional treatment.

- Puncture wounds
- Gaping wounds that require stitches
- Wounds that have exposed fatty tissue, white tissue, or muscle
- Wounds with visible foreign material (plant, material, glass, metal, or gravel)
- Wounds that are spurting blood
- Wounds causing severe pain or resulting in numbness or inability to move structures below the wound
- Nonhealing wounds
- Infected wounds (Pray, 2006)

## PATIENT EDUCATION

Advise patients to call or see a health care provider if:

- The wound continues to bleed after 10 minutes of direct pressure
- The abrasion or cut is gaping, deep, jagged, or at least a half inch long
- The wound is over a joint or the bone is visible
- The abrasion or cut is on the face
- The wound has foreign material in it
- The wound is a puncture wound
- They think that they may have damaged a nerve or tendon
- The abrasion or tear is greater than 4 by 4 inches
- The part that was injured (e.g., a finger) cannot be moved
- They have not had a tetanus shot within the past 5 years
- Exposure to rabies is possible
- They have questions about wound care (Richards, 2012)

## CLINICAL PEARLS

- When teaching patients about self-care, consider possible concerns of patients and parents, includings scarring, ability to resume normal activities, and cost of treatment (Chardon, 2011).
- For dirty wounds, patients should obtain a tetanus booster within 24 hours (booster is needed every 5 years; Kifer, 2012).
- For minor clean wounds, recommend that patients obtain a booster tetanus shot within 72 hours (a booster is needed every 10 years).

# REFERENCES

Chardon, Z. (2011). *Abrasion care in healthy young adults.* Retrieved from http://www.Nursing2011.com

Kifer, Z. A. (2012). *Fast facts for wound care nursing. Practical wound management in a nutshell.* New York, NY: Springer Publishing Company.

LeBlanc, K., & Baranoski, S. (2011). Skin tears: A state of the science: Consensus statements for the prevention, assessment, and treatment of skin tears. *Advances in Skin & Wound Care, 24,* 2–15.

Pray, W. S. (2006). *When to refer wounds.* Retrieved from http://www.medscape.com/viewarticle/530793

Richards, T. (2012). Cuts, scrapes, and scratches. *Adult Health Advisor,* 1(1).

# Acne

## OVERVIEW

Acne is a common skin condition that affects all ages and both sexes; however, 80% of adolescents are affected by acne at some point (Ramanathan & Hebert, 2011). Acne represents the most common dermatologic diagnosis in the United States (Knutsen-Larson, Dawson, Dunnick, & Dellavalle, 2012). In recent years, treatment guidelines for acne have been revised with the greater understanding of its pathophysiology, and therapy is targeted at treating as many pathogenic factors as possible.

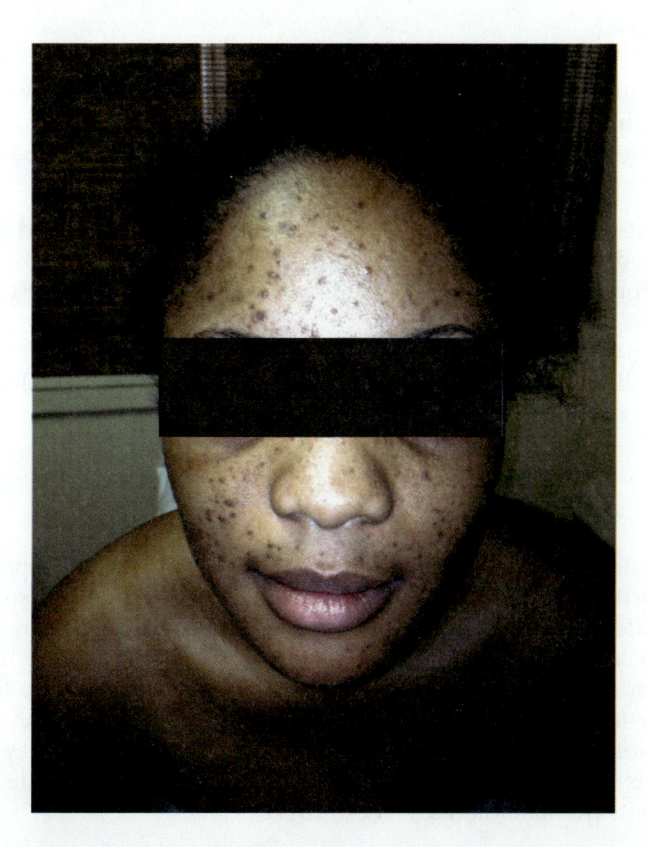

FIGURE III.2  Inflammatory acne

## EPIDEMIOLOGY

There are approximately 5 million physician visits for acne each year in the United States, leading to an annual direct cost in excess of $2 billion. The annual cost of acne treatment is also high because of frequency and chronicity of the disease (Knutsen-Larson et al., 2012).

The average age of onset of acne is 11 years, although reports indicate children have been affected as early as 9 years. This is attributed to the earlier onset of puberty that has been observed in the United States in recent years. Acne is more common in male than female adolescents, but this reverses with age and acne becomes more common in women than in men (Knutsen-Larson et al., 2012).

## PATHOLOGY/HISTOLOGY

Normally, *sebum*, an oily waxy matter that lubricates the skin, is produced by sebaceous glands at the base of the hair follicle and is released at the skin surface. In acne, hyperkeratinization blocks the hair follicle, trapping the sebum. This entrapment results in blockage and inflammation of the hair follicle and the production of a *comedo* (plural: comedones), which is the precursor of an acne lesion. Closed comedones are referred to as whiteheads, and open comedones are referred to as blackheads. These clogged, inflamed lesions are populated with *Propionibacterium acnes (P. acnes)*, a bacterium that is part of the normal flora found on the skin surface that can invade and cause inflammation. Inflammatory acne lesions can often result in papules, pustules, or cysts (Ramanathan & Hebert, 2011; Webster, 2005).

## CLINICAL PRESENTATION

From age 10 through 17 years, pubertal production of androgens, which control sebum secretion, increases. The female clinical course of acne will wax and wane depending on menses (Selway, 2010). There are typically three types of classifications for acne.

- *Mild acne* consists of whiteheads (open comedones), blackheads (closed comedones), and few scattered papules on the face, chest, or back.
- *Moderate acne* consists of extensive comedones, papules, and pustules on the face, chest, or back.
- *Severe acne* consists of nodules and cysts that can cause scarring; comedones, papules, and pustules will be present on the face, chest, and/or back (Ramanathan & Hebert, 2011).

## DIAGNOSTIC TESTS

Individual differences in the distribution, type, and severity of acne depend on one's sensitivity to *P. acnes* and genetic factors (Yan, 2006). The typical signs of androgen excess typically affect females and include hirsutism, alopecia, premature adrenarche, body odor, and accelerated growth. If androgen excess is suspected, the management plan should include diagnostic blood work to determine total and free testosterone, dehydroepiandrosterone (DHEA), DHEA-S, prolactin, luteinizing hormone, follicle-stimulating hormone, and thyroid-stimulating hormone levels. If polycystic ovarian syndrome (POS) is suspected, a hand film should be obtained to evaluate bone age in prepubertal patients (Ramanathan & Hebert, 2011).

## DIFFERENTIAL DIAGNOSIS

- Anabolic steroid use
- Cortisone-induced acne
- Folliculitis
- Perioral dermatitis
- Rosacea
- Seborrheic dermatitis

## TREATMENT/MANAGEMENT

The treatment of acne includes many therapies and depends on several clinical features. Determining the appropriate treatment requires a thorough assessment that includes (Graber, 2011):

- Type of acne (comedonal, inflammatory, or nodular)
- Severity of acne (presence of scarring or postinflammatory hyperpigmentation)
- Skin type (dry vs. oily; topical medications are typically in a cream or gel form, gels have more of a drying effect than creams)
- Menstrual history or signs of hyperandrogenism in women
- Psychological impact of acne on the patient
- Patient compliance

The treatment of acne is meant to decrease follicular hyperproliferation, sebum production, *P. acne* excess, and inflammation (Graber, 2011).

### Cleansers and Abrasives

Retinoids are a class of topical medication that are used to dry up oiliness/treat comedones. Examples include: Retin-A, Atralin, Avita, Renova. Each of these is available in cream and gel form. Creams are not as drying to the skin, gels are more drying because they contain alcohol.

*Salicylic acid* is less irritating than topical retinoids but is considered less effective (Ramanathan & Hebert, 2011). Salicylic acid is useful in patients who do not tolerate retinoids or in patients with comedonal acne of the trunk, where it may be expensive to use a retinoid. Examples of salicylic acid products include Acnex, Acnevir, Condylax, Oxy Balance Deep Pore Cleanser, Neutrogena, Clearasil, and Salex Cream.

- Other cleansers: Graber (2011) recommended that patients use cleansers gently and avoid irritating skin care products. Noncomedogenic (water-based) skin care products and cosmetics are preferred. Examples of water-based skin products include OLAY facial cleansers, Neutrogena facial cleanser, Clinique facial cleansing products.

### Topical Treatments

*Topical benzoyl peroxide* or *topical antibiotics* (erythromycin and clindamycin) used in combination with topical retinoids can improve inflammatory acne caused by *P. acnes* (Grade 2A). They can be used in monotherapy or in combination with benzoyl peroxide or retinoids. Topical benzoyl peroxide and retinoids can be mixed with antibiotics. Examples of such combination products include Duac Gel, Epiduo Gel, Benzamycin Pak, and Ziana. Sulfacetamide topical agents inhibit *P. acnes* but are usually not considered a first-line therapy option.

Topical retinoids are recommended for use as maintenance therapy for long-term prevention of acne. Daily application of these products can help prevent flare ups of acne (Grade 2A; Graber, 2011; Onselen, 2010; Strauss et al., 2007; Zaenglein & Thiboutot, 2006).

## Antibiotics

Systematic antibiotics are the standard of care for the management of moderate to severe acne and for the treatment of resistant forms of inflammatory acne.

- Doxycycline and minocycline are more effective than tetracycline, and there is evidence that minocycline is superior to doxycycline in reducing *P. acnes*.
- Erythromycin is effective but is not recommended because of side effects.
- Bactrim is recommended if other antibiotics fail or cannot be used (Graber, 2011; Strauss et al., 2007).

## Hormonal Agents

Androgens stimulate increased sebum production, which aids in the formation of acne.

- Endocrinologic testing (androgen) is recommended for young children who experience signs of androgen excess (body odor, axillary or pubic hair, and clitoromegaly).
- Young women with symptoms of hyperandrogenism may present with stubborn or late-onset acne, abnormal menses, hirsutism, male and female pattern alopecia, infertility, acanthosis nigricans, and truncal obesity.
- Hormonal therapy may benefit women with moderate to severe acne, even in the absence of a hyperandrogenic state (Graber, 2011; Strauss et al., 2007).
- Examples of hormonal agents used in acne therapy includes Spironolactone and Aldactone.

In the presence of associated polycystic ovarian syndrome (POS), acne can be treated with low androgenic oral contraceptives such as Yaz, Yasmine, or Loryna.

- Spironolactone (Aldactone) may be effective for women who are seeking contraception or antiandrogen therapy.
- Metformin has demonstrated effectiveness equal to oral contraceptives in reducing acne (Smith & Taylor, 2011).

## Other Options

- Isotretinoin use is approved for the treatment of severe resistant nodular acne. Oral isotretinoin can be used for the management of lesser degrees of acne if the individual is resistant to previous treatment or showing signs of scarring (Strauss et al., 2007). *Caution:* Mood disorders, depression, and suicide have been reported in patients taking this drug. Because of teratogenicity, female patients of childbearing potential may be treated only if approved pregnancy prevention and management is used. It is now mandatory that providers be enrolled in the iPLEDGE program when prescribing isotretinoin (Graber, 2011; Strauss et al., 2007). According to the iPLEDGE website (https://www.ipledgeprogram.com/AboutiPLEDGE.aspx).
- The iPLEDGE program is a computer-based, risk-management program designed to further the public health goal of eliminating fetal exposure to isotretinoin through a special restricted distribution program approved by the Food and Drug Administration. The program strives to ensure that no female patient starts isotretinoin therapy if pregnant and no female patient on isotretinoin therapy becomes pregnant.

- Dapsone 5% gel is effective in the treatment of inflammatory acne vulgaris (Graber, 2011).
- Echinacea has shown antibacterial and anti-inflammatory properties in the treatment of acne (Sharma, Schoop, Suter, & Hudson, 2011).
- Laser treatments, chemical peels, and dermabrasion have been used for the treatment of acne scarring; however, there are no well-accepted guidelines for treatment (Knutsen-Larson et al., 2012).
- Smoking increases acne risk and severity (Knutsen-Larson et al., 2012).

An association between milk and acne has been suggested, based on the increased levels of insulin-like growth factor 1 in milk, which causes an increase in circulating androgens. Associations of omega-3 fatty acids, antioxidants, zinc, vitamin A, and iodine also have been proposed, but research is weak (Knutsen-Larson et al., 2012).

The role of the provider in the treatment of acne calls for continuous patient education, motivation, and frequent follow-up. Addressing patient concerns, evaluating treatment efficacy and tolerability, and monitoring adherence to treatment are critical components of acne management (Selway, 2010).

## SPECIAL CONSIDERATIONS

Acne should be considered more than a dermatologic problem. Depression and anxiety can be associated with acne; therefore, clinicians should repeatedly assess for evidence of emotional problems, and reported symptoms should be taken seriously. Acne has been associated with greater psychological burden than many other chronic disorders. An evidence-based review indicated that effective acne treatment resulted in improved self-esteem and affect, improvements in obsessive-compulsive disorder symptoms, less shame and embarrassment, and improved body image, social assertiveness, and self-confidence (Steventon & Cowdell, 2013; Tan, 2004).

## WHEN TO REFER

Resistant and cystic acne should be referred to a dermatologist. Patients with this degree of acne require close follow-up and possibly oral isotretinoin to prevent scarring.

## PATIENT EDUCATION

Before a treatment plan is started, adherence issues and expectations should be addressed. Parents and adolescents should be involved in the education and treatment plan.

- Explain the following to patients and parents.
  - Acne is a slow-responding disorder; it will take approximately 8 weeks before improvement will be visible. The duration of an acne lesion is 2 months from the time it develops under the skin to the full-blown pustule stage; thus even after treatment initiation, new acne lesions may appear.
  - Benzoyl peroxide agents can bleach sheets and clothing. Old T-shirts, sheets, towels, and the like, should be used if applying topical medications to the back and face at night.
  - Smoking increases acne risk.
  - Dairy intake can increase acne.

- Explain when to apply topical medications and when to take oral medications.
- Educate patients to:
  - Wash the face twice daily with a mild cleanse; explain that comedones are not caused by dirt
  - Avoid scrubbing, picking, or squeezing acne lesions
  - Apply a pea-sized amount of topical medications to the face (retinoids cause skin irritation if too much is applied); use a mild, nongreasy moisturizer if skin becomes dry
  - Use oil-free and noncomedogenic (water-based) cosmetics
  - Minimize sun exposure, especially if using medications that increase the risk of sunburn, such as doxycycline

## CLINICAL PEARLS

- Acne vulgaris: ICD-10, L70.0; Other acne: ICD-9, 706.1
- Educate patients to expect acne to worsen for the first 2 weeks of treatment, with full resolution occurring normally in 8 to 12 weeks (Levine, 2013)

## REFERENCES

Graber, E. (2011). *Treatment of acne vulgaris.* Retrieved from http://www.uptodate.com/contents/treatment-of-acne-vulgaris

Knutsen-Larson, S., Dawson, A. L., Dunnick, C. A., & Dellavalle, R. P. (2012). Acne vulgaris: Pathogenesis, treatment, and needs assessment. *Dermatology Clinics, 30,* 99–106.

Levine, G. I. (2013). *Acne vulgaris.* Retrieved from http://www.unboundmedicine.com/5-minute/view/5-minute-clinical-consultation

Onselen, J. V. (2010). Prescribing for mild to moderate acne. *Nurse Prescribing, 8,* 424–431.

Ramanathan, S., & Hebert, A. A. (2011). Management of acne vulgaris. *Journal of Pediatric Health Care, 25,* 332–337.

Selway, J. (2010). Case review in adolescent acne: Multifactorial considerations to optimizing management. *Dermatology Nursing, 22,* 1–8.

Sharma, M., Schoop, R., Suter, A., & Hudson, J. B. (2011). The potential use of echinacea in acne: Control of Propionibacterium acnes growth and inflammation. *Phytotherapy Research, 25,* 517–521.

Smith, J. W., & Taylor, J. S. (2011). Polycystic ovary syndrome. *Nursing for Women's Health, 15,* 404–411.

Steventon, K., & Cowdell, F. (2013). Psychological impact of facial acne in adult women. *Journal of the Dermatology Nurses' Association, 5,* 148–152.

Strauss, J. S., Krowchuk, D. P., Leyden, J. J., Lucky, A. W., Shalita, A. R., & Siegfried, E. C., . . . Bhushan, R. (2007, April 1). *National Guidelines Clearinghouse: Guidelines of care for acne vulgaris management.* Retrieved from http://www.guideline.gov/search.aspx?/term=acne

Tan, J. K. (2004). Psychosocial impact of acne vulgaris: Evaluating the evidence. *Skin Therapy Letter, 9,* 1–3.

Webster, G. (2005). The pathophysiology of acne. *Cutis, 76*(2), 4–7.

Yan, A. C. (2006). Current concepts in acne management. *Adolescent Medicine Clinics, 17,* 613–637.

Zaenglein, A. L., & Thiboutot, D. M. (2006). Expert committee recommendations for acne management. *Pediatrics, 118,* 1188–1199.

# Alopecia

## OVERVIEW

Hair loss, or alopecia, is a common problem that can affect males and females of all ages throughout their lives (Mounsey & Reed, 2009; Figure III.3). The human scalp contains approximately 150,000 hair follicles. Each hair follicle sits above a dermal papilla, which induces the development of hair follicles in the fetus and may play an important role in follicular cycling and hair growth (Shapiro, Otberg, & Horkinsky, 2013).

The two types of hair follicles on the human body are *terminal hair* and *vellus hair* follicles. Terminal hair follicles are larger than vellus hair follicles and grow into the subcutaneous fat during hair growth. Vellus hair follicles, however, generally extend into the reticular dermis only. Terminal hair follicles produce hair that is 0.06 mm in diameter, whereas vellus hairs are short, fine, and usually less than 0.03 mm in diameter. At birth, terminal hairs are found on the scalp, eyebrows, and eyelashes, and vellus hairs populate the rest of the hair-bearing areas. During puberty, the vellus hairs in the genital and axillary areas change to terminal hair. Women with *hirsutism* (abnormal growth of hair) experience an abnormal transition from vellus hair to terminal hair (Shapiro et al., 2013). Hair-loss disorders may occur as a result of disorders of hair cycling, inflammatory conditions that damage hair follicles, or inherited disorders of the hair shaft.

Hair follicles have a continuous cycle of growth (anagen phase), transformation (catagen phase), and rest (telogen phase) (Shapiro et al., 2013).

- *Anagen Phase*: The growth phase; at any given time, approximately 90% of scalp hair follicles are in this phase.
- *Catagen Phase*: The phase in which the lower portion of the hair follicle regresses, and hair production ceases.
- *Telogen Phase*: The resting phase. Normally about 10% of hair follicles on the scalp are in the telogen phase. The anagen phase follows this phase, which results in new hair growth.

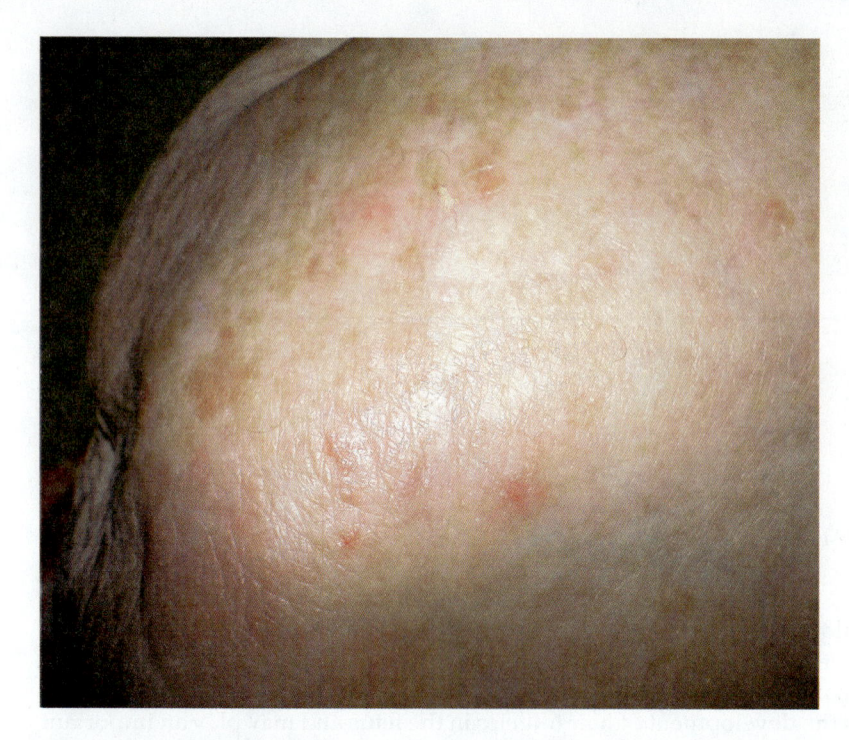

FIGURE III.3  Alopecia or hair loss

# ALOPECIA AREATA

## EPIDEMIOLOGY

In the United States, alopecia areata (AA) is a common nonscarring hair disorder that is responsible for approximately 3.8% of dermatology clinic visits (Alkhalifah, 2013; Figure III.3). Alopecia affects men and women equally and can occur at any age, with the most common occurrence being in children and young adults; almost 50% of cases occur before 20 years of age (Mounsey & Reed, 2009). Approximately 10% to 20% of patients with AA have a positive family history (Monroe, 2013a). The lifetime risk of developing AA is 1.7%, and there appears to be a genetic predisposition with a polygenic pattern of inheritance (Mounsey & Reed, 2009).

## PATHOLOGY/HISTOLOGY

In AA, the body's immune system mistakenly attacks the hair follicles for unknown reasons. AA is thought to be a tissue-specific, T-cell-mediated autoimmune disease of the hair follicle. The leading theory at this time points to a T-cell-mediated attack on anagen hair follicles after loss of immunity in genetically susceptible individuals (Kos & Conlon, 2009).

## CLINICAL PRESENTATION

Most frequently, hair loss occurs in patches, but occasionally it can occur all over the scalp and body. When the entire body is affected, the term used is *alopecia universalis* (Shapiro et al., 2013). AA usually manifests acutely and leads to complete hair loss in a well-defined annular pattern. It may resolve with or without treatment (Monroe, 2013b). Alopecia can be associated with autoimmune conditions, such as vitiligo, diabetes, thyroid disease, rheumatoid arthritis, and discoid lupus erythematous (Mounsey & Reed, 2009).

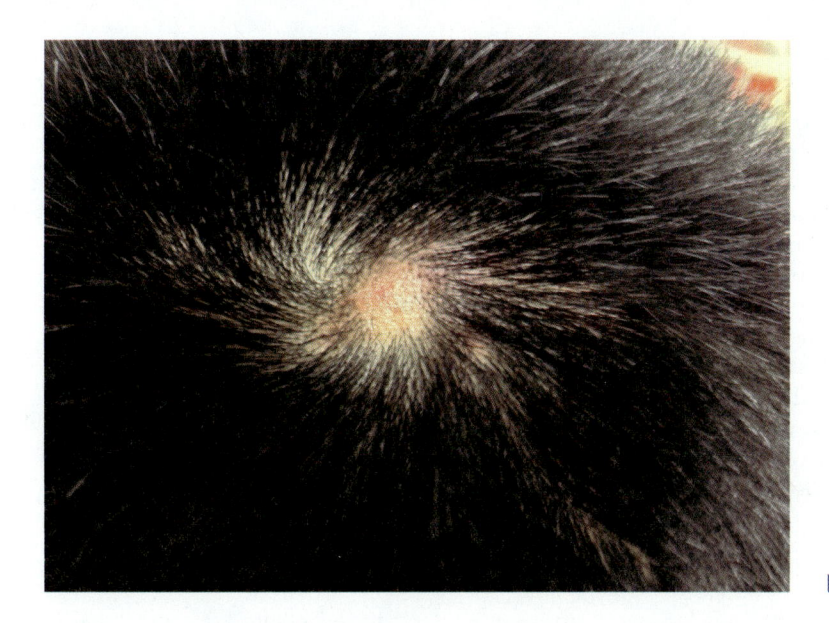

FIGURE III.4  Alopecia areata

# TELOGEN EFFLUVIUM

## PATHOLOGY/HISTOLOGY

The major histologic finding in *telogen effluvium* is the increase in the percentage of catagen/telogen hairs. The total number of hairs and follicular size are normal, and the terminal/vellus (T/V) ratio is preserved; there are fibrous streamers below telogen hairs with no significant inflammation or miniaturization. In absolute telogen effluvium, the only abnormality is the increase in percentage of terminal telogen hairs (typically 20%–50%); with regard to the patient's normal telogen percentage, a percentage of telogen hairs less than 20% could be abnormal. Although the total number of hairs is normal when viewed at the level of the mid-dermis, when evaluating transverse sections at the level of the subcutis, the number of terminal hairs will appear to be reduced, owing to the presence of fibrous streamers replacing the lower segments of the telogen hairs. The gradual but progressive course of the disease allows for increased sun exposure with solar elastosis seen in some cases (Childs & Sperling, 2013). Solar elastosis can be observed in patients with long-term sun exposure. This condition includes both a yellow hue in the exposed skin and skin thickening.

## CLINICAL PRESENTATION

Telogen effluvium is a common cause of diffuse hair shedding that occurs when an increased number of hairs enter the telogen phase prematurely from the anagen phase, and these hairs are lost approximately 3 months later (Mounsey & Reed, 2009). Factors that can contribute to early or prolonged telogen shedding are physical or psychological stressors, childbirth, dietary restriction, and medications that induce hair loss, which usually occurs 2 to 3 months after the event. Arsenic, thallium, or mercury poisoning can also result in telogen effluvium (Shapiro et al., 2013). Telogen hair loss involves generalized hair loss without a pattern. The hair is actually lost, and often seen in the sink, bathtub, or in a brush or comb. The scalp is often visible, but usually no more than 50% of the person's hair is affected (Habif, 2004; Monroe, 2013b).

# ANDROGENIC ALOPECIA

## PATHOLOGY/HISTOLOGY

In *androgenic alopecia* (AGA), the hair follicles contain androgen receptors, which then stimulate genes that shorten the anagen phase. With continuous anagen cycles, the follicles become smaller, and nonpigmented vellus hairs replace pigmented terminal hairs. Women with AGA do not have higher levels of circulating androgens, but they do have higher levels of 5α-reductase (an enzyme that converts testosterone to dihydrotestosterone), more androgen receptors, and lower levels of cytochrome P450 (which converts testosterone to estrogen) (Thiedke, 2003). Biopsies from affected areas (vertex, crown, and frontal) show a normal amount of follicles when counted at the superficial dermis, with scattered vellus hairs. The terminal/vellus ratio is decreased to less than two to one, and because each follicle cycles independently, the miniaturized hairs are randomly scattered among normal follicles (Childs & Sperling, 2013).

## CLINICAL PRESENTATION

AGA affects both men and women, although women begin to develop AGA when they are about 10 years older than affected males. Among women, only 13% develop AGA before menopause, whereas the majority note the appearance after menopause (Monroe, 2013b). AGA in men is characterized by the slow, progressive loss of hair in a characteristic distribution (Shapiro et al., 2013). In both sexes, AGA results from the gradual conversion of terminal hairs to vellus hairs, with miniaturization of the follicles. Hair loss in men starts at the vertex, followed by bitemporal recession; in women, AGA primarily affects the crown of the scalp, often with partial preservation of the frontal hairline (Monroe, 2013b).

## DIFFERENTIAL DIAGNOSIS

Multiple disorders and diseases can cause hair loss. A skin biopsy on the scalp is recommended to determine the etiology of the hair loss (Shapiro et al., 2013). Possible causes include:

- Acne keloidalis nuchae
- Acne necrotica
- Cicatricial alopecia
- Neutrophilic primary cicatricial alopecia (two types: dissecting cellulitis of the scalp and folliculitis decalvans)
- Nonscarring alopecia
- Pseudopelade of Brocq
- Tinea capitis (ringworm; Figure III.5)

## TREATMENT/MANAGEMENT

Obtaining patient history can provide valuable clues for diagnosis. Questions should address:

- Duration and rate of progression of hair loss
- Location and pattern of hair loss
- Extent of hair loss
- Associated symptoms

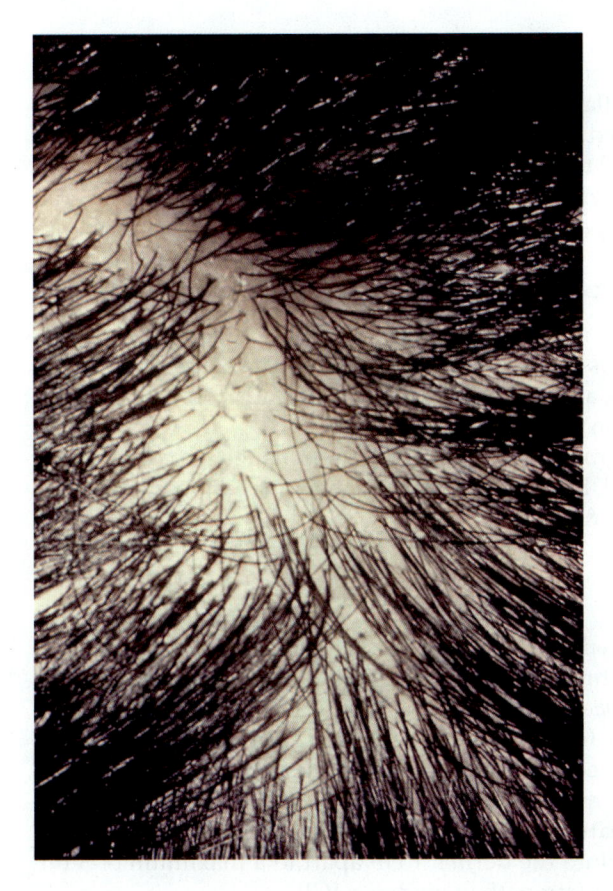

**FIGURE III.5** Alopecia caused by tinea capitis or ringworm.
Courtesy of Dr. Lucille K. George, Centers for Disease Control (CDC)

- Differentiation of hair shedding from hair breakage
- Hair-care practices
- Medical and family history
- Drug use, including those prescribed, over the counter, and illegal (drugs that can cause telogen effluvium include antithyroid agents, hormones, anticonvulsants, anticoagulants, beta-blockers, angiotensin-converting enzyme inhibitors, and lithium.)
- Diet, in particular caloric or protein restriction
- Medical disorders or recent medical events (surgery) (Shapiro et al., 2013)

Physical assessment of the entire body should include all hair-bearing areas, nails, and teeth. Examine the scalp and pattern of hair loss, evaluate the area affected, and perform the hair-pull test. The hair-pull test aids in the assessment of active loss and should be done on every patient who presents with hair-loss complaints. To perform the test, grasp 50 to 60 hair fibers close to the skin surface and tug from the base. The easy extraction of more than six hair fibers is suggestive of a hair-loss disorder (Shapiro et al., 2013). The following routine laboratory tests help to determine the presence of underlying causes and risk factors associated with hair loss (Grimes, Blankenship, Kremer, Reece, & Sonstein, 2011):

- Chemistry panel
- Thyroid panel
- Complete blood count (CBC) with differential
- Ferritin/total iron-binding capacity levels
- HIV-1 and HIV-2 screen

- Rapid plasma regain to rule out syphilis
- Antinuclear antibodies (ANA), rheumatoid factor, C-reactive protein, and erythrocyte sedimentation rate to rule out inflammatory or autoimmune disorders
- If hormonal causes are suspected (menstrual irregularities, infertility, cystic acne, virilization, or galactorrhea), total testosterone, free testosterone, dehydroepiandrosterone sulfate (DHEA-S), luteinizing hormone, follicle-stimulating hormone, and prolactin levels (be sure to have patient stop exogenous hormones at least 1 month before endocrine evaluation)
- Nutritional assessment, including albumin levels, zinc, and vitamin $B_{12}$

Most women with AGA have normal menses, fertility, and endocrine function, including gender-appropriate levels of circulating androgens. The signs of an endocrine disorder are irregular menses, abrupt hair loss, hirsutism, and acne. If these signs are present, an endocrine evaluation is warranted (Thiedke, 2003).

Treatment may prompt hair growth but usually does not change the course of the disease. When treatment is stopped, hair loss recurs. Treatment for hair loss is detailed in the following sections (Mounsey & Reed, 2009).

## Alopecia Areata

- *Topical Steroids*: A treatment applied twice daily to the scalp (strength of evidence [B])
- *Topical Minoxidil (Rogaine)*: A treatment applied twice daily (strength of evidence [B])
- *Topical Immunotherapy with Diphenylcyclopropenone or Squaric Acid*: A treatment applied by a dermatologist every few weeks (strength of evidence [B])
- *Oral Steroids*: A treatment prescribed as a 6-week tapering course of prednisone starting at 40 mg per day (strength of evidence [B])
- *Intralesional Corticosteroids*: A treatment using 5 to 10 mg/mL of Kenalog; 0.1 m is injected with a 30-gauge needle into the dermis 1 cm apart to a maximum of 3 mL (can be repeated every 4–6 weeks) (strength of evidence [C])
- *Anthralin Cream*: A 0.5% to 1% cream applied once daily for 20 to 30 minutes, increasing by 10 to 15 minutes every 2 weeks (strength of evidence [C])

## Telogen Effluvium

Treatment includes removal of the known stressors or resolving any precipitating medical conditions (Mounsey & Reed, 2009). Additionally, Watkins (2009a) discussed the prevention of hair loss with chemotherapy with the "cold-cap" treatment. This procedure involves placing a cool cap on the scalp for 15 minutes before chemotherapy and wearing it for 1 to 2 hours after, thus restricting blood flow to the hair follicles.

## Androgenic Alopecia

Treatment with spironolactone (Aldactone), 100 to 200 mg daily, may slow the rate of hair loss. Women with evidence of a hyperandrogenic state requesting combined oral contraceptives would benefit from using antiandrogenic progesterones, such as drospirenone (Messenger, 2012; Mounsey & Reed, 2009).

## SPECIAL CONSIDERATIONS

People may find it difficult to accept a diagnosis of alopecia because of the unpredictable nature of the disease. This can lead to emotional stress and an altered body image.

Teasing by others unfamiliar with the disease is damaging, especially among children, adolescents, and young adults. Losing one's hair can be a devastating experience if it develops suddenly and the loss is difficult to hide. Patients who are experiencing the psychosocial effects of losing their hair should consult with a health care provider. Providers can offer support and advise consult with a psychologist. In the United States, patients can contact the National Alopecia Areata Foundation, a national support group that publishes a newsletter and provides names of local support groups (Messenger, 2012).

## WHEN TO REFER

Most primary care providers can manage hair loss; however, when an autoimmune disorder or endocrine disorder is responsible for hair loss, a referral to a specialist is recommended. If nutrition imbalance is the cause of hair loss, consider a nutritionist. Psychiatric counseling may be warranted if stress is the cause of the hair loss or if patients are experiencing emotional issues with the disease.

## PATIENT EDUCATION

Hairpieces, hair-integrated systems, wigs, head scarves, and semipermanent makeup are all effective ways to cope psychologically with hair loss, as is choosing to wear nothing. However, depending on the person's emotional state, personal budget, and environment or climate, the choices may be limited (McKillop, 2010).

Prevention of sun damage is better than having to treat its effects. People with alopecia should be advised to wear a hat or a wig when out or apply sunscreen, particularly in the summer months (Watkins, 2009b).

## CLINICAL PEARLS

- Alopecia, unspecified: ICD-9, 704.00; Alopecia areata: 704.01; Other alopecia: 704.09; Telogen effluvium: 704.02
- Nonscarring hair loss, unspecified: ICD-10, L65.9; Androgenic alopecia, unspecified: L64.9; Alopecia areata, unspecified: L63.9; Alopecia (capitis) totalis: L63.0; Alopecia universalis: L63.1; Telogen effluvium: L65.0
- Taking a history and performing a physical aids in determination of the type of alopecia
- Treatment of the cause of alopecia will usually cause hair regrowth without need for further treatment (DeCastro, 2013)

## REFERENCES

Alkhalifah, A. (2013). Alopecia areata update. *Dermatology Clinics, 31*, 93–108.

Childs, J. M., & Sperling, L. C. (2013). Histopathy of scarring and nonscarring hair loss. *Dermatologic Clinics, 31*(1), 43–56.

DeCastro, A. (2013). *Alopecia*. Retrieved from http://www.unboundmedicine.com/5-minute/view/5-minute-clinical-consultation

Grimes, D. A., Blankenship, O., Kremer, C., Reece, S., & Sonstein, F. (2011). Initial office evaluation of hair loss in adult women. *Journal for Nurse Practitioners, 7*(6), 456–462.

Habif, T. P. (2004). *Clinical dermatology* (4th ed.). Philadelphia, PA: Mosby.
Kos, L., & Conlon, J. (2009). An update on alopecia areata. *Current Opinion in Pediatrics, 21*, 475–480.
McKillop, J. (2010). Management of autoimmune associated alopecia areata. *Nursing Standard, 24*(36), 42–46.
Messenger, A. G. (2012). *Patient information: Alopecia areata (Beyond the basics)*. Retrieved from http://www.uptodate.com/contents/alopecia-areata-beyond-the-basics
Monroe, J. R. (2013a). After 15 years, still losing hair, only faster. *Clinician Reviews, 23*, 13.
Monroe, J. R. (2013b). Is man balding "just like dad"? *Clinician Reviews, 23*, 9–10.
Mounsey, A. I., & Reed, S. W. (2009). Diagnosing and treating hair loss. *American Family Physician, 80*(4), 356–362.
Shapiro, J., Otberg, N., & Horkinsky, M. (2013). *Evaluation and diagnosis of hair loss*. Retrieved from http://www.uptodate.com/contents/evaluation-and-diagnosis-of-hair-loss
Thiedke, C. C. (2003). Alopecia in women. *American Family Physician, 67*(5), 923–924.
Watkins, J. (2009a). Alopecia, part 1: Non-scarring forms. *Practice Nursing, 20*(7), 358–363.
Watkins, J. (2009b). Alopecia, part 2: Scarring forms. *Practice Nursing, 20*(9), 454–459.

# Aphthous Stomatitis

## OVERVIEW

Recurrent aphthous stomatitis (RAS) is one of the most frequent painful oral mucosal conditions (Preeti, Magesh, Rajkumar, & Karthik, 2011; Figure III.6). RAS is not contagious and is not caused by a viral, bacterial, or fungal infection. Instead, it is considered an unusual type of autoimmune reaction (American Academy of Oral & Maxillofacial Pathology, 2013).

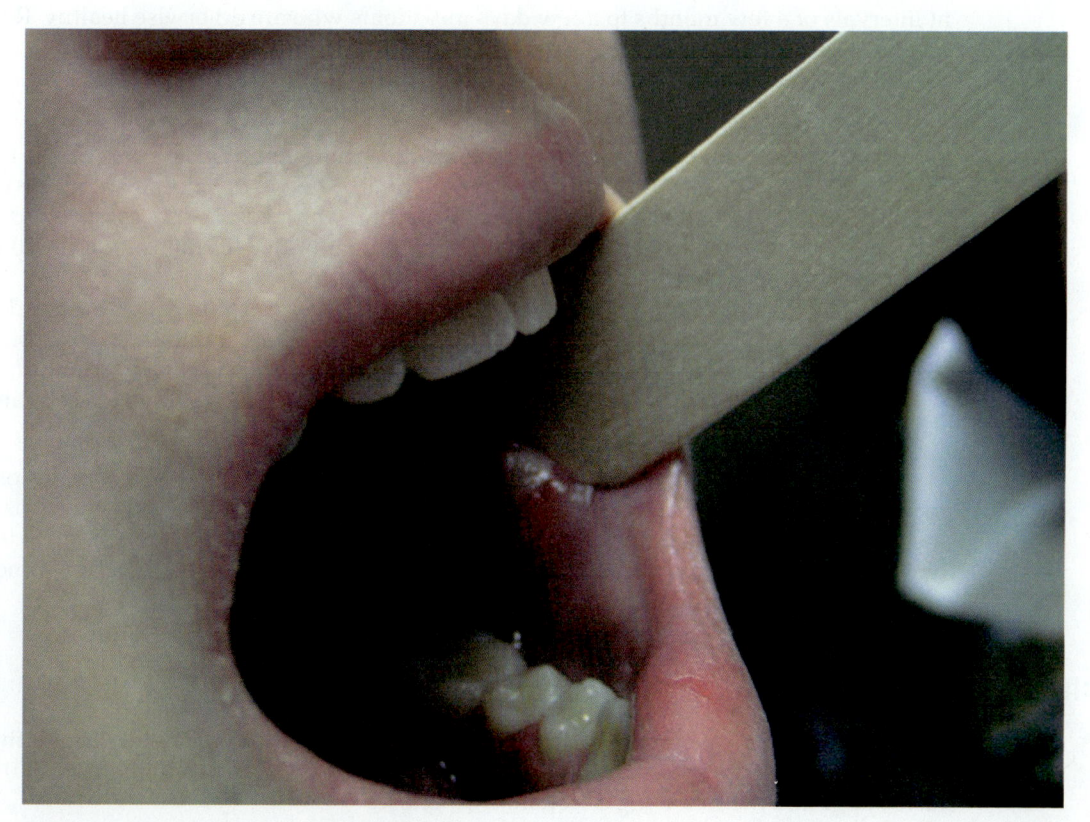

FIGURE III.6   An ulcer caused by RAS.

## EPIDEMIOLOGY

Aphthous ulcers are the most common oral lesion, affecting 25% of the general population with a 3-month recurrence rate as high as 50% (Barrons, 2001). Anyone is susceptible to developing the lesions, which can occur at any age and in both sexes but seem to affect young adults and women more frequently (American Academy of Oral & Maxillofacial Pathology, 2013).

## PATHOLOGY/HISTOLOGY

Diagnosis of RAS is often made by history and clinical examination. Microscopically, the mucous membrane of an aphthous ulcer reveals superficial tissue necrosis with a fibrinopurulent membrane covering the ulcerated area. The necrosis is covered by tissue debris and neutrophils. The epithelium has an abundance of lymphocytes and few neutrophils. The adjacent areas have inflammatory cell infiltration, with neutrophils present immediately below the ulcer (Preeti et al., 2011).

Tumor necrosis factor-alpha (TNF-α) is an inflammatory cytokine that is one of the most important cytokines in the development of new aphthous ulcers. This is supported by the fact that immunomodulatory drugs such as thalidomide and pentoxifylline have been found effective in the treatment of RAS (Preeti et al., 2011).

## CLINICAL PRESENTATION

RAS is characterized by recurrent attacks of solitary or multiple shallow painful ulcers at intervals of a few months to a few days in patients who are otherwise healthy. RAS begins as small, red, discrete or grouped papules; within a few hours, they become necrotizing ulcerations (James, Berger, & Elston, 2006). There are three clinical variations (McBride, 2000; Preeti et al., 2011):

- Minor RAS is also known as Miculiz's aphthae or mild aphthous ulcers. This is the most common type, representing about 80% of all RAS cases. Ulcer size can be up to 10 mm and is frequently seen in the nonkeratinized mucosal surfaces, such as the labial mucosa, buccal mucosa, and the floor of the mouth. Ulcers heal within 10 to 14 days without scarring.
- Major RAS is also known as periadenitis mucosa necrotica recurrens or Sutton disease. Ulcers can be larger than 1 cm in diameter and most commonly involve sites on the lips, soft palate, and fauces, although masticatory mucosa like the dorsum of the tongue or gingiva may also be involved. The ulcers persist for up to 6 weeks and heal with scarring.

*Herpetiform ulceration* appears as recurrent crops of ulcers (>100), but lesions may merge to form large, irregular ulcers as well. The individual lesions are small, measuring 2 to 3 mm in diameter. These ulcers last 10 to 14 days and are not preceded by vesicles, and unlike herpetic ulcers, they do not contain viral-infected cells. Women are affected more frequently than men and at a later age of onset.

## DIFFERENTIAL DIAGNOSIS

Infections causing ulcerations of the mouth should be considered when evaluating patients with oral symptoms. McBride (2000) and Morelli, Calmet, and Jhingade (2010) have suggested the following differential diagnoses:

- Viral etiology includes herpesvirus, cytomegalovirus, varicella, and coxsackievirus
- Treponemal etiology includes syphilis

- Fungal etiology includes cryptosporidium, mucormycosis, and histoplasma
- Autoimmune etiology includes Behçet syndrome, Reiter syndrome, inflammatory bowel disease, Crohn's disease, and lupus erythematosus
- Hematologic etiology includes cyclic neutropenia, anemia, and leukemia
- Neoplastic etiology includes squamous cell carcinoma
- Cutaneous etiology includes lichen planus, erythema multiforme, pemphigus vulgaris, and bullous pemphigoid

## TREATMENT/MANAGEMENT

Predisposing factors of RAS include the following (Barrons, 2001; Preeti et al., 2011):

- *Food allergies:* Examples include allergies to spicy or acidic foods, fresh pineapple, or walnuts.
- *Genetics:* Forty percent of patients have a family history of RAS, and these patients develop more severe ulcers at a younger age than other patients.
- *Trauma to the oral mucosa:* This may result from local anesthetic injections, sharp tools, dental treatments, or toothbrush injury.
- *Tobacco:* Several studies reveal a positive association between cigarette smoking or smokeless tobacco and RAS. A possible explanation is increased mucosal keratinization, which provides a protective barrier against trauma and bacteria.
- *Drugs:* Examples include the angiotensin converting enzyme inhibitor captopril, gold salts, nicorandil, phenindione, phenobarbital, sodium hypochlorite, and nonsteroidal anti-inflammatories such as propionic acid, diclofenac, and piroxicam.
- *Anemias:* Examples include deficiencies in iron, vitamin $B_{12}$, and folic acid.
- *Gastrointestinal diseases:* This includes celiac disease, inflammatory bowel disease, and *Helicobacter pylori* infection.
- *Hormonal changes:* Conflicting reports exist regarding the association between hormonal changes in women and RAS. Some studies described an association of oral ulcerations and the phases of the menstrual cycle.
- *Stress:* Examples include stress caused by habitual lip or cheek biting.
- *Immune disorders:* Examples include HIV infection and systemic lupus.

Correct any iron or vitamin deficiency once the cause has been identified and treated. If there is a dietary cause for RAS, the nutrient responsible should be excluded from diet. If there seems to be a relationship between menstrual cycle and RAS, oral contraceptives that contain progesterone may help suppress ovulation (Scully, 2013).

Treatment for RAS can be divided into five categories (McBride, 2000; Scully, 2013).

- *Topical and systemic antibiotics:* These treatments are often used because of the belief that some as-of-yet-undiscovered infection may cause RAS. Tetracycline and minocycline are the agents most commonly used. A 250-mg antibiotic capsule of tetracycline can be dissolved in 180 mL of water and used as a "swish-and-swallow" or "swish-and-spit" treatment four times per day for several days in adult patients. A minocycline 100-mg tablet dissolved in 180 mL of water can be used in the same fashion. Tetracycline and minocycline should be avoided in children younger than 12 years of age and pregnant women because of their tendency to stain the teeth.
- *Local anti-inflammatory agents:* These may help speed healing and relieve symptoms in the management of RAS. Triamcinolone 0.1% (Kenalog in Orabase) can be applied to ulcers four times per day until the ulcer is healed. Dexamethasone elixir, at 0.5 mg per 5 mL, may be used as a rinse and spit. Patients should be warned of the potential for a secondary fungal infection when using a steroid topically or as a rinse.
- *Immune modulators:* Thalidomide is the agent used most frequently in this category. Thalidomide at 200 mg once or twice daily for 3 to 8 weeks is often tried.

Thalidomide is teratogenic, and patients using this should be using birth control options. Amlexanox 5% paste (Aphthasol) has been examined in several studies. The paste was applied two to four times per day, and healing time was improved. James et al. (2006) stated that Dapsone in doses of 25 to 50 mg per day or colchicine at 0.6 mg two to three times a day may also be tried.

- *Symptomatic treatments:* Pain relief may be achieved with 2% viscous lidocaine applied with a cotton swab several times daily. Over-the-counter preparations such as Orabase or Zilactin-B may also be beneficial. The use of over-the-counter magnesium hydroxide antacid and diphenhydramine hydrochloride (Benadryl) at 5 mg per 5 mL mixed half and half and used four to six times per day will bring symptom relief; however, swallowing this mixture can cause sedation, which is a side effect of Benadryl.
- *Alternative therapies:* The following may provide symptom relief and speed the healing process:
    - Zinc gluconate lozenges
    - Vitamin C, vitamin B complex, lysine
    - Sage and chamomile mouthwash, created by infusing equal amounts of the two herbs in water, may be helpful when used four to six times per day
    - Echinacea
    - Carrot, celery, and cantaloupe juices

## SPECIAL CONSIDERATIONS

Evaluation of the effects of aphthous ulcers should include considering the effects on the patient's oral functions, such as tasting, speaking, and eating and swallowing (Preeti et al., 2011). The goals of therapy for RAS should include pain relief, reduction of ulcer duration, and restoration of normal oral function (Barrons, 2001). Patients should understand that there is no cure for RAS, only symptomatic treatment to provide relief.

It is important to:

- Assess pain associated with RAS.
- Monitor nutritional intake and hydration because of pain that occurs with eating. Suggesting frequent sips of cool water or crushed ice, the use of topical and systemic analgesics, and selecting soft, bland, nonacidic foods is helpful.
- Because the patient's body image may be affected as a result of the appearance of ulcerations or altered speech, provide emotional and supportive feedback, and encourage compliance with treatment regimens.

## WHEN TO REFER

Consultation should be considered with a gastroenterologist, immunologist/allergist, hematologist, or a rheumatologist for recurrent/chronic episodes of RAS to rule out other etiologies (Scully, 2013).

## PATIENT EDUCATION

Patients should be instructed on the management of RAS as follows:

- Brush teeth gently by using a small-headed, soft toothbrush
- Identify and correct predisposing factors
- Avoid eating particularly hard or sharp food, such as potato chips or toast
- Avoid trauma to oral mucosa (Scully, 2013)

## CLINICAL PEARLS

- RAS: ICD-9, 528.2; ICD-10, K12.0
- Recommend that patients keep a detailed journal of diet, activities, hobbies, and menstrual cycle (including ovulation). This may help with determining the cause of RAS.

## REFERENCES

American Academy of Oral & Maxillofacial Pathology. (2013). *Aphthous ulcerations*. Retrieved from http://www.aaomp.org/public/aphthous-ulcerations.php

Barrons, R. W. (2001). Treatment strategies for recurrent oral aphthous ulcers. *American Journal of Health-System Pharmacy, 58*(1), 41–50.

James, W. D., Berger, T. G., & Elston, D. M. (2006). *Andrews' diseases of the skin. Clinical dermatology* (10th ed.). Philadelphia, PA: Saunders/Elsevier.

McBride, D. R. (2000). Management of aphthous ulcers. *American Family Physician, 62*(1), 149–154.

Morelli, V., Calmet, E., & Jhingade, V. (2010). Alternative therapies for common dermatologic disorders, part 2. *Primary Care Clinic Office Practice, 37*, 285–296.

Preeti, L., Magesh, K. T., Rajkumar, K., & Karthik, R. (2011). Recurrent aphthous stomatitis. *Journal of Oral Maxillofacial Pathology, 15*(3), 252–256.

Scully, C. (2013). *Aphthous ulcers: Treatment & management*. Retrieved from http://emedicine.medscape.com/article/867080-treatment

# Bruise and Contusion

## OVERVIEW

A *bruise* is defined as a discoloration resulting from injury through the skin to its underlying structures causing bleeding from ruptured blood vessels. Bruises are usually accompanied by pain, swelling, and inflammation (Carlson, 2007; Nash & Sheridan, 2009). Bruise is synonymous with *contusion*. Ecchymosis, petechiae, and purpura are not classified as bruises because these cutaneous hemorrhages are better categorized as rashes or leakages of blood under the skin not directly caused by blunt force trauma (Nash & Sheridan, 2009).

## EPIDEMIOLOGY

In the United States, studies indicate the frequency of easy bruising in healthy individuals ranges from 12% to 55%. Women are more likely than men to report easy bruising (Kraut, 2012).

## PATHOLOGY/HISTOLOGY

The red or purple discoloration in a bruise/contusion following trauma is caused by the release of red blood cells and hemoglobin from the damaged vessels into subcutaneous tissue. The occurrence of inflammation causes vasodilation and attracts macrophages to the site of injury. The erythema is quickly replaced by a blue or purple appearance caused by the further release of deoxygenated venous blood into the interstitial tissue (Nash & Sheridan, 2009).

With time, the macrophages ingest the escaped erythrocytes and break down the attached hemoglobin. As a bruise heals, hemoglobin is first broken down into biliverdin, which causes the green discoloration, then biliverdin is broken down into bilirubin, which accounts for the yellow color. As hemoglobin is further broken down, some of the iron contained therein is released and combines with ferritin. This causes hemosiderin, which appears brown in the tissue, explaining why many bruises take on a yellow-brown to pure brown tone late in the healing process (Nash & Sheridan, 2009).

## CLINICAL PRESENTATION

The typical appearance of a bruise is that of unbroken skin with discoloration ranging from red-purple to yellow-green. There also may be associated redness and swelling (Carlson, 2007). Numerous factors contribute to a bruise's appearance (Nash & Sheridan, 2009).

- Increased adipose tissue, compared with muscle, can contribute to increased bleeding.
- Skin color affects how bruise discoloration is perceived.
- The depth of injury can affect how soon bruise discoloration appears. Superficial bruises may appear immediately, but deeper bruises may take several hours or days to appear.
- The characteristics of the inflicting object, including its surface and force of impact against the body, can also affect the bruise's size, shape, and pattern.
- Age can affect bruising because of changes typical of different age groups.
- Gender can play a role in bruising.
- Certain diseases can increase the tendency to bruise.
- Medications can affect coagulation, macrophage production, and hemoglobin degradation. Medications that cause bleeding and bruising include aspirin, Plavix, heparin, nonsteroidal anti-inflammatory drugs, and warfarin. Less common causes include cephalosporins, ginkgo biloba, gold, interferon, metaxalone, penicillins, propylthiouracil, selective serotonin reuptake inhibitors, testosterone replacement therapy drugs, and tricyclic antidepressants.

## DIFFERENTIAL DIAGNOSIS

- Alcohol abuse
- Bleeding disorders such as platelet disorders, hemophilia, factor inhibitors, vasculitis, leukemia, or vitamin K deficiency
- Cushing disease
- Marfan syndrome
- Physical abuse
- Purpura
- Senile purpura
- Vitamin C deficiency

## TREATMENT/MANAGEMENT

Health care providers are encouraged to document bruising well, especially on children and the elderly. When assessing a bruise, document the following (Nash & Sheridan, 2009):

- Complete history of how the injury occurred that caused the bruise
- Size of the bruise (measure length and width)
- Shape of the bruise
- Location of the bruise
- Color(s) of the bruise
- Distinction of margins
- Whether the bruise is indurated or painful

- Whether the bruises are patterned (various stages of healing, known as a *pattern injury*)
- A body diagram if possible

Plan to reexamine the patient at a later date to evaluate for the appearance of new bruises either from deep injury now visible or new injuries.

Treatment of bruising includes ice and compression, acetaminophen for pain, and assessment of causes of the bruise. Consider laboratory testing if other causes of bruising are suspected (e.g., complete blood count with differential, prothrombin time, and partial thromboplastin time, and comprehensive metabolic panel) (Ballas & Kraut, 2008).

## SPECIAL CONSIDERATIONS

The elderly, particularly those who are frail, tend to bruise easily because of thinning skin, weakening of the tissue surrounding and supporting blood vessels, and side effects of medication. Children also bruise easily because of delicate skin and less adipose tissue. Women tend to bruise more easily because of increased adipose tissue distribution. Women with red hair have been found to report higher levels of bruising compared with women with black or brown hair, although coagulation tests do not differ between the two groups (Nash & Sheridan, 2009).

## WHEN TO REFER

If the laboratory workup is negative for bruising etiology but there is still high suspicion based on personal and family history, the patient should be referred to a hematologist (Ballas & Kraut, 2008).

Nonambulatory babies (usually younger than 6 months of age) cannot crawl or pull up to a stand but may still be able to roll. If bruising is noted, these babies should be referred immediately to a pediatrician and social services for evaluation (Learner, 2010).

## PATIENT EDUCATION

Typical bruises last about 2 weeks, but providers should inform patients that it may take months for a bruise to fade, especially if skin color is darker. To aid in reducing the duration and size of a bruise apply ice and elevate site if possible. If signs and symptoms of infection (additional redness and tenderness surrounding the bruise) occur, notify a health care provider (MedlinePlus, 2013).

## REFERENCES

Ballas, M., & Kraut, E. H. (2008). Bleeding and bruising: A diagnostic work-up. *American Family Physician, 77*(8), 1117–1124.
Carlson, S. (2007). A bruise by any other name would be … an ecchymosis? *Outlook, 30*(1), 17–20.
Kraut, E. H. (2012). *Easy bruising*. Retrieved from http://www.uptodate.com/contents/easy-bruising
Learner, S. (2010). The mark of responsibility. *Nursing Standard, 25*(11), 20–21.
MedlinePlus. (2013). *Bruises*. Retrieved from http://www.nlm.nih.gov/medlineplus/bruises.html
Nash, K. R., & Sheridan, D. J. (2009). Can one accurately date a bruise? State of the science. *Journal of Forensic Nursing, 5*, 31–37.

# Burns

## OVERVIEW

Burns can result from heat (thermal), chemical exposure, and radiation. Burns are classified as follows:

- First-degree: involve the epidermis
- Second-degree: involve the epidermis and parts of the dermis
- Third-degree (full-thickness): affect the epidermis and all of the dermis

Morbidity and mortality depend on the depth and location of the burn, as well as the percentage of body surface area affected. Complications such as pneumonia and other infections can arise from moderate to severe burns (Gaby, 2010).

Thermal burn severity is determined by the depth of the burn injury related to duration of exposure to the heat source, contact temperature, and the thickness of the skin. The thermal conductivity of skin is low, so most thermal burns only involve the epidermis and part of the dermis. The most common thermal burns are associated with flames, hot liquids, hot solid objects, and steam. The depth of the burn largely determines the healing potential and the treatment involved (Rice & Orgill, 2012).

Chemical burns are injuries caused by various caustic reactions, including an alteration in pH, a disruption of cellular membranes, and direct toxic effects on metabolic processes. The injury severity is determined by the duration of exposure and the nature of the agent. Contact with acid produces tissue coagulation, whereas alkaline burns generate colliquation necrosis. Systemic absorption of some chemicals can be life threatening (Rice & Orgill, 2012).

Sunburn occurs as an injury to the skin caused by overexposure to ultraviolet (UV) rays by natural and artificial means (Figure III.7). There are three types of UV rays: UVA, UVB, and UVC. UVA rays have the longest waveforms and penetrate the dermis, which causes premature aging of the skin. UVB rays are known as the burning rays and have shorter wavelengths. These rays are absorbed in the upper layers of the skin, which can result in sunburn and skin cancer. UVC rays have the shortest wavelength but are the most damaging. Fortunately, UVC rays are filtered by the ozone layer surrounding the Earth (Land & Small, 2009).

90 ■ III. Common Dermatologic Conditions

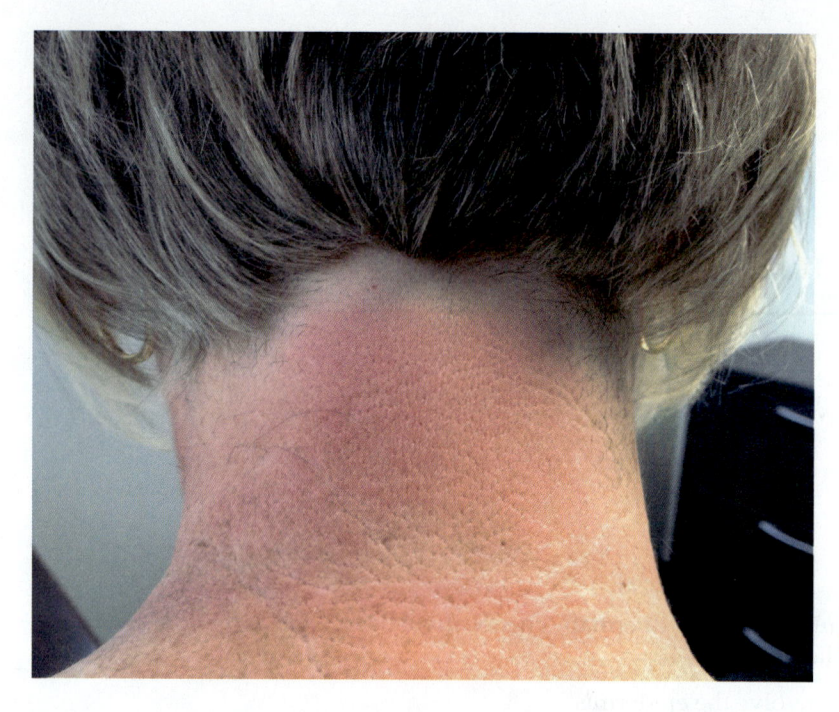

FIGURE III.7   Sunburn of the neck

## EPIDEMIOLOGY

In the United States, more than half a million people go to the emergency department annually with burn injuries, and approximately 400,000 of those patients are hospitalized. The majority of patients with burn wounds are treated in the outpatient setting, making primary care providers the main treatment source for thousands of burn patients each year (Lloyd, Rodgers, Michener, & Williams, 2012).

Burn injuries are most common in children. Scalding accounts for 80% of burns in young children caused by touching hot objects or pulling hot liquids off of a stovetop or counter. Flame-related injuries occur more in children 6 to 16 years of age and usually relate to experimenting with lighters, lighter fluid, firecrackers, and gasoline (Lloyd et al., 2012).

Hardwicke, Hunter, Staruch, and Moiemen (2012) found that chemical burns accounted for a small proportion of burns with reported incidences of up to 10.7% but are attributed to 30% of all burn deaths. Most chemical burns occur in a domestic or industrial setting. Acids caused 26% of all chemical burns, and alkalis caused 55%.

In 2000, 2005, and 2010, sunburn prevalence was highest among Whites (65.6% in 2010) and lowest among Blacks (10.9% in 2010). The prevalence of sunburn in 2010 among men (49.1%) and women (51.3%) was not significantly different. In 2000, sunburn prevalence was 50.9%; in 2005, it was down to 45.5%. It then increased over the next 5 years to 50.1% in 2010 (U.S. Department of Health and Human Services, 2012).

## PATHOLOGY/HISTOLOGY

The skin's three layers (epidermis, dermis, and subcutaneous tissue) lose valuable functions after a burn injury. The epidermis serves as a barrier to bacteria and moisture loss. The dermis provides elasticity and protection from mechanical trauma, and it contains blood vessels that supply blood to all skin layers. When the skin is damaged, epidermal cells regenerate from cells deep within the dermal layer, which explains why deep dermal injury causes significant scarring and permanent skin damage (Lloyd et al., 2012).

Different chemical exposures to the skin induce different reactions (Butcher & Swales, 2012).

- Exposure of skin proteins to some chemicals (e.g., phosphorus burns) will incite an exothermic reaction, generating high levels of local heat.
- Corrosive agents such as acids and alkalis cause coagulative necrosis of the tissues.
- Some chemicals, such as hydrofluoric acid, will produce a chemical reaction that may cause local or systemic electrolyte imbalance, resulting in local or systemic toxicity.
- Seemingly innocuous chemicals, such as cement, can produce burns that may progress to full-thickness loss if contact is maintained and treatment is not administered.

Sunburns produce erythema, edema, blisters, ulcerations, and pain. This results in vasodilation and increased vascular permeability of blood vessels in the upper dermis and irreversible DNA damage. It is the DNA damage that leads to skin cancer (Miners, 2010).

## CLINICAL PRESENTATION

The classification of burns (Butcher & Swales, 2012; Lloyd et al., 2012) is:

1. Superficial (first-degree) burns involve the epidermis. Symptoms include erythema, pain, and dryness of the skin. These burns usually heal in 5 to 10 days. Examples include sunburn and minor thermal injuries.
2. Superficial partial-thickness (superficial second-degree) burns involve all of the epidermis and part of the underlying dermis. Symptoms are clear blisters that weep and erythema, and the skin will blanch painfully when touched. These burns heal within 2 weeks and generally do not scar, but pigment changes are possible.
3. Deep partial-thickness (deep second-degree) burns involve deeper layers of the dermis. The skin is white and does not blanch. These burns can take up to 4 to 6 weeks to heal and often result in scarring and contractures.
4. Full-thickness (third-degree) burns destroy all skin layers (epidermis, dermis, and subcutaneous fat). These burns are tan to dark brown and have a thick leathery appearance with a lack of sensitivity to touch. These wounds often require skin grafts and result in contractures.
5. Fourth-degree burns cause all of the skin layers to be destroyed, and the damage can extend into the muscle, tendon, or bone.

## DIFFERENTIAL DIAGNOSIS

- Cellulitis
- Staphylococcal scalded skin syndrome
- Toxic epidermal necrolysis

## TREATMENT/MANAGEMENT

Burn size is determined by evaluating the percentage of the patient's body surface area that is covered by a burn. The hand is often used to measure small burn areas, correlating to approximately 1% of total body surface area (TBSA; Butcher & Swales; 2012; Lloyd et al., 2012).

Rice and Orgill (2012) described the *Rule of Nines* for the adult assessment of TBSA involved in burn injury.

- Each leg represents 9% TBSA
- Each arm represents 9% TBSA
- The anterior and posterior trunk each represent 18% TBSA
- The head represents 9% TBSA

Treatment of burns varies according to severity and may include debridement of damaged tissue, topical applications of antibiotics, pain medication, intravenous fluids, and dietary and nutritional supplements (Gaby, 2010). All burns should be treated as follows (Butcher & Swales, 2012; Lloyd et al., 2012; Tenenhaus, 2013).

- Cleaning the wound with sterile water is sufficient to remove debris. Scrubbing the wound with povidone/iodine solution (Betadine), chlorhexidine (Peridex), or other cleaning agents is not recommended.
- Management of blisters in partial-thickness burns is controversial, but data have shown that small blisters (< 6 mm) should be left intact, whereas large blisters with thin walls should be debrided to prevent infection. Blisters that prevent proper movement of a joint or can rupture should also be debrided. Necrotic tissue is often debrided by gentle techniques (brushing, scraping, curetting, and cutting).
- Topical burn care is recommended because burns heal best in moist environments that foster reepithelialization and prevent cellular dehydration. Topical agents provide pain control, promote healing, and prevent wound infection and desiccation. Topical honey has been used as a folk remedy for burns. Honey has antibacterial activity, provides a barrier to fluid loss and bacterial invasion, and provides a moist environment that promotes epithelialization (Gaby, 2010).
- Superficial burns can be treated effectively with the topical application of lotion, honey, aloe vera, or antibiotic ointment. The lipid part of these treatments quickens the repair of damaged skin and reduces drying. Topical nonsteroidal anti-inflammatory drugs (NSAIDs) and aloe vera may reduce pain. Topical corticosteroids do not show anti-inflammatory properties.
- Partial-thickness burns should be treated with a topical antimicrobial agent or absorptive occlusive dressing to reduce pain, promote healing, and prevent wound dryness. Topical silver sulfadiazine 1% (Silvadene) is the usual antimicrobial treatment used; however, it cannot be used in patients with sulfa allergy, pregnant and lactating woman, or newborns. Combination antibiotics such as Polysporin are often used, especially for burns on the face and perineum.
- Pruritus and neuropathic pain are common postburn complications. Histamine H-1 receptor antagonists such as Zyrtec are the safest pharmacologic treatment for postburn pruritus. Topical doxycycline, aloe vera, petroleum oil–based creams, cocoa butter, mineral oil, hydrogel sheets, colloidal oatmeal in liquid paraffin, Unna boots, EMLA cream, silicone gel sheeting, compression garments, and massage therapy are also used to treat pruritus. Do not use products that contain lanolin, which increases pruritus. Lyrica has also been found to reduce postburn neuropathic pain in 69% of patients.

If antimicrobial activity is not required, semipermeable film dressings and hydrocolloid dressings can be used to provide protection and a moist wound environment. However, they have limited absorbency and tend to be reserved for small, localized burns or low-exuding wounds (Butcher & Swales, 2012).

Three types of dressings can be used for burn management (Tenenhaus, 2013):

1. *Compresses*: These include fine-mesh gauze, hydrocolloid dressings, and silver-containing dressings.

2. *Biosynthetics*: These include Biobrane and similar dressings as well as bio-cellulose-containing Polyhexanide.
3. *Biologics*: These include allogenic skin grafts, human amnion, and skin xenografts.

Deficiencies of zinc, copper, and selenium occur after burns as a result of renal excretion of these minerals, losses through the burned skin, and sloughing of necrotic skin. During the first 7 days of a major burn, potentially 5% to 10% of total body zinc content and 20% to 40% of the total body copper content is lost through the skin. Intravenous fluid administration with these minerals has been shown to decrease incidence of pneumonia and promote tissue healing (Gaby, 2010).

Sunburn treatment includes subduing inflammatory mediators by means of corticosteroids and NSAIDs. Other treatments include symptom relief with emollients (e.g., aloe vera), cool compresses, elevation, cool baths, oatmeal soaks, moisturizers, analgesics, and increased fluid intake (Land & Small, 2009).

## SPECIAL CONSIDERATIONS

The very young and elderly persons are at the greatest risk of experiencing burns because of physical impairment, reduced mobility, inability to remove themselves from danger, and impaired risk decision making (Butcher & Swales, 2012). Children younger than age 5 and adults older than age 55 are at increased risk of deeper burns because of thinner skin (Rice & Orgill, 2012).

## WHEN TO REFER

Burn depth and size are significant elements in deciding how a burn will be classified and in determining the initial steps of burn assessment and management. The following conditions require referral to a burn specialist (Butcher & Swales, 2012; Lloyd et al., 2012).

- Patients with full-thickness burns; burns to hands, feet, perineum, or genital areas; or circumferential burns (because of the risk of compartment burns)
- Patients with burns to the face (may result in significant psychological trauma and identity issues)
- Children with second-degree burns involving more than 10% of TBSA or suspicious burns requiring the opinion of a specialist need referral to a burn center
- Any unwell or febrile child with a burn
- Burns that do not start healing after 2 weeks
- Patients who will need special social, emotional, or rehabilitative care
- Patients with comorbidities that could complicate management, prolong recovery, and affect mortality
- Chemical burns
- Electrical or friction burns
- Inhalation injury
- Any cold injury
- Partial-thickness burns on more than 10% of the TBSA
- Third-degree burns in any age group

Superficial burns can often be managed on an outpatient basis, whereas full-thickness burns must be evaluated by a specialist for possible excision and grafting. Frequent evaluation and assessment are necessary for all categories of burns because the determination of burn depth can be difficult as a result of the conversion of burns to a higher burn category within the first several days. Conversion occurs when the damaged skin continues to spread and burn depth increases because thermal injury was not evident on initial assessment (Lloyd et al., 2012).

Investigate all burns with detailed history and assessment. If physical abuse is suspected, proper authorities should be notified for a full investigation. If self-harm is suspected, a psychiatric evaluation is warranted (Butcher & Swales, 2012).

## PATIENT EDUCATION

To promote burn prevention in children, instruct parents and guardians to:

- Test the bathwater.
- Check household smoke alarms.
- Cook on the back burners of the stove.
- Avoid leaving a child alone in the bathtub or near water faucets.
- Avoid leaving a child alone near a fireplace.
- Keep matches, firecrackers, gasoline, and other explosives out of reach of children and adolescents.
- Set household water heaters to less than 120°F.
- Keep children away from exercise treadmills unless supervised. (Lloyd et al., 2012)

Sunburn prevention starts with education. Simple behavioral measures, such as minimizing sun exposure, wearing protective clothing, and using topical sunscreens, have been proved to minimize the risk of becoming sunburned. It is generally recommended that the minimum level of sunscreen protection used is a sun protective factor (SPF) of 15; however, longer sun exposure times will necessitate higher levels of protection and repeated applications (Miners, 2010).

## REFERENCES

Butcher, M., & Swales, B. (2012). Assessment and management of patients with burns. *Nursing Standard*, 27(2), 50–56.

Gaby, A. (2010). Nutritional treatment for burns. *Integrative Medicine*, 9(3), 46–51.

Hardwicke, J., Hunter, T., Staruch, R., & Moiemen, N. (2012). Chemical burns—An historical comparison and review of the literature. *Burns*, 38, 383–387.

Land, V., & Small, L. (2009). The evidence on how to best treat sunburn in children: A common treatment dilemma. *Dermatology Nursing*, 21(3), 126–137.

Lloyd, E. C., Rodgers, B. C., Michener, M., & Williams, M. S. (2012). Outpatient burns: Prevention and care. *American Family Physician*, 85(1), 25–32.

Miners, A. L. (2010). The diagnosis and emergency care of heat related illness and sunburn in athletes: A retrospective case series. *Journal of the Canadian Chiropractic Association*, 54(2), 107–117.

Rice, P. L., & Orgill, D. P. (2012). *Classification of burns*. Retrieved from http://uptodate.com/contents/classification-of-burns

Tenenhaus, M. (2013). *Local treatment of burns: Topical antimicrobial agents and dressings*. Retrieved from http://uptodate.com/contents/local-treatment-of-burns-topical-antimicrobial-agents-and-dressings

U.S. Department of Health and Human Services. (2012). Sunburn and sun protective behaviors among adults aged 18–29 years—United States, 2000–2010. *Morbidity and Mortality Weekly Report*, 61(18), 317–322.

# Candidiasis

*Candida* is a genus of yeast that is currently the most common cause of fungal infections worldwide. The variations of infection with *Candida* species range from local mucous membrane infections to widespread dissemination and multisystem organ failure. Most *Candida* infections are characterized by local overgrowth on mucous membranes (oropharyngeal or vaginal) or superficial cutaneous sites as a result of changes in the normal flora (Fitzpatrick, Johnson, Wolff, Polano, & Suurmond, 1997). Extensive chronic mucous membrane infections occur in individuals with deficiencies in cell-mediated immunity, such as AIDS (Kauffman, 2012).

The following sections will discuss various types of *Candida* infections. Cutaneous candidiasis is a common secondary and at times primary cause of intertrigo in patients who are elderly, diabetic, and/or immunocompromised (Goodheart, 2011). The majority of cuntaneous candidal infections occur in skin folds. Vaginitis is very frequently caused by candidiasis. Also, *Candida albicans*, present in the mouths of up to 50% of all people globally, causes the majority of oral fungal infections (Goodheart, 2011).

## ANGULAR CHEILITIS

### OVERVIEW

*Angular cheilitis* or *perleche* is an acute or chronic inflammation of the oral commissures caused by mechanical trauma and/or fungal or bacterial infection. It is often associated with ill-fitting dentures, change in bony structure or bite, dry mouth, poor oral hygiene, and secondary *Candida albicans*, or rarely, *Staphylococcus aureus* infection. Less common causes include nutritional deficiencies, immune deficiency, or irritant or allergic reactions to oral hygiene products or denture materials (Goldstein & Goldstein, 2012).

### EPIDEMIOLOGY

The prevalence rate of this condition is 7 per 1,000, and it is seen most often in older people. The incidence is increased about threefold in denture wearers and almost twofold in men. Angular cheilitis was detected in 7.8% of patients with Crohn's disease, 5% of patients with ulcerative colitis, and 10% of patients with HIV (BMJ Group, 2012).

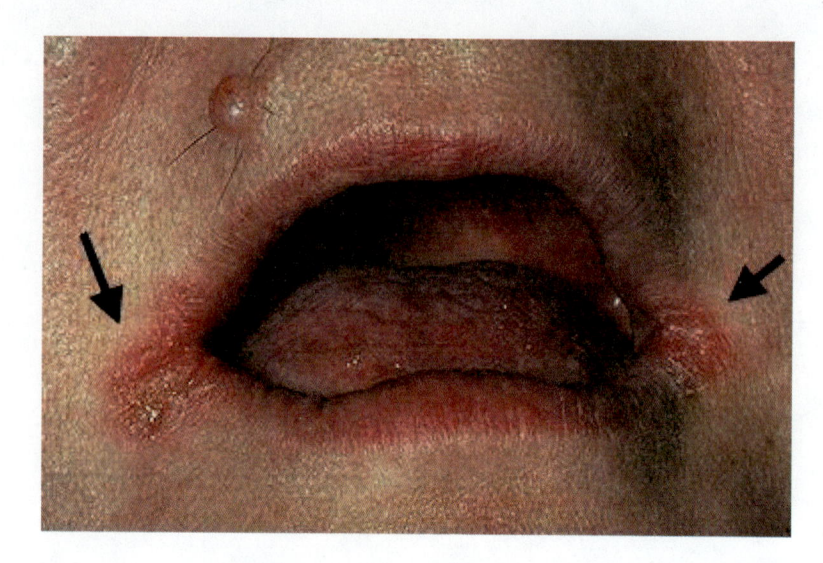

**FIGURE III.8** Angular cheilitis
Courtesy of Dr. Martin Spiller

Other causes of angular cheilitis include:

- Mechanical factors such as destruction of the commissural epithelium brought on by dental trauma, flossing, excessive salivation, drooling, habitual licking, and ill-fitting dentures
- Nutritional deficiencies of riboflavin, niacin, folate, iron, vitamin $B_{12}$, and zinc; general protein malnutrition; eating disorders; or a history of total parenteral nutrition
- Chronic inflammatory skin diseases such as atopic dermatitis, perioral dermatitis, and allergic contact dermatitis at the oral commissures
- Crohn's disease or orofacial granulomatosis may be found in a small minority of patients
- Rarely, the presence of sinuses of developmental origin at the angles of the mouth (BMJ Group, 2012)

## PATHOLOGY/HISTOLOGY

The diagnosis of angular cheilitis is usually uncomplicated. A positive potassium hydroxide (KOH) preparation from lesions and oral mucosa beneath the dentures is needed to confirm the diagnosis of *Candida* infection (Goldstein & Goldstein, 2012).

## CLINICAL PRESENTATION

Appearance may vary from a bluish white to a pale pink color and may be adjoining a wedge-shaped erythematous scaling dermatitis of the skin portion of the oral commissure. Fissures, maceration, and crust formation may be present with soft, pinhead-sized papules. Involvement is usually bilateral (James, Berger, & Elston, 2006).

## DIFFERENTIAL DIAGNOSIS

- For recurrent cheilitis, a lesion swab should be done to rule out bacterial and fungal etiology (Goldstein & Goldstein, 2012).

- Similar changes may occur in riboflavin deficiency or other nutritional deficiencies (James et al., 2006).
- Another possibility is the herpes simplex virus.

## TREATMENT/MANAGEMENT

Treatment options include measures such as improving denture fit and cleaning, proper oral hygiene, and the use of salivary alternatives when needed. For patients with negative KOH results, barrier creams (e.g., zinc oxide paste) or petrolatum applied twice daily can be helpful. For *Candida* infection, topical antifungal therapy with azole (miconazole or clotrimazole) ointment is applied two times per day for 1 to 3 weeks (Goldstein & Goldstein, 2012). James et al. (2006) recommended using the azole cream in combination with a mid-strength topical corticosteroid for a faster response to treatment.

## SPECIAL CONSIDERATIONS

- The aging process leads to facial changes, such as larger skin folds that hold moisture surrounding the mouth, which can lead to angular cheilitis.
- In Down syndrome, prognathism (jaw protrusion) and increased salivation may lead to cheilitis.
- Xerostomia from medications and illnesses may lead to angular cheilitis.
- In children, lip-licking and thumb-sucking behavior are frequent causes of angular cheilitis.

## WHEN TO REFER

- If angular cheilitis is a result of vertical shortening of the lower third of the face, referral to a dentist or oral surgeon may be beneficial.
- Injections of collagen into the oral commissures can be helpful. Referral to a dermatologist who provides these services is recommended.

## PATIENT EDUCATION

Patients should be instructed to rinse the mouth with water before going to bed to prevent oral-hygiene products from remaining in the mouth. This will prevent irritation from the products if the patient drools when sleeping.

### CLINICAL PEARLS

- Candidiasis: ICD-9, 112.0; ICD-10, B 37.8
- Patients should also be assessed for gastroesophageal reflux disease (GERD). Stomach acid entering the mouth during sleep can cause irritation in oral commissures if patient drools in sleep.
- Washing skin with benzoyl peroxide can reduce *Candida* colonization (Fitzpatrick et al., 1997).

# BLACK HAIRY TONGUE

## OVERVIEW

*Black hairy tongue (lingua villosa nigra)* is often a benign condition associated with antibiotic use, *C. albicans*, or poor hygiene (Goldstein & Goldstein, 2012).

## EPIDEMIOLOGY

In the United States, the prevalence of hairy tongue varies from 8.3% in children and young adults to 57% in persons who are addicted to drugs or incarcerated. The prevalence increases with age. Hairy tongue has been reported more frequently in males, those who use tobacco, those who drink coffee and tea, patients infected with HIV, and HIV-negative persons who use intravenous drugs. No racial predilection is associated with hairy tongue (Lynch, 2012).

## PATHOLOGY/HISTOLOGY

Histopathologic findings in hairy tongue show elongated filiform papillae, with mild hyperkeratosis and occasional inflammatory cells. Often there is accumulated debris intermingled among the papillae and candidal pseudohyphae (Lynch, 2012).

## CLINICAL PRESENTATION

Those affected have a surplus of keratin on the filiform papillae of the dorsal tongue that leads to the formation of elongated strands that resemble hair. The color of the tongue ranges from a yellowish white to a brown or black dorsal tongue surface. The darker color results from the trapping of food and bacteria in the elongated strands. Occurrence is more common in smokers and persons with poor hygiene (Goldstein & Goldstein, 2012; Reamy, Derby, & Bunt, 2010).

Hairy tongue is asymptomatic, although overgrowth of *C. albicans* may result in glossopyrosis (burning tongue). Patients often complain of a tickling sensation in the soft palate and the oral pharynx during swallowing or, in more severe cases, a gagging sensation (Lynch, 2012).

## DIFFERENTIAL DIAGNOSIS

- Lichen planus
- Mucosal candidiasis
- Oral leukoplakia

## TREATMENT/MANAGEMENT

A culture of the tongue's dorsal surface should be taken if oral candidiasis or other specific oral infection is suspected. Cytologic smears stained with Gram stain or periodic acid–Schiff stain may reveal candidal organisms. Potassium hydroxide preparations are useful for rapid diagnosis of oral candidiasis (Lynch, 2012). Therapy consists of brushing the area of the tongue with a soft-bristle toothbrush and toothpaste two or three times per day (Goldstein & Goldstein, 2012).

## SPECIAL CONSIDERATIONS

Patients who are on a continuous soft diet occasionally develop hairy tongue because the texture of the diet does not aid in mechanically debriding the dorsal surface of the tongue during eating and swallowing. Elderly patients and ill patients who are not able to complete oral activities of daily living and are on soft diets are at greatest risk (Lynch, 2012).

Most patients are asymptomatic, but some experience halitosis or abnormal taste (Reamy et al., 2010). Poor self-esteem may be present as a result of oral appearance; patients may be withdrawn and not speak for fear of others noticing their tongue.

## WHEN TO REFER

Referral to a general dentist may be indicated if the etiology of a patient's hairy tongue appears to be primarily caused by poor oral hygiene.

## PATIENT EDUCATION

Inform the patient of the following tips:

- Add roughage to the diet when possible
- Brush or scrape the tongue two to three times daily
- Mouthwash can help halitosis

# DIAPER DERMATITIS

## OVERVIEW

Diaper dermatitis is a form of irritant contact dermatitis that can affect anyone who is incontinent and wears diapers or disposable briefs (Figure III.9). Diaper dermatitis is caused by (Agrawal, 2011):

- Overhydration of the skin
- Maceration
- Prolonged contact with urine and feces
- Retained diaper soaps
- Topical preparations
- More than three diarrheal stools per day
- Side effects of oral antibiotics

## EPIDEMIOLOGY

Diaper dermatitis commonly affects infants, with peak incidence at age 9 to 12 months. At any given time, diaper dermatitis is prevalent in 7% to 35% of the infant population (Agrawal, 2011).

## PATHOLOGY/HISTOLOGY

Diaper dermatitis affects the areas that are covered by a diaper. The moisture in the diaper causes the skin to be more susceptible to irritation by physical, chemical, and enzymatic mechanisms. Moist skin aids in the penetration of irritant substances. The urease enzyme found in the stratum corneum releases ammonia from cutaneous bacteria, which causes irritation to nonintact skin. Lipases and proteases in stool mix with urine on irritated skin and cause an alkaline surface pH, which adds to the skin breakdown. The bile salts in the stools enhance the activity of fecal enzymes, adding to the effect (Agrawal, 2011).

*C. albicans* has been recognized as another causative factor in diaper dermatitis and infection often occurs after 48 to 72 hours of active eruption. *Candida* is isolated from the diaper area in approximately 92% of children with diaper dermatitis (Agrawal, 2011).

## CLINICAL PRESENTATION

The diagnosis of candidiasis is suspected if there are multiple small, erythematous desquamating "satellite" lesions scattered along the edges of larger erythematous macules (James et al., 2006). Patients with diaper dermatitis present with an erythematous scaly perineal area often associated with papulovesicular or bullous lesions, fissures, and erosions. The rash can be patchy or confluent, affecting the abdomen from the umbilicus down to the thighs and encompassing the genitalia, perineum, and buttocks. Genital skin folds are spared in irritant dermatitis but often involved in primary candidal dermatitis (Agrawal, 2011).

## DIFFERENTIAL DIAGNOSIS

There are a number of differential diagnoses, including the following (Agrawal, 2011; Habif, 2004):

- Acrodermatitis enteropathica (zinc deficiency)
- Atopic dermatitis
- Biotin deficiency
- Child/elder abuse (physical and sexual)
- Contact dermatitis
- HIV infection
- Kawasaki disease
- Langerhans cell histiocytosis (Letterer-Siwe disease)
- Psoriasis
- Scabies
- Seborrheic dermatitis
- Varicella

## TREATMENT/MANAGEMENT

Dryness should be maintained by changing the diaper frequently or leaving it off for short periods. Habif (2004) recommends the following:

- Antifungal creams should be applied twice daily until eruption is clear (i.e., for approximately 10 days).

- Some erythema may be present after 10 days, which can be treated with 1% hydrocortisone cream followed in a few hours by creams active against yeast. Apply each twice daily.
- Baby powder may help prevent recurrence by absorbing moisture.
- Mupirocin ointment 2% (Bactroban) applied three to four times daily is effective for severe *Candida* and bacterial diaper dermatitis.
- Combination creams of azole, zinc, and petroleum are effective in the treatment of diaper dermatitis.

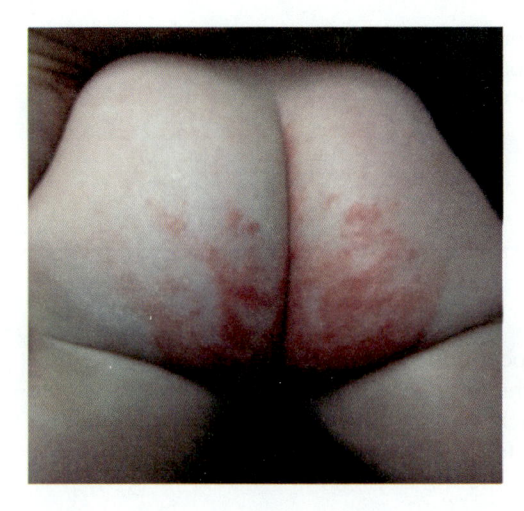

FIGURE III.9  Diaper dermatitis

## SPECIAL CONSIDERATIONS

Immunocompromised individuals may have increased prevalence of diaper dermatitis. Additionally, providers should consider the emotional state of young adults and the elderly who frequently have diaper dermatitis and be aware that recurrent infections can be embarrassing for patients.

## WHEN TO REFER

A dermatologist consultation may be indicated for the following:

- Atypical incidents of diaper dermatitis
- Patients who are immunocompromised
- Individuals who present with comorbidities
- Diaper dermatitis that is not responding to treatment

If signs of neglect are present, contact social services.

## PATIENT EDUCATION

Keeping the patient clean and dry will help heal diaper dermatitis and prevent recurrences. Whenever possible, leave the diaper off of the patient. The following are recommendations for maintenance of diaper dermatitis (U.S. National Library of Medicine/National Institutes of Health, 2012).

- Change the diaper as soon as the patient urinates or passes stool.
- Use water and a soft cloth or cotton ball to gently clean the diaper area with every diaper change. Avoid rubbing or scrubbing the area.
- Pat the area dry or allow air drying.
- Leave diapers loose to allow air to flow in the diaper.
- Use highly absorbent diapers to keep the skin dry and reduce the chance of infection.
- Wash hands before and after diaper changes.
- Zinc oxide or petroleum jelly–based products can act as a barrier to keep moisture away from the skin.
- Do not use wipes that have alcohol or perfume.
- Do not use cornstarch. It can make a yeast diaper rash worse.
- Do not use talc (talcum powder) on a baby.

## ORAL CANDIDIASIS/THRUSH

### OVERVIEW

*Oropharyngeal candidiasis*, or thrush, is a local infection often seen in infants; denture wearers; those treated with antibiotics, chemotherapy, or radiation therapy; people with cellular immunodeficiency states such as AIDS; patients with xerostomia; and those treated with inhaled glucocorticoids for asthma or rhinitis (Kauffman, 2012).

### EPIDEMIOLOGY

The infection is very common. It is estimated that approximately 7% of babies younger than 1 month old will develop oral candidiasis. The prevalence among patients with AIDS is estimated to be between 9% and 31%, and studies have documented clinical evidence of oral candidiasis in nearly 20% of cancer patients (Centers for Disease Control and Prevention, 2012).

### PATHOLOGY/HISTOLOGY

The diagnosis is confirmed by performing a Gram stain or KOH preparation on the lesions. Samples can be obtained by using a tongue depressor and scrapping the lesions. Budding yeast with or without pseudohyphae are often seen (Kauffman, 2012).
   The diagnosis of *Candida* esophagitis is usually made when white mucosal plaque-like lesions are noted on endoscopy. Biopsy results will show the presence of yeast and pseudohyphae invading mucosal cells, and cultures will reveal *Candida* (Kauffman, 2012).

### CLINICAL PRESENTATION

The usual symptoms of thrush are a dry feeling in the mouth, loss of taste, and a possible presence of pain when eating and swallowing. The diagnosis is usually made by the clinical presence of white plaques on the buccal mucosa, palate, tongue, or the oropharynx. There is usually erythema without plaques under dentures (Kauffman, 2012).

Esophageal candidiasis is most common in HIV-infected patients and in patients with hematologic malignancies. Coexistent thrush may or may not be present. The hallmark of esophageal candidiasis is odynophagia or pain on swallowing, and patients will usually localize their pain to a discrete area on the sternum (Kauffman, 2012).

## DIFFERENTIAL DIAGNOSIS

Tolan (2013) listed the following as differential diagnoses of oral thrush:

- Aphthous ulcers
- Blastomycosis
- Candidiasis
- Cytomegalovirus infection
- Diphtheria
- Enteroviral infection
- Esophagitis
- Herpes simplex virus infection
- HIV infection
- Lymphohistiocytosis
- Pharyngitis
- Syphilis

## TREATMENT/MANAGEMENT

Goldstein and Goldstein (2012) recommended topical therapy for treatment, which is usually effective; however, relapses in immunosuppressed patients are common. Treatments include the following:

- A nystatin troche (200,000–400,000 units four to five times per day) can be used.
- A clotrimazole troche (10-mg troche dissolved five times per day) for 7 to 14 days can be used. Clotrimazole troches are more palatable and potentially more effective.
- Nystatin suspension (400,000–600,000 units four times per day) can be used. Nystatin suspension is the least expensive option.

## SPECIAL CONSIDERATIONS

Healthy, newborn infants, especially if premature, are susceptible to thrush. In healthy newborns, thrush is a self-limited infection but should be treated to avoid interference with eating. The mother should be examined for vaginal candidiasis. In older infants, thrush usually occurs in the presence of predisposing factors such as antibiotic treatment or illness (Habif, 2004).

Patients using asthmatic inhalers should be instructed to rinse the mouth with water after inhaler use to prevent thrush.

## WHEN TO REFER

Chronic infection warrants further workup.

## PATIENT EDUCATION

Elderly patients with dentures should be reminded to clean their dentures carefully and frequently to reduce the likelihood of developing candidiasis (Goldstein & Goldstein, 2012). Chronic infections may occur from mechanical trauma of cheek biting, poor hygiene of dental prostheses, pipe smoking, or irritation from dentures (Habif, 2004).

### CLINICAL PEARLS

- Oropharyngeal candidiasis: ICD-9, 112.0; ICD-10, B37.0
- Patients with oral thrush are encouraged to change their toothbrush when receiving treatment to prevent recurrence.
- Diaper dermatitis: ICD-10, B37.2L22

## VULVOVAGINAL CANDIDIASIS

### OVERVIEW

Vulvovaginal candidiasis (VVC) is the most common form of mucosal candidiasis (Kauffman, 2012). VVC refers to a disorder characterized by signs and symptoms of vulvovaginal inflammation in the presence of *Candida* species. VVC is the second most common cause of vaginitis symptoms, after bacterial vaginitis, and accounts for approximately one third of vaginitis cases (Sobel, 2013).

Women who have *Candida* organisms in their vaginas have VVC, which has a variety of appearances ranging from an asymptomatic presence of yeast to severe acute systemic infection. Yeast colonization occurs relatively frequently, with up to 30% of healthy asymptomatic women having a positive culture for yeast at any single point in time (Cooper, 2010; Nyirjesy, 2008). VVC can be identified in the lower genital tract in 10% to 20% of healthy women of reproductive age, 6% to 7% of menopausal women, and 3% to 6% of prepubertal girls (Sobel, 2013).

### EPIDEMIOLOGY

For the treatment of VVC, an estimated $275 million is spent annually on over-the-counter (OTC) antifungal medications, and these number in the top 10 of all OTC medications sold in the United States. The total cost of VVC in the United States, including medical and treatment expenses, travel cost, and time missed from work, was estimated in 1995 to be $1.8 million (Nyirjesy, 2008).

When antifungal drugs became available for OTC use, advertisers described benefits such as convenience, ability to initiate therapy rapidly, patient empowerment, and potential health care cost savings, estimated at $63.8 million from 1990 to 1994 alone. However, data showed that only 34.5% of women who have had a previous diagnosis of VVC and only 11% of women without a history of VVC could accurately self-diagnose the infection (Nyirjesy, 2008).

## PATHOLOGY/HISTOLOGY

Two components are important in the development of a symptomatic episode of VVC. The first is vaginal colonization by *Candida* species, followed in turn by the transformation from the asymptomatic state to a symptomatic infection. *Candida* can enter the vagina through multiple sources, including local spread from the perineum and gastrointestinal tract, digital introduction, and sexual transmission (Nyirjesy, 2008).

*C. albicans* is responsible for 80% to 92% of episodes of VVC. Of the non–*C. albicans* yeast species, *Candida glabrata* is considered the most common (Sobel, 2013). In a review of vaginal yeast isolates obtained from more than 1,300 women across the United States, *C. albicans* accounted for 80.2%, *C. glabrata* for 14.3%, *Candida parapsilosis* for 5.9%, and *Candida tropicalis* for 8.0% (Nyirjesy, 2008). Studies indicated increased frequency of non–*C. albicans* species, particularly *C. glabrata*, likely because of increased use of OTC drugs, long-term use of suppressive azoles, and the use of short courses of antifungal drugs (Cooper, 2010; Sobel, 2013).

## CLINICAL PRESENTATION

The diagnosis of VVC is usually made clinically, but confirmation is easily made by observing budding yeast, with or without pseudohyphae, on a wet mount or KOH preparation of vaginal secretions (Kauffman, 2012). The most common symptoms of VVC include vaginal itching, irritation, soreness, burning, or dyspareunia. On vulvar examination, patients may exhibit erythema, edema, and excoriations and have a thick curdy discharge (Kauffman, 2012; Nyirjesy, 2008). The intensity of the signs and symptoms ranges from mild to severe, except in women with *C. glabrata* or *C. parapsilosis* infection, who tend to have mild or minimal clinical symptoms (Sobel, 2013).

## DIFFERENTIAL DIAGNOSIS

- Allergic or chemical reactions
- Atopic dermatitis
- Atrophic vaginitis
- Bacterial vaginitis
- Chlamydia or gonorrhea
- Contact dermatitis
- Herpes simplex
- Hypersensitivity reactions
- Lichen sclerosus et atrophicus
- Trichomoniasis
- Urinary tract infection
- Vulval psoriasis

## TREATMENT/MANAGEMENT

Treatment is indicated for relief of symptoms. From 10% to 20% of women of reproductive age who harbor *Candida* species are asymptomatic; these women do not require therapy (Sobel, 2013).

The following discuss topical and oral antifungal treatments for symptomatic infections:

- Nurbhai, Grimshaw, Watson, Bond, Mollison, & Ludbrook (2007) found no statistically significant differences between oral and intravaginal antifungal treatment for clinical cure in the short term. However, there was a significant difference for long-term follow-up in favor of oral treatment.
- Nyirjesy (2008) recommended treatments that include topical and oral therapy varying from 1 to 7 days. For severe VVC, one or two doses of oral fluconazole (150 mg) is recommended. For recurrent VVC, recommended treatment options include ketoconazole (100 mg oral daily), clotrimazole (500-mg suppositories weekly), and fluconazole (150 mg orally once weekly) for 6 to 12 months.
- Pappas et al. (2009) recommended a single 150-mg dose of fluconazole in the treatment of uncomplicated VVC. For recurrent VVC, the authors recommended 10 to 14 days of induction therapy with a topical or oral azole, followed by fluconazole at a dosage of 150 mg once weekly for 6 months.
- Sobel (2013) recommended the use of oral fluconazole in a 150-mg single-dose tablet because most women prefer oral drugs to topical or intravaginal applications. However, topical antifungal treatments have fewer side effects, such as nausea, headache, and potential for elevated liver function test; topical therapy also tends to relieve irritation more quickly.
- For pregnant patients, topical therapy with clotrimazole or miconazole vaginally for 7 days is recommended. Administration of oral azoles during the first trimester is contraindicated. After the first trimester, the use of a single, low-dose fluconazole 150-mg tablet to treat VVC has not shown increased risk for birth defects. In Germany, third-trimester treatment of VVC is recommended to prevent oral thrush and diaper dermatitis in newborns (Sobel, 2013).
- There is no substantial evidence to support the use of probiotics, boric acid, or immunotherapy for the treatment and prevention of VVC (Powell, 2010; Sobel, 2013).

## SPECIAL CONSIDERATIONS

- Many women experience at least one episode of VCC by age 25, primarily because of initiation of sexual activity. Among college women, VVC is more common among Black women than White women (Nyirjesy, 2008).
- Diabetic patients are less likely to respond to therapy and may be more prone to developing infections caused by *C. glabrata* (Nyirjesy, 2008).
- In HIV-infected women, vaginal colonization with *Candida* is vastly increased (Nyirjesy, 2008).
- Treatment of pregnant women is primarily for relief of symptoms. VVC is not associated with adverse pregnancy outcomes.

## WHEN TO REFER

Recurrent VVC is defined as four or more episodes of symptomatic candidiasis a year and warrants a complete workup to rule out diabetes, HIV, and autoimmune diseases. If cause of recurrent infections is not determined, then prompt referral to an infectious disease specialist is warranted (Powell, 2010; Pritchard, 2010).

## PATIENT EDUCATION

Risk factors for the development of *C. albicans* are as follows (Cooper, 2010; Duncan, 2012; Nyirjesy, 2008; Powell, 2010; Pritchard, 2010; Sobel, 2013):

- Sexual factors—in particular, orogenital sex—contribute to the introduction of microorganisms or may facilitate symptomatic disease because of microtrauma to the vulva.
- Oral contraceptives, use of a diaphragm and spermicide, and the use of an intrauterine device (IUD) are associated with an increased risk of *Candida* infection.
- Hygienic habits such as using tampons or menstrual pads, wearing tight clothing, using perfumed soaps or feminine hygiene sprays, and douching have been associated with increased risk for VVC.
- Women with diabetes mellitus, especially type 2 diabetes, who have poor glycemic control, are more prone to VVC.
- The use of broad-spectrum antibiotics significantly increases risk for VVC.
- VVC appears to occur more often in women with increased estrogen levels, such as that caused by oral contraceptives, pregnancy, and hormone-replacement therapy.
- Immunosuppression increases the risk for VVC. People taking glucocorticoids, chemotherapy, or other immunosuppressive drugs and people with HIV are at higher risk.
- During pregnancy, there is increased risk because of changing vaginal pH caused by hormonal changes.

## CLINICAL PEARLS

- Genital candidiasis: ICD-9, 112.2; ICD-10, B37.3/B37.4
- Providers should always encourage women to self-examine and, perhaps more important, follow up for consultation if symptoms of VVC occur.

## REFERENCES

Agrawal, R. (2011). *Diaper dermatitis*. Retrieved from http://emedicine.medscape.com/article/911985-overview

BMJ Group. (2012). *Angular cheilitis*. Retrieved from http://bestpractice.bmj.com/best-practice/monograph/619/basics/epidemiology.html

Centers for Disease Control and Prevention. (2012). *Oral candidiasis statistics*. Retrieved from http://www.cdc.gov/fungal/candidiasis/thrush/statistics.html

Cooper, M. (2010). Assessment and diagnosis. *Practice Nursing, 21*(7), 366–370.

Duncan, D. (2012). Assessing and managing persistent thrush. *Practice Nursing, 23*(2), 78–81.

Fitzpatrick, T., Johnson, R., Wolff, K., Polano, M., & Suurmond, D. (1997). *Color atlas and synopsis of clinical dermatology common and serious disease* (3rd ed.). New York, NY: McGraw-Hill.

Goldstein, B., & Goldstein, A. (2012). *Oral lesions*. Retrieved from http://www.uptodate.com/contents/oral-lesions

Goodheart, H. (2011). *Goodheart's same-site differential diagnosis: A rapid method of diagnosing and treating common skin disorders*. Philadelphia, PA: Lippincott Williams & Wilkins.

Habif, T. P. (2004). *Clinical dermatology* (4th ed.). Philadelphia, PA: Mosby.

James, W. D., Berger, T. G., & Elston, D. M. (2006). *Andrews' diseases of the skin. Clinical dermatology* (10th ed.). Philadelphia, PA: Saunders.

Kauffman, C. A. (2012). *Overview of Candida infections*. Retrieved from http://www.uptodate.com/contents/overview-of-candida-infections

Lynch, D. P. (2012). *Hairy tongue.* Retrieved from http://emedicine.medscape.com/article/1075886-overview#a0199

Nurbhai, M., Grimshaw, J., Watson, M., Bond, C. M., Mollison, J. A., & Ludbrook, A. (2007). Oral versus intra-vaginal imidazole and triazole anti-fungal treatment of uncomplicated vulvovaginal candidiasis (thrush). *Cochrane Database of Systematic Reviews*, (4). doi:10.1002/14651858.CD002845.pub2

Nyirjesy, P. (2008). Vulvovaginal candidiasis and bacterial vaginosis. *Infectious Disease Clinics of North America, 22,* 637–652.

Pappas, P. G., Kauffman, C. A., Andes, D., Benjamin, D. K., Calandra, T. F., Edwards, J. E., ... Sobel, J. D. (2009). Clinical practice guidelines for the management of candidiasis: 2009 update by the Infectious Diseases Society of America. *Clinical Infectious Diseases, 48*(5), 503–535.

Powell, K. (2010). Vaginal thrush: Quality of life and treatments. *British Journal of Nursing, 19*(17), 1106–1111.

Pritchard, J. (2010). Appropriate treatment choice. *Practice Nursing, 21*(9), 484–487.

Reamy, B. V., Derby, R., & Bunt, C. W. (2010). Common tongue conditions in primary care. *American Family Physician, 81*(5), 627–634.

Sobel, J. D. (2013). *Candida vulvovaginitis.* Retrieved from http://www.uptodate.com/contents/candida-vulvovaginitis

Tolan, R. W. (2013). *Thrush differential diagnosis.* Retrieved from http://emedicine.medscape.com/article/969147-differential

U.S. National Library of Medicine/National Institutes of Health. (2012). *Diaper rash.* Retrieved from http://nlm.nih.gov/medlineplus/ency/article/000964.htm

# Cellulitis/Erysipelas

## OVERVIEW

*Cellulitis* is an acute, dispersing infection of dermal and subcutaneous tissues, distinguished by a red, hot, tender area of skin, often at the site of bacterial entry (Fitzpatrick, Johnson, Wolff, Polano, & Suurmond, 1997; Habif, 2004; Figure III.10a and III.10b). Inducing factors include disturbance to the skin barrier as a result of trauma, inflammation, or a preexisting skin infection, as well as edema. The most common cause of cellulitis is beta-hemolytic *Streptococcus* (Groups A, B, C, G, and F) and other pathogens, including *Staphylococcus aureus* and gram-negative aerobic bacilli (Baddour, 2013; Fitzpatrick et al., 1997). Cellulitis in children younger than age 3 is typically caused by *Haemophilus influenza* type B (Habif, 2004).

*Erysipelas*, also known as *St. Anthony's fire* and *ignis sacer*, is an acute beta-hemolytic Group A streptococcal infection of the skin involving the superficial dermal lymphatics. Occasional cases caused by streptococcal Group C or G are reported in adults, but Group B *Streptococcus* is often responsible in the newborn and may be the cause of abdominal or perineal erysipelas in postpartum women (James, Berger, & Elston, 2006).

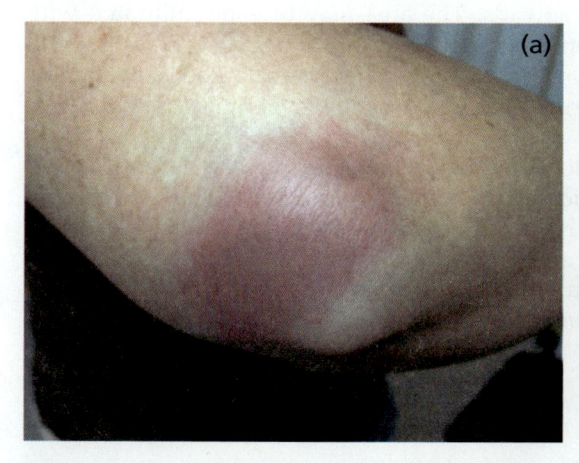

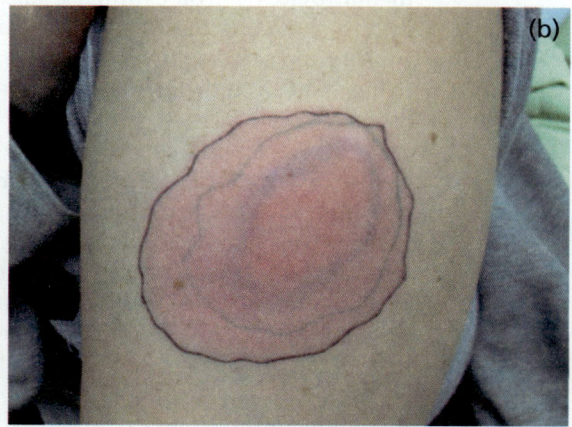

FIGURE III.10  (a) An example of cellulitis. (b) Cellulitis resulting from a vaccination for varicella.

## EPIDEMIOLOGY

Cellulitis occurs most frequently among middle-aged and elderly individuals, whereas erysipelas occurs more often in young children and the elderly (Baddour, 2013). The incidence of cellulitis and erysipelas is about 200 cases per 100,000 patients in a year (Baddour, 2013). The number of people admitted to the hospital for treatment of cellulitis has increased by 77% in recent years, with 87,000 patients being admitted to the hospital in 2010, costing approximately $254 million for inpatient treatment (Nazarko, 2012).

Cellulitis affects all racial and ethnic groups, both men and women, and people of all ages. The following age groups are at higher risk for cellulitis (Herchline, 2013):

- Previously, buccal cellulitis caused by *H. influenzae* type B was more common in children younger than 3 years; vaccination against this organism has helped decrease incidence.
- Facial cellulitis is more common in adults older than 50 years; however, pneumococcal facial cellulitis occurs primarily in young children who are at risk for pneumococcal bacteremia.
- Perianal cellulitis, usually with Group A beta-hemolytic *Streptococcus*, occurs in children younger than 3 years.
- Elderly patients with cellulitis are at an increased risk for thrombophlebitis.

## PATHOLOGY/HISTOLOGY

Cellulitis is most commonly seen in the lower extremities and caused by beta-hemolytic streptococci. The release of enzymes causes the infection to spread locally, causing erythema and edema. The skin becomes hot and tender to the touch, and lymphangitic streaks may develop, which is also common in erysipelas. Typically, cellulitis occurs near surgical wounds or cutaneous ulcers, but it may occur in normal skin (Hill, 2003).

## CLINICAL PRESENTATION

Cellulitis is inflammation involving particularly the subcutaneous tissue, caused most frequently by *Streptococcus pyogenes* or *S. aureus* and usually follows some apparent wound. On the lower extremities, tinea pedis is the most common portal of entry and is characterized by mild local erythema and tenderness, malaise, and chills. The erythema rapidly becomes intense and spreads. The area may become infiltrated with pitting skin, and the area may become nodular with a centralized vesicle that will rupture and secrete pus and necrotic material. This produces streaks and lymphangitis that spread from the area to neighboring lymph nodes (Habif, 2004; James et al., 2006; Scheinfeld, 2013).

Erysipelas is characterized by local redness, heat, swelling, and a classic raised border (Figure III.11). The lymphatic system is usually involved, and streaking is pronounced. The onset is preceded by prodromal symptoms of malaise for several hours, which may be accompanied by a severe reaction with chills, high fever, headache, vomiting, and joint pains. There is commonly a polymorphonuclear leukocytosis of 20,000/mm$^3$ or more (Habif, 2004; James et al., 2006; Scheinfeld, 2013).

## DIFFERENTIAL DIAGNOSIS

- Angioneurotic edema
- Bursitis

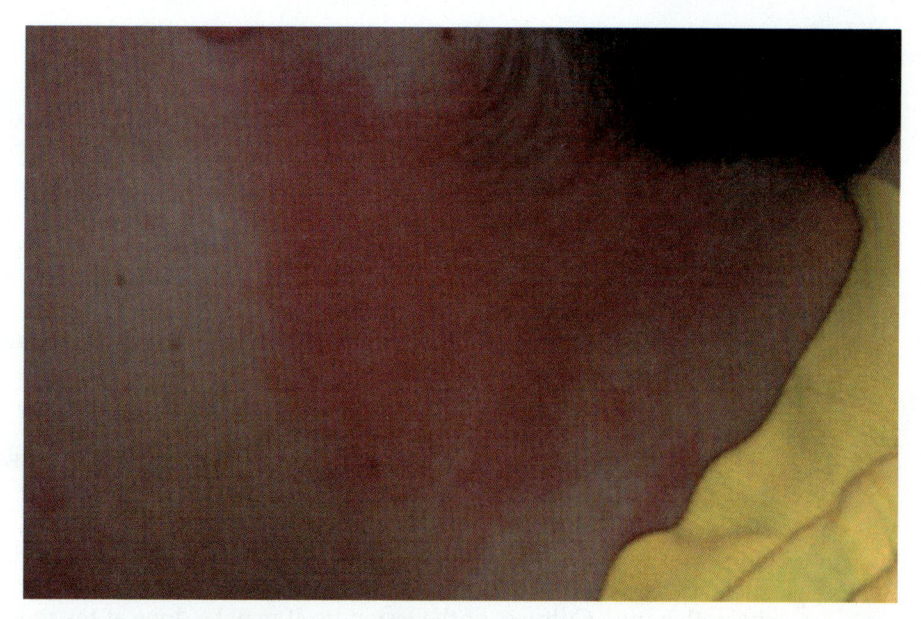

**FIGURE III.11** An example of erysipelas
Courtesy of Nancy Seal, FNP

- Contact dermatitis from plants, drugs, or dyes
- Deep vein thrombosis (DVT)
- Erythema migrans
- Gas gangrene
- Gout
- Herpes zoster
- Insect bites
- Lipodermatosclerosis
- Lymphedema
- Necrotizing fasciitis
- Nummular eczema
- Osteomyelitis
- Polychondritis (ear involvement)
- Scarlet fever
- Systemic lupus (facial cellulitis/erysipelas)
- Toxic shock syndrome
- Vasculitis
- Venous eczema

## TREATMENT/MANAGEMENT

Assessment of cellulitis should include (Hill, 2003):

1. History
   a. When did the symptoms start? Has this happened before?
   b. Has the affected area changed since it began?
   c. Are there symptoms of pruritus or pain?
   d. What is the patient's occupation or hobbies?

2. Evaluation of the patient's health status
3. Physical examination
   a. Pain
   b. Erythema
   c. Warmth
   d. Edema
   e. Fever
   f. Presence of preexisting lesion
   g. Lymphadenopathy
4. Diagnostic tests
   a. Obtain a complete blood count with differential; the provider may see mild leukocytosis with a shift to the left.
   b. Assess sedimentation rate; it may be mildly elevated.
   c. Perform a C-reactive protein test; it may be elevated.
   d. Obtain a comprehensive metabolic panel; if planning to use antibiotics, assess liver and kidney functions, nutritional status, and assess for diabetes if not already diagnosed.
   e. Blood cultures are recommended, especially in adults with underlying diseases (diabetes, hematologic malignancies, intravenous drug abuse, HIV infection, and chemotherapy). Cultures of the lesion itself may be done at the point of maximal inflammation (Habif, 2004).

The approach to treatment for cellulitis or erysipelas is dependent on whether there is purulent cellulitis present. Many patients have underlying conditions that predispose them to developing cellulitis (tinea pedis, lymphedema, chronic venous insufficiency), and these underlying conditions must also be addressed (Baddour, 2013). The following are some cellulitis treatment options:

■ Nonantibiotic therapy

1. Baddour (2013) recommended hydration of skin, elevation to prevent edema, and treating underlying conditions that predispose the skin to cellulitis.
2. Beasley (2011) discussed the HAMMMER acronym as a helpful tool for nonantibiotic treatment: hydrate, analgesia, monitor pyrexia, mark off the area, measure the circumference of the limb, elevate the limb, and record the site.

■ Antibiotics

1. Baddour (2013) recommended that patients with purulent cellulitis be managed empirically with antibiotics until culture results are available because of the risk of methicillin-resistant *Staphylococcus aureus* (MRSA) infection. Options for empiric oral therapy for treatment of MRSA include clindamycin, Bactrim DS, tetracycline, and linezolid. The duration of therapy should be individualized depending on response for 5 to 10 days.
2. Nazarko (2012) recommended that patients who do not have contraindications for antibiotic therapy take oral antibiotics. The usual prescription is flucloxacillin 500 mg to be taken every 6 hours. For patients who are allergic to penicillin, clarithromycin 500 mg twice daily is recommended.
3. Hill (2003) recommends that staphylococcal or streptococcal cellulitis be treated with penicillinase-resistant penicillin, dicloxacillin, or cephalosporin. Intravenous antibiotics may be used for advanced infections. Recurrent diseases should be treated with prophylactic antibiotics.
4. James et al. (2006) recommended intravenous penicillin for erysipelas and cellulitis for the initial 24 to 48 hours, followed by oral antibiotics for at least 10 days.

Erythromycin is also used, although some macrolide-resistant streptococci are possible. In lack of response to antibiotics, MRSA should be considered and treatment strategies chosen. Leg involvement, especially when bullae are present, will require hospitalization and intravenous antibiotics.

5. Habif (2004) recommended treating adults with antibiotics aimed at staphylococcal and streptococcal organisms. Treatments include penicillinase-resistant penicillin (dicloxacillin 500–1,000 mg orally every 6 hours) or a cephalosporin. For more severe infections, intravenous penicillinase-resistant penicillin should be used. An aminoglycoside (gentamicin or tobramycin) should be considered in patients at risk for gram-negative infection. In children, *H. influenza* cellulitis therapy should be prompt. All family members should be treated. Cefuroxime is effective against all of the major etiologic agents and is especially effective against *H. influenza*.
6. Scheinfeld (2013) stated that for streptococcal cellulitis or erysipelas, treatment should consist of penicillin or cephalosporin. Cephalexin 500 mg four times a day for 10 to 14 days or Cefdinir 300 mg two times a day is used. For those allergic to penicillin, prescribe azithromycin 500 mg on the first day, followed by 250 mg for the next 4 days. Quinolones are used as a third-line therapy.

## SPECIAL CONSIDERATIONS

The elderly, patients with diabetes, and children often require hospitalization and intravenous antibiotics for erysipelas infections (Habif, 2004). In elderly patients and in patients with diabetes, temperature and white blood cell counts cannot dictate treatment because these are sensitive, as opposed to specific, markers of infection (Scheinfeld, 2013). Previous episodes of cellulitis, surgery with lymph node resection, and radiation therapy can compromise the lymphatic system (Habif, 2004). A number of factors contribute to the increase in cellulitis (Nazarko, 2012).

- Obesity
- Diabetes
- Leg ulcerations
- Older age (Elderly people are at a greater risk of developing cellulitis than younger people. This may be because of weakening immune systems and poorer circulation.)
- Skin breakdown (This can promote bacterial invasion through the skin.)

## WHEN TO REFER

If the signs and symptoms of sepsis are present, quick referral to a specialist or hospital admission is warranted (Nazarko, 2012). Other referable conditions include the following:

- Cold/clammy skin
- Confusion/disorientation
- Diarrhea
- Elevated white blood cell count
- Hypotension
- Increased respirations
- Pyrexia
- Reduced urine output
- Tachycardia

## PATIENT EDUCATION

If cellulitis is affecting the lower extremities, the patient should decrease physical activity and elevate the extremity. Over-the-counter medications such as acetaminophen (Tylenol) or ibuprofen (Advil, Motrin) can help with pain (Herchline, 2013).

Patients should seek medical care if the following conditions occur (Herchline, 2013):

- Fever (> 100.5°F)
- Cellulitis with surrounding soft areas that are suggestive of abscess formation
- Red streaking from an area of cellulitis or a rapidly expanding erythema
- Significant pain not relieved by acetaminophen or ibuprofen
- Inability to move an extremity or joint because of pain

In addition, patients with diabetes, cancer, chronic lymphedema, or immunosuppression should be made aware that they are at higher risk for serious infections from cellulitis and that minor skin infections can lead to cellulitis.

## CLINICAL PEARLS

- Cellulitis, unspecified: ICD-10, L03.90
- *Staphylococcus aureus* and Group A *Streptococcus* are the most common causes of cellulitis.
- Cellulitis is predominantly unilateral.
- Tinea pedia is a common portal of entry for bacteria. It is imperative that patients with recurrent leg cellulitis be assessed and appropriately treated for tinea pedis.

## REFERENCES

Baddour, L. M. (2013). *Cellulitis and erysipelas*. Retrieved from http://www.uptodate.com/contents/cellulitis-and-erysipelas

Beasley, A. (2011). Management of patients with cellulitis of the lower limb. *Nursing Standard, 26*(11), 50–55.

Fitzpatrick, T. B., Johnson, R. A., Wolff, K., Polano, M. K., & Suurmond, D. (1997). *Color atlas and synopsis of clinical dermatology. Common and serious diseases* (3rd ed.). New York, NY: McGraw-Hill.

Habif, T. P. (2004). *Clinical dermatology: A color guide to diagnosis and therapy* (4th ed.). Philadelphia, PA: Mosby.

Herchline, T. E. (2013, April 14). *Cellulitis*. Retrieved from http://emedicine.medscape.com/article/214222-overview#a0156

Hill, M. J. (2003). *Dermatologic nursing essentials* (2nd ed.). Pitman, NJ: Dermatology Nurses Association.

James, W. D., Berger, T. G., & Elston, D. M. (2006). *Andrews' diseases of the skin: Clinical dermatology* (10th ed.). Philadelphia, PA: Elsevier/Saunders.

Nazarko, L. (2012). An evidence-based approach to diagnosis and management of cellulitis. *British Journal of Community Nursing, 17*(1), 6–12.

Scheinfeld, N. S. (2013, July). Bacterial skin infections in the elderly. *Consultant*, 505b–505j.

# Cysts

A cyst is a nodule that measures greater than 0.5 cm and contains fluid or semisolid material composed of keratin and lipid-rich debris. Cysts, derived from epithelium of a hair follicle, connect to the surface of the skin by a central core (Goodheart, 2011). Epidermoid cysts, also referred to as sebaceous cysts, occur most commonly on the face, behind the ears, neck, trunk, scrotum, and labia. Pilar cyst, the second most common, occur on the scalp.

## EPIDERMAL INCLUSION CYST/SEBACCEOUS CYST

### OVERVIEW

*Epidermoid cysts* are the most common cutaneous cysts (Figure III.12). They most frequently occur on the face, scalp, neck, and trunk. In the past, epidermoid cysts have been referred to by various terms, including *follicular infundibular cysts, epidermal cysts, epidermal inclusion cysts*, and *sebaceous cysts,* but because most lesions originate from the follicular infundibulum, the general term *epidermoid cyst* is favored. Epidermoid cysts are benign lesions; although rare cases of associated malignancies have been noted (Fromm, 2012; Goldstein & Goldstein, 2012).

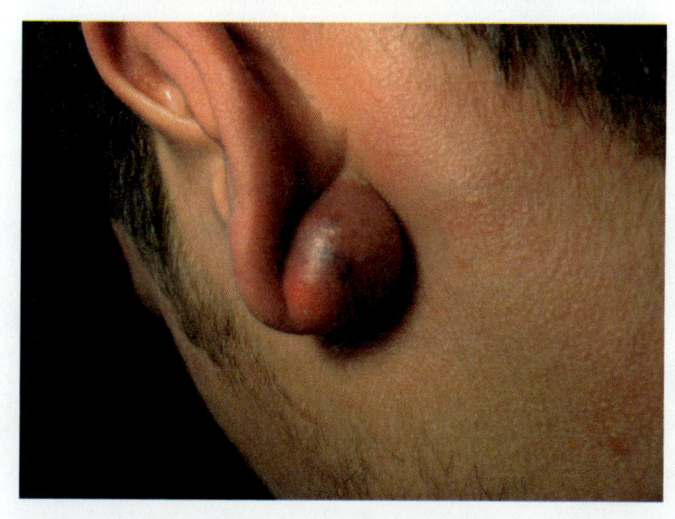

FIGURE III.12    Sebaceous cyst

## EPIDEMIOLOGY

No racial prevalence has been found for epidermoid cysts. Pigmentation changes associated with epidermoid cysts are common in individuals with dark skin. Epidermoid cysts affect men twice as often as women and can occur at any age; however, they most commonly arise in the third and fourth decades of life. Small epidermoid cysts known as *milia* are common in the neonatal period and on the faces of individuals with oily complexions (Fromm, 2012).

## PATHOLOGY/HISTOLOGY

The cyst wall consists of normal epidermis that produces keratin. A *comedo* or trauma may cause the epidermis to become lodged in the dermis. Lesions remain stable and enlarge with time (Goldstein & Goldstein, 2012). The skin surface has a small opening filled with keratin that is connected through a narrow channel to the cyst in the dermis (Habif, 2004).

## CLINICAL PRESENTATION

The surface of the overlying skin is usually smooth and shiny from the upward pressure of the cyst. Epidermoid cysts are asymptomatic, and palpation of the cyst reveals a discrete, freely moveable cyst or nodule. The cysts are located above the underlying tissue and are attached to the normal skin above by a comedo-like central infundibular, or funnel-shaped, structure or punctum. Before rupture there is a sudden onset of redness, pain, swelling, and local heat (James, Berger, & Elston, 2006). Discharge of a foul-smelling, cottage cheese–like material may occur with rupture. Sometimes cysts can become infected, resulting in pain and tenderness. In the rare event of malignancy, rapid growth, friability, and bleeding may be reported (Fromm, 2012; Goldstein & Goldstein, 2012; Habif, 2004).

Epidermoid cysts are most common on the face, trunk, neck, extremities, and scalp; cysts in the breast or genital area are also not uncommon in the general population. Rarely, the ocular and oral mucosae can also be affected, as well as the palpebral conjunctivae, lips, buccal mucosa, tongue, and uvula. Cysts on the distal portions of the digits may extend into the terminal phalanx, which can create changes in the nails, such as pincer nails, erythema, edema, tenderness, and pain (Fromm, 2012).

## DIFFERENTIAL DIAGNOSIS

- Branchial cleft cyst
- Calcinosis cutis
- Dermoid cyst
- Gardner syndrome
- Lipomas
- Milia
- Pachyonychia congenita
- Pilar cyst
- Steatocystoma multiplex

## TREATMENT/MANAGEMENT

Fromm (2012) and Goldstein and Goldstein (2012) have stated that laboratory studies are usually not necessary; however, with recurrent infection or lack of response to antibiotics, a culture and sensitivity should be obtained. Asymptomatic epidermoid cysts do not require treatment. Injection of Kenalog, 3 mg/mL for the face and 10 mg/mL for the trunk into the surrounding inflamed dermis can reduce inflammation, lessen the chance of infection, and decrease the need for incision and drainage. Oral antibiotics may be used if erythema or signs of infection are present. Epidermoid cysts may be removed by simple excision with removal of entire cyst and cyst wall. If the cyst wall is not removed, there may be reoccurrence. Excision with punch biopsy technique may be used if the size of the lesion permits.

## SPECIAL CONSIDERATIONS

The causes of epidermoid cysts are as follows (Fromm, 2012):

- Congenital epidermoid cysts of the anterior fontanelle or those that are orogenital in location likely result from the trapping of epidermal nests along embryonic fusion planes during development. Lip and lingual lesions may be related to abnormal fusion of the branchial arches, and genital lesions may result from abnormal closure of the genital folds.
- Any abnormal process that affects or grows near the pilosebaceous unit may cause occlusion or impingement of the follicular ostia, which will lead to the formation of a cyst. Cystic acne is most likely the result of follicular occlusion. Years of sun damage can damage the pilosebaceous unit causing abnormalities such as comedo occlusion, which can lead to cyst formation. This is referred to as Favre-Racouchot syndrome.
- Epidermal inclusion cysts can result from the attaching of epithelial elements to the dermis. Crushing-type injuries have been associated with subungual or terminal phalanx epidermoid cysts. Any surgical procedure can result in epidermoid cysts; examples include the formation of multiple epidermoid cysts after rhinoplasty, breast augmentation, and liposuction. Dermal and myocutaneous grafts and needle biopsies have also been linked to the development of epidermoid cysts.
- Hereditary syndromes are associated with epidermoid cysts, including Gardner syndrome, basal cell nevus syndrome, and pachyonychia congenita.

## WHEN TO REFER

Cysts located in atypical areas warrant consultation.

## PATIENT EDUCATION

Patients should be educated not to squeeze or manipulate cysts. Warm compresses to an inflamed cyst can assist with opening and drainage of the cyst without the need for incision.

## CLINICAL PEARLS

- Epidermal inclusion cyst: ICD-9, 706.2; ICD-10, L72.01
- Wolff, Johnson, and Saavedra, (2013) recommended excision for epidermal inclusion cysts, that occur on the palms, soles, and fingers. A variant of an epidermal cyst is a giant comedo, which should be excised and drained (Habif, Campbell, Chapman, Dinulos, & Zug, 2011).
- According to Habif, Campbell, Chapman, Dinulos, and Zug (2011), complete surgical incision with narrow margins is curative.

# HIDRADENITIS SUPPURATIVA

## OVERVIEW

*Hidradenitis suppurativa* (HS) is a chronic, follicular, and occlusive disease characterized by recurrent boils or abscesses primarily affecting the intertriginous skin of the axillae, groin, genital, perianal, and inframammary areas (Danby & Margesson, 2010; Figure III.13). HS was once associated with the apocrine sweat (*hidros*) glands (*aden*), as first described in 1921 (Revuz, 2010). Since then, follicular occlusion has been shown to be the cause in HS.

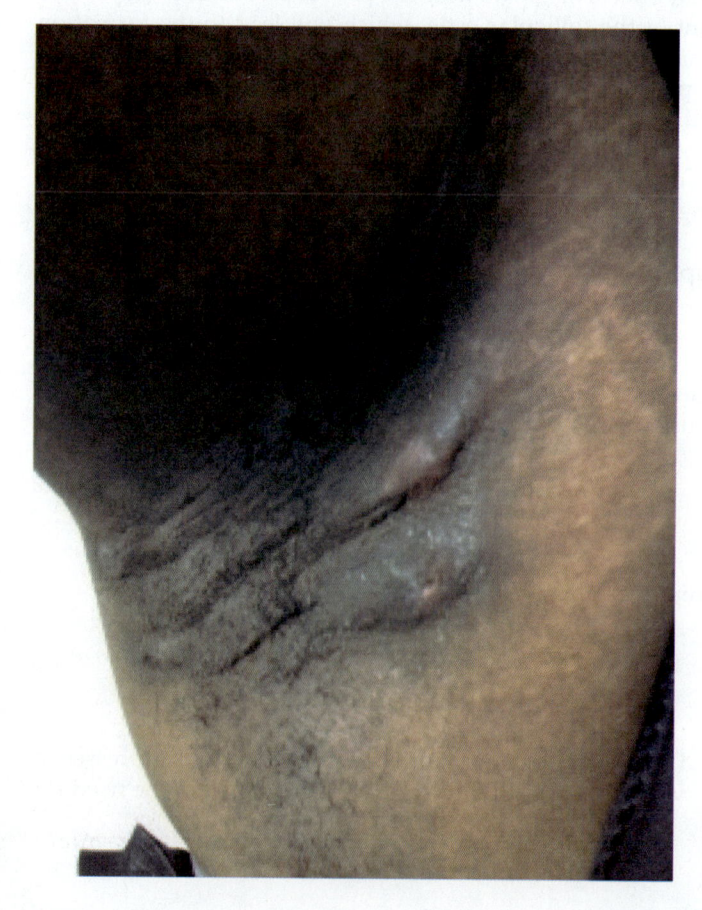

FIGURE III.13  Hidradenitis suppurativa on the axilla

## EPIDEMIOLOGY

HS is often considered a rare disease. However, the prevalence of HS in the United States and globally is approximately 4%, with higher incidence in hot and humid climates (Danby & Margesson, 2010; Krbec, 2007).

HS is more common in women than men, at a ratio of 3.3 to 1.4 and affects genders differently, being more common under the breast (22%) and in the groin (93%) in women and on the buttocks (40%) and perianal area (51%) in men. The average age of onset is 23 years and it rarely occurs before puberty, but can occur prior to puberty if there is a family history of HS. HS is unusual after menopause, but in men HS can continue into old age (Danby & Margesson, 2010; Krbec, 2007).

## PATHOLOGY/HISTOLOGY

HS is thought to develop in the following sequence (Krbec, 2007):

1. Keratin plugs the apocrine duct and hair follicle, and dilation occurs.
2. Inflammation develops, causing bacterial growth in the dilated duct.
3. The duct ruptures, extending the inflammation and infection.
4. Localized tissue destruction, ulceration, fibrosis, and sinus tract formation occurs.

Other theories include failure of the apocrine ducts to drain properly and immunosuppression.

HS is affected by hormonal, mechanical, genetic, and other influences. With increased hormonal stimulation, the ductal keratinocytes that line the ducts fail to separate from one another, causing a buildup of keratinocytes, also known as a comedo. The comedo causes a tight plug in the duct. Genetic weaknesses or lack of the periodic acid–Schiff positive glassy membrane glycoprotein material that supports the duct under pressure of a bulging follicular canal permits the wall of the duct to weaken. Small follicular material leaks out, which activates the immune system and causes the rupture of the duct wall. The pilosebaceous unit attempts to heal, but the failure of the inflammatory contents to rise to the surface and then heal is what differentiates HS from acne, folliculitis, or a simple boil. After rupturing beneath the surface, the follicular fragments and their growth cause the extensive lateral spread and the characteristic inflammatory response. The epithelial material still in the dermis remains alive and exposed to hormones and growth factors that sustain the initial production of the keratinocytes. Continuous growth of these hormonally stimulated fragments beneath the surface produces the connecting sinuses and causes increasing amounts of irritating debris (Danby & Margesson, 2010).

## CLINICAL PRESENTATION

Patients with HS may have early signs of pruritus, erythema, and local hyperhidrosis (Krbec, 2007). The lesions occur in areas of the skin that contain apocrine glands: axillae, inguinal areas, inner thighs, perianal and perineal areas, mammary and inframammary areas, buttocks, pubic area, scrotum, vulva, chest, scalp, and retroauricular region. The onset can be deceptive, with indiscriminate small nodules that develop as a red, indurated papule, pustule, or cyst that may heal without leaving a scar (Danby & Margesson, 2010; James et al., 2006; Krbec, 2007; Smith, Chao, & Teitelbaum, 2010). The hallmark of HS is the double comedo in the form of a blackhead with two or sometimes several surface openings that interconnect under the skin (Habif, 2004).

The Second International Hidradenitis Suppurativa Research Symposium adapted the following three diagnostic criteria, which must be met to establish a diagnosis of HS (Danby & Margesson, 2010):

1. Typical lesions: In the early stages, primary lesions are deep painful nodules that lead to draining sinuses, bridged scars, and tombstone open comedones in secondary lesions.
2. Typical sites affected: Axillae, groin, genitals, perineal and perianal region, buttocks, and inframammary and intermammary folds are commonly affected.
3. Chronicity and recurrences: The mean age of onset is at 22 years, and HS typically lasts about 19 years. It may lessen with pregnancy and breastfeeding.

## DIFFERENTIAL DIAGNOSIS

Danby and Margesson (2010); James, Berger, and Elston (2006); Krbec (2007); and Smith, Chao, and Teitelbaum (2010) noted the following considerations and associated conditions for differential diagnosis:

- Acanthosis nigricans
- Actinomycosis
- Anal or vulvovaginal fistulae
- Bartholin abscess
- Boils
- Cat-scratch disease
- Crohn's disease
- Deep fungi (e.g., blastomyces, *Nocardia*)
- Down syndrome
- Epidermal cyst
- Erysipelas
- Folliculitis
- Furuncles/carbuncles
- Granuloma inguinale
- Graves disease
- Hashimoto thyroiditis
- Herpes simplex
- Hyperandrogenism
- Infected Bartholin glands
- Lymphogranuloma venereum
- Sjogren's syndrome
- Squamous cell carcinoma
- Ulcerative colitis

## TREATMENT/MANAGEMENT

HS is diagnosed by clinical appearance in typical locations. The pattern of recurrent boils in one area that do not respond to antibiotic therapy is a good indicator of HS (Danby & Margesson, 2010).

There is no single effective treatment for HS. The only permanent cure that has been reported for severe HS is wide excision surgery. Most patients with HS require a combination of medical and surgical strategies. Recommended treatments for HS include antibiotics, antiandrogens, corticosteroids, cyclosporine, and tumor necrosis factor-alpha (TNF-α) inhibitors. Isotretinoin is used although not always effectively (Danby & Margesson, 2010; Habif, 2004; Krbec, 2007; Smith et al., 2010).

1. Antibiotics
   a. Topical clindamycin 1% solution twice a day reduces abscesses and pustules.
   b. Oral antibiotics (doxycycline, minocycline, erythromycin, cephalosporins, and amoxicillin-clavulanate [Augmentin]) are recommended for short- and long-term therapy.
   c. Dapsone has also been used effectively.
2. Antiandrogens
   a. Finasteride 5 mg daily has been used effectively in a few studies.
   b. If oral contraceptives are used, those containing estradiol and drospirenone are recommended, combined with the antiandrogen spironolactone 50 to 100 mg.
3. Dietary and metabolic management
   a. Restriction of dairy products and a low-glycemic diet is recommended. This is thought to decrease hormonal stimulation of genetically susceptible pilosebaceous ducts.
4. Immunosuppressives
   a. Corticosteroids have been used successfully intralesionally and systemically for symptomatic care. High dosages of systemic steroids, rapidly tapered, can be effective in stopping acute HS lesions by quickly reducing pain and inflammation.
   b. Cyclosporine (4–5 mg/kg/day) has been reported to help in a few cases.
   c. Methotrexate has not been shown to be effective.
5. Retinoids
   a. Isotretinoin
6. TNF-α inhibitors
   a. Infliximab, which is used to treat Crohn's disease, has been reported to improve HS.
   b. Adalimumab has also been used successfully.
7. Miscellaneous therapies
   a. Zinc salts have been found to be anti-inflammatory and have been used for mild to moderate acne. Zinc is also antiandrogenic.
   b. Photodynamic therapy has shown controversial results.
   c. Botulinum toxin has been shown to decrease the apocrine output, leading to less stress on the plugged orifice.
   d. Radiotherapy has shown variable response and was used in the past. Good information if patient had therapy in past provider needs to be aware.
   e. Cryotherapy has been effective in patients with limited but persistent lesions.

## SPECIAL CONSIDERATIONS

Several factors are related to the development of HS (Danby & Margesson, 2010; James et al., 2006):

- Genetic factors: Thirty-five percent to 40% of patients with HS have a positive family history of HS.
- Infection: Bacterial infections are considered secondary causes. The general consensus is that bacteria do not cause HS but may contribute to the pathogenesis of chronic relapsing lesions.
- Hormonal factors: Androgens play a strong role in the development of HS.
- Immune factors: Even in its most severe form, HS does not produce acute systemic inflammatory effects. There is no fever, no lymphadenopathy, no septicemia, and no local cellulitis, and cultures are often sterile.
- Diabetics have an increased risk for HS related to insulin resistance.

- Hypercholesterolemia, specifically hypertriglyceridemia and low high-density lipoproteins (HDL) are more common in HS patients. Obesity is associated with HS risk.
- Lithium can enhance neutrophil migration, increase epithelial cell proliferation, and cause follicular plugging, triggering HS.
- Sirolimus has been related to new onset of HS, and medroxyprogesterone acetate acting as an androgen has precipitated or aggravated HS.
- Smoking: Seventy percent to 89% of patients with HS are current or past smokers, and nicotine has been shown to activate nonneuronal acetylcholine receptors, causing increased keratinization of the pilosebaceous duct, suggesting that nicotine plays a role in causing HS.

HS patients have a significantly lower quality of life than patients with other chronic skin conditions because the pain associated with the disease can make everyday tasks such as walking, exercising, or wearing fitted or light-colored clothing extremely difficult (Lovegrove, 2013).

## WHEN TO REFER

HS has been associated with other diseases that may require prompt referral to a specialist (Danby & Margesson, 2010).

- Severe acne
- Cellulitis of the scalp
- Pilonidal cyst
- Rheumatoid arthritis
- Pityriasis rubra pilaris
- HIV
- Pyoderma gangrenosum

Practitioners should consider referring to a dermatologist, general surgeon, and/or gynecologic oncologist if patients do not respond to oral therapy or if lesions recur after incision and drainage (Krbec, 2007).

## PATIENT EDUCATION

Practitioners should provide reassurance and psychological support to patients, stressing that their condition is not caused by poor hygiene and is not contagious. Patients may become depressed because of concerns related to living with HS, such as pain, odor, or soiled clothing from discharge (Krbec, 2007).

Education for the patient and family should include the pathology of HS and explanation that the actual cause is unknown. Patients should be instructed that shaving, antiperspirants, and deodorant have not been shown to cause the disease (Krbec, 2007).

General care includes the following:

- Gentle washing with a mild nonsoap cleansing bar is recommended. If an odor is present, the use of an antiseptic cleanser with triclosan is advised. Wash with hands only; washcloths can induce friction and irritation.
- Reduce trauma by decreasing heat, humidity, sweating, and friction. Avoid tight clothing.
- Stop smoking and avoid all nicotine and nicotine-replacement products.
- Nonsteroidal anti-inflammatories, as well as warm compresses, baths, and hydrotherapy, can help with pain and inflammation. (Danby & Margesson, 2010)

## CLINICAL PEARLS

- Hidradenitis suppurativa: ICD-9, 705.83; ICD-10, L73.2
- Patients can seek support through organizations such as HS-USA (http://www.hs-usa.org/home.htm).
- Early HS can present with small tender pustules in the groin and axillae (Habif et al., 2011).
- This disease can lead to depression in patients dealing with drainage, odor, and the specific lesion sites (genitals/anal); aggressive treatment should be provided to maximize disease management (Wolff et al., 2013).
- HS can occur in prepubertal children, including children who are not obese (Habif et al., 2011).
- If a woman complains of boils in groin, suspect hidradenitis (Habif et al., 2011).
- The best treatment for severe refractory HS is complete surgical excision of the affected area (Fitzpatrick & Morelli, 2011).

## KERATOSIS PILARIS

### OVERVIEW

Keratosis pilaris (KP) is a common, autosomal dominant (Morelli, 2011) skin condition manifested by the appearance of rough, white or red bumps on the skin. It generally appears on the back and outer sides of the arm (although the forearm can be affected) and can also occur on the thighs, hands, and tops of legs, sides, buttocks, or any body part except the palms or soles of feet (Figure III.14). This disease is common and seems to occur more often and extensively in patients with atopic dermatitis (Habif, 2004). KP has also been associated with xerosis, abnormal dryness of the skin or mucus membranes (Morelli, 2011).

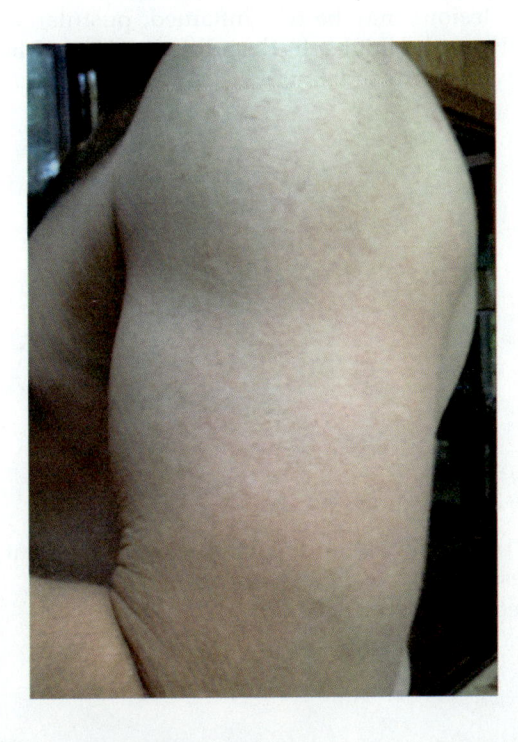

FIGURE III.14  Keratosis pilaris on the arm

## EPIDEMIOLOGY

KP appears at any age but is more common in children. The incidence peaks at adolescence, with an estimated 50% to 60% affected, and seems to improve with age (Habif, 2004). In the United States, KP affects approximately 42% of the population, and a significant variation in severity is observed between individuals. There is no evidence of racial predilection; however, the inflammatory form of KP is more prevalent in females (Crowe, 2012).

Risk factors for KP are:

- Familial indications consistent with autosomal dominant transmission
- Ichthyosis vulgaris
- Hormonal influence (a high prevalence and intensity of KP is noted during puberty and in women with hyperandrogenism) (Crowe, 2012)

## PATHOLOGY/HISTOLOGY

The etiology is unknown, although theories suggest that KP may be caused by a disorder of corneocyte adhesion that prevents normal break down in the area around the follicle. The follicular orifice becomes plugged with keratin and results in a keratotic papule because of a lack of proper desquamation of keratinocytes (Crowe, 2012).

## CLINICAL PRESENTATION

KP presents most often on the triceps and anterior thighs, but, as noted earlier, can occur on any part of the body other than the palms and soles. KP on the face may be confused with acne, but the uniform small size and association with dry skin and chapping differentiate KP from acne. Lesions on the triceps appear as a horny plug in each hair follicle. KP may be generalized, resembling a heat rash or miliaria. Usually KP is asymptomatic, but the lesions may be red, inflamed, pustular, and resemble bacterial folliculitis, especially on the thighs. In the adult form, a red halo may surround the keratotic papule that persists indefinitely (Crowe, 2012; Habif, 2004; James et al., 2006).

## DIFFERENTIAL DIAGNOSIS

- Acne
- Bacterial folliculitis
- Heat rash
- Milia

## TREATMENT/MANAGEMENT

Treatments of KP include the following:

- Topical retinoids (Retin-A or Tazorac cream) may induce improvement but usually causes irritation and redness.
- Topical calcipotriene is effective in some patients.

- Short courses of Group II to V topical steroids help reduce redness.
- Application of 12% ammonium lactate or lotion (e.g., Lac-Hydrin, AmLactin) or Vanamide cream (urea) is the most practical and effective way to reduce roughness and is routinely used. (Habif, 2004; James et al., 2006)

## SPECIAL CONSIDERATIONS

Children and adolescence may be concerned with appearance of KP, especially if it is on the face. Girls may be embarrassed if KP occurs on triceps, especially if wearing sleeveless garments.

## WHEN TO REFER

Dermatology referral may be needed if patient does not respond to recommended therapy.

## PATIENT EDUCATION

Education and reassurance are the foundations of therapy for KP. In young children, gentle skin care is all that is recommended. The noninflamed horny papules resolve with age and are typically resistant to therapy (Crowe, 2012).

### CLINICAL PEARLS

- Keratosis pilaris: ICD-9, 757.39; ICD-10, L85.8
- KP occurs on the face of children and adolescents and is often misdiagnosed for acne.
- Patients seek treatment for KP (which is asymptomatic) because of the cosmetic issues.
- Daily emollient application can lessen the appearance of KP (Habif et al., 2011).

# MILIA CYST

## OVERVIEW

*Milia* are tiny white cysts commonly found on the skin of people of all ages. They form when keratin (a substance produced by the skin) becomes entrapped beneath the outer layer of the skin, forming a cyst.

## EPIDEMIOLOGY

Milia cysts are most common in newborns and in middle-aged women but can occur at any age and in any race (Cooper, 2012; James et al., 2006).

## PATHOLOGY/HISTOLOGY

Milia are tiny epidermoid cysts that originated from the pilosebaceous follicle. Primary milia arise on facial skin bearing vellus hair follicles, and secondary milia result from damage to the pilosebaceous unit. The histologic features are identical to those of epidermoid cysts, but milia cysts are much smaller. The milia are usually located in the superficial dermis, have a complete epithelial lining, and contain lamellated keratin (Cooper, 2012).

## CLINICAL PRESENTATION

Milia are tiny, white, pea-shaped cysts that commonly occur on the face. There are two types of milia (Habif, 2004; James et al., 2006): (1) Primary milia arise spontaneously, most often on the eyelids and cheeks, and arise from the lowest portion of the infundibulum of the vellus hairs; (2) secondary milia may represent retention cysts following injury to the skin. Milia may occur spontaneously or after habitual rubbing of the eyelids. They are seen in blistering dermatosis, such as epidermolysis bullosa, porphyria cutanea tarda, and bullous pemphigoid; after dermabrasion or topical treatment with fluorouracil; in the area of chronic cortisone-induced atrophy; and after burns or radiation therapy. Secondary milia are morphologically and histologically identical to primary milia.

## DIFFERENTIAL DIAGNOSIS

- Acne vulgaris
- Comedonal acne
- Syringoma
- Trichoepithelioma

## TREATMENT/MANAGEMENT

Milia have no opening on the surface and cannot be expressed like blackheads. A number 11 pointed surgical blade tip is inserted with a sharp edge up and advanced laterally approximately 1 mm. Apply pressure with the Schamberg extractor to remove the soft, white material. Other treatments include electrocautery for adults (Goodheart, 2011), laser ablation, and electrodesiccation (Habif, 2004; James et al., 2006).

## SPECIAL CONSIDERATIONS

A skin biopsy is necessary only if the diagnosis is in question for milia cyst. If milia en plaque is suspected, a skin biopsy is vital to exclude follicular mucinosis and multiple trichoepitheliomata. In an elderly person with sun-damaged skin, Favre-Racouchot syndrome (nodular elastosis of the skin) should be excluded (Cooper, 2012).

## WHEN TO REFER

Referral to a dermatologist is warranted if biopsy reveals diagnosis other than milia.

## PATIENT EDUCATION

- Do not squeeze or scrub milia cysts.
- Noncomedogenic makeup and moisturizers may help decrease the development of milia cysts.

## CLINICAL PEARLS

- Milia cyst: ICD-9, 706.2; ICD-10, L72.83
- Milia can occur at any age, including infancy (Wolff et al., 2013).
- The treatment of milia is incision and expression of contents (Wolff et al., 2013).
- Electrocautery is also a treatment modality for adults (Goodheart, 2011.

## REFERENCES

Cooper, S. (2012). *Milia*. Retrieved from http://emedicine.medscape.com/article/1058063-overview

Crowe, M. A. (2012). *Pediatric keratosis pilaris*. Retrieved from http://emedicine.medscape.com/article/910223-overview

Danby, F. W., & Margesson, L. J. (2010). Hidradenitis suppurativa. *Dermatology Clinic, 28*, 779–793.

Fitzpatrick, J. E., & Morelli, J. G. (2011). *Dermatology secrets plus* (4th ed.). Philadelphia, PA: Elsevier/Saunders.

Fromm, L. (2012). *Epidermal inclusion cyst*. Retrieved from http://emedicine.medscape.com/article/1061582

Goldstein, B. G., & Goldstein, A. O. (2012). *Overview of benign lesions of the skin*. Retrieved from http://uptodate.com/contents/overveiw-of-benign-lesions-of-the-skin

Goodheart, H. (2011). *Goodheart's same-site differential diagnosis: A rapid method of diagnosing and treating common skin disorders*. Philadelphia, PA: Lippincott Williams & Wilkins.

Habif, T. P. (2004). *Clinical dermatology: A color guide to diagnosis and therapy* (4th ed.). Philadelphia, PA: Mosby.

Habif, T., Campbell, J., Chapman, M., Dinulos, J., & Zug, K. (2011). *Skin disease diagnosis and treatment* (3rd ed.). Philadelphia, PA: Elsevier/Saunders.

James, W. D., Berger, T. G., & Elston, D. M. (2006). *Andrews' diseases of the skin: Clinical dermatology* (10th ed.). Philadelphia, PA: Elsevier/Saunders.

Krbec, A. C. (2007). Current understanding and management of hidradenitis suppurativa. *American Academy of Nurse Practitioners, 19*, 228–234.

Lovegrove, F. (2013). Sexual well-being in patients with hidradenitis suppurativa. *Journal of the Dermatology Nurses' Association, 5*(1), 51–52.

Morelli, J. (2011). Pediatric dermatology. In J. Fitzpatrick & J. Morelli (Eds.), *Dermatology secrets plus* (pp. 154, 404). Philadelphia, PA: Elsevier/Saunders.

Revuz, J. (2010). Hidradenitis suppurativa. *La Presse Médicale, 39*(12), 1254–1264. doi: 10.1016/j.lpm.2010.08.003

Smith, H. S., Chao, J. D., & Teitelbaum, J. (2010). Painful hidradenitis suppurativa. *Clinical Journal of Pain, 26*(5), 435–444.

Wolff, K., Johnson, R., & Saavedra, A. (2013). *Fitzpatrick's color atlas and synopsis of clinical dermatology* (7th ed.). Philadelphia, PA: McGraw-Hill Medical.

# Dermatitis

*Dermatitis* comprises a group of diseases that involve inflammation, erythema, and papulovesicular lesions of the skin with acute disease and scaling of the skin with chronic disease. The most common dermatitis presentations are allergic/contact dermatitis, atopic dermatitis, and seborrheic dermatitis (SD).

## ALLERGIC/CONTACT DERMATITIS

### OVERVIEW

*Contact dermatitis* (CD) refers to a dermatoses that is caused by an external agent. The major types are *irritant contact dermatitis* (ICD) and *allergic contact dermatitis* (ACD), which make up more than 95% of the total cases of CD (Herro & Jacob, 2011; Figure III.15).

ICD is the more common of the two types. It occurs when the skin comes in contact with a substance that is harsh to the skin. The severity of inflammation is dependent on the concentration of the irritant and the exposure time (Hill, 2003). The most frequent causes of ICD include contaminated water, soaps and detergents, fiberglass and particulate dusts, food products, cleaning agents, solvents, plastics, resins, petrolatum products, lubricants, metals, and machine oils and coolants (Beltrani, 2003; Nijhawen, Matiz, & Jacob, 2009). The top 10 specific offending allergens are poison ivy/oak and sumac, rubber compounds, nickel, cobalt, thimerosal, gold, fragrance mix, neomycin, balsam of Peru, colophony, formaldehyde, and lanolin (Herro & Jacob, 2011; James, Berger, & Elston, 2006).

ACD is characterized by a complex immunologic event. ACD is an acquired sensitivity to numerous substances that produce inflammatory reactions in persons who have been previously sensitized to the allergen (James et al., 2006). Clinically, ACD presents as a delayed type IV hypersensitivity reaction with a 2- to 3-day dormancy period between contact with the substance and a reaction on the skin. It may take several weeks to resolve (Militello, Jacob, & Crawford, 2006).

130 ■ III. Common Dermatologic Conditions

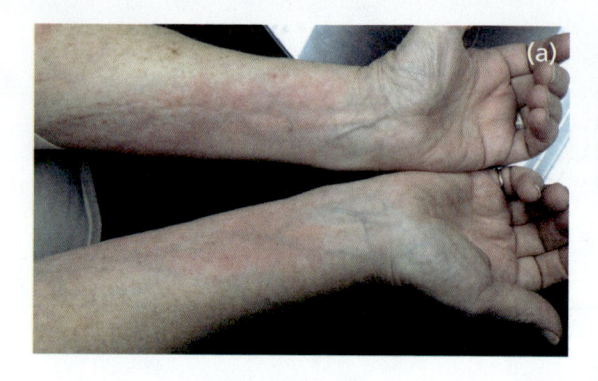

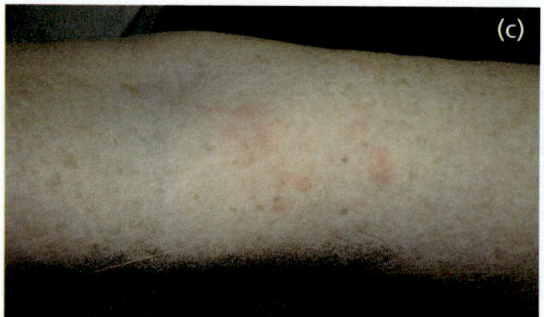

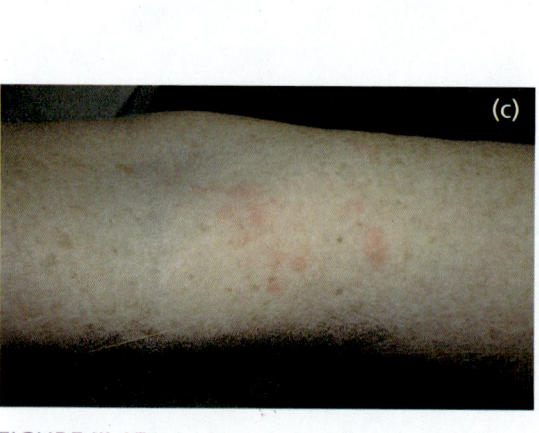

FIGURE III.15 (a-c) Examples of contact dermatitis

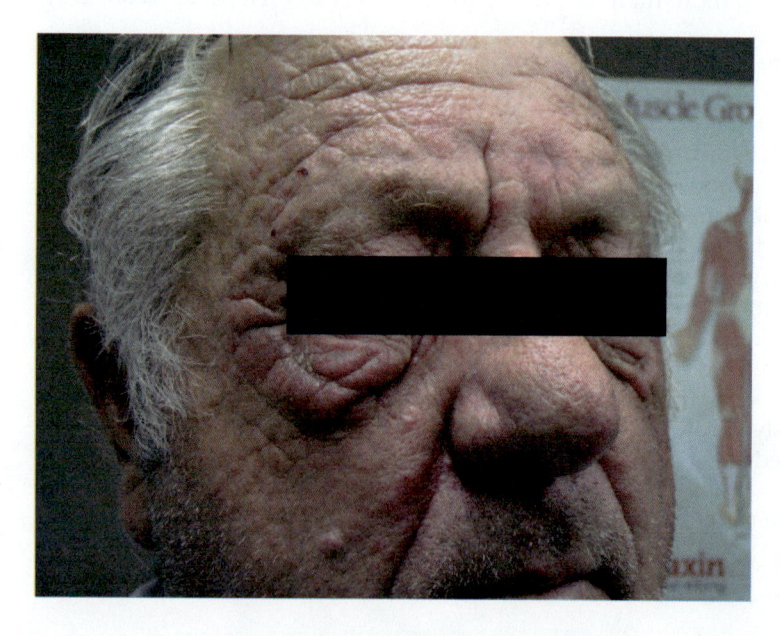

FIGURE III.16 Facial contact dermatitis

## EPIDEMIOLOGY

CD has been found to be highly related to occupation, attributable to approximately 30% of all occupational conditions (Diepgen & Weisshaar, 2007). Because of exposure incidence, the hand is the most commonly affected site of dermatitis, with an estimated prevalence of 2% to 10% of hand dermatitis in the general population (Yang & Zirwas, 2009). Those at risk for dermatitis include hairdressers, dental technicians, health care workers, construction workers, and food service workers (Koch, 2001; Van Coevorden, Diepgen, & Coenraads, 2008). ACD has become a more recognized pediatric disease in the United States, responsible for an estimated 20% of all cases of dermatitis in children (Herro & Jacob, 2011).

## PATHOLOGY/HISTOLOGY

ICD is a nonallergic response that occurs when contact with an irritant results in direct skin damage by disrupting the outer layer of the epidermis, the cells, and aids in the production of inflammatory cytokines, such as tumor necrosis factor and interleukin (IL) from the keratinocyte. The inflammatory process continues until the irritant is removed and the skin heals (Yang & Zirwas, 2009).

ACD results when an allergen comes in contact with skin that has been previously sensitized to the allergen. The resultant reaction is a specific acquired hypersensitivity of the delayed type, also known as *cell-mediated hypersensitivity* or *immunity*. Sometimes dermatitis will occur when an allergen—for example, cinnamon or various medications—is taken internally by a patient first sensitized by a topical application. This response is known as *systemic contact dermatitis* (SCD) (James et al., 2006). SCD occurs in two main stages (Herro & Jacob, 2011).

1. The sensitization stage involves the exposure of allergens into the epidermis, where they bond to keratinocytes and are recognized by the antigen-presenting cells. These cells then process these antigens and present them to naive T cells, resulting in memory T-cell clonal expansion.
2. The elicitation stage occurs after repeated exposure to an environmental allergen. When the body recognizes the allergen, there is a cloning of memory T cells and release of inflammatory cytokines. This results in the appearance of the dermatitis at the site of exposure to the allergen and potentially at previous sites of reactivity.

## CLINICAL PRESENTATION

ICD and ACD appear the same: pruritic, eczematous plaques that may blister, erode, scale, crust, or shed. However, distinguishing between the two can be done by clinical time course. ICD can be either acute or chronic but usually resolves in 3 to 4 days, whereas ACD may just be peaking in intensity at this time. ICD is typically confined to areas of contact exposure and appears as well-demarcated erythematous and sometimes follicular reaction and may have an associated burning sensation. ACD often develops beyond the area of contact, has induration and/or papulovesicular eruptions, and is very pruritic (Herro & Jacob, 2011; Yang & Zirwas, 2009).

## DIFFERENTIAL DIAGNOSIS

- Atopic dermatitis/eczema
- Atopic hand dermatitis

- Herpes zoster
- Psoriasis
- Tinea manuum

## TREATMENT/MANAGEMENT

A complete history should be obtained to include:

- Occupation (exposures to chemicals, work habits)
- Exposures at home
- Activities or hobbies (e.g., gardening)
- Cleansing habits
- Does the individual wear protective gloves, have latex allergies?
- Over-the-counter products
- Pets
- Recent vacation, hiking, or exposure to plants

In 2008, the result of the first reported patch-testing studies in the U.S.-based populations were made available, confirming that CD was equally prevalent in all ages and that patch testing was safe and efficacious (Herro & Jacob, 2011). Bourke, Coulson, and English (2009) stated that the mainstay of diagnosis in allergic CD is the patch test. The test has a sensitivity of 70% and a specificity of 80%. Standardized prepared tests are more reliable than operator-prepared tests. The optimal timing for reading the test is on Days 2 and 4. The test should be confrimed on Days 2 and 4 for optical results; however, an additional 10% positive results can be observed on Days 6 and 7. The most common allergens that may become positive after Day 4 are neomycin, tixocortol pivalate, and nickel.

Nichols and Cook-Bolden (2009) recommended the Thin Rapid Use Epicutaneous Test (TRUE) test with readings to occur on Days 3 and 5 and again on Day 7 if allergies to metals, topical antibiotics, and purified protein derivative (PPD) are suspected. Herro and Jacob (2011) also recommended the TRUE test but note that it is currently only approved by the Food and Drug Administration for use in patients aged 18 and older.

For a skin disorder to qualify as an occupational skin disease, Beltrani (2003) defined the following criteria: (1) the skin disorder should have developed for the first time when the patient was on a job, (2) the skin disorder should improve when the patient is away from the work environment, and (3) there should be a reasonable etiology in the workplace that can be linked to the presence of the disease. Bourke et al. (2009) recommended asking patients to bring in samples of lubricants, oils, fabrics, or material that they are exposed to in the workplace to help identify potential allergens and irritants.

Treatments for ACD include the following:

1. Bourke et al. (2009) found that barrier creams alone are questionable against ACD. After-work creams and the use of soap substitutes benefit the incidence of ACD. Evidence supports the use of soap substitutes and emollients in the treatment of ACD.
2. Nichols and Cook-Bolden (2009) recommended the use of gloves on the job.
3. Yang and Zirwas (2009) recommended the use of mild soap and moisturizers as a first-line therapy for ACD.
4. Herro and Jacob (2011) recommended the use of emollients or barrier creams for first-line management and prophylaxis of ACD.

5. Bourke et al. (2009), Weston and Howe (2011c), and Yang and Zirwas (2009) recommended treatment with medium to high-potency topical steroids for patients with mild to moderate ACD. For patients with more that 10% of the body surface area involved, a course of systemic oral steroids may be warranted.
6. Bourke et al. (2009) and Yang and Zirwas (2009) stated that topical tacrolimus has been shown to be effective in a nickel model of ACD.
7. Bourke et al. (2009) supported the use of psoralen plus ultraviolet A, azathioprine, and cyclosporine for steroid-resistant CD. Oral retinoids have also been used for chronic hand eczema.

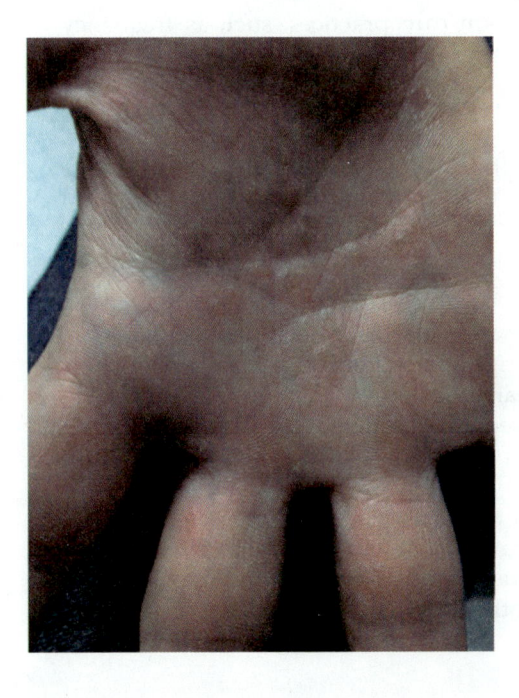

FIGURE III.17  Eczema of the hand

## SPECIAL CONSIDERATIONS

1. Diabetic and immunocompromised patients have increased risk of infection at the sites of ICD and ACD.
2. Patients may need to consider a change of occupation if the allergic reaction is a result of work exposure (Figure III.17). Recommend that they consult with their human resources or occupational health care clinician for potential options.
3. Dermatitis can be devastating for affected children and adults. Children can experience stress, anxiety, and low self-esteem from bullying by other children or may not take part in sports or other activities. Parents of children who are affected with dermatitis experience increased financial stress because of frequent doctor visits, lost wages caused by missing work for an ill child, and the cost of medications (Fleischer, 2008).

## WHEN TO REFER

If the history and clinical findings are suggestive of ACD, or if the patient has been diagnosed with ICD but does not respond to treatment, then referral to dermatology or an allergist may be warranted for patch testing and allergy prevention.

## PATIENT EDUCATION

- Provide basic knowledge about skin structure and function.
- Discuss risk factors.
- Describe the different forms of contact dermatitis.
- Remove causative agent.
- Instruct patient to wear gloves, mask, and goggles if necessary.
- Teach patient the proper way to apply topical medications (see Part II, Chapter 6, Topical Treatment).
- Teach patient about skin care. Discuss skin care practices, such as frequency of hand washing, soap choices, and correct application of skin care products (e.g., moisturizers).

## ATOPIC DERMATITIS/ECZEMA

### OVERVIEW

*Atopic dermatitis* (AD), also known as eczema, is a skin disease of unknown origin that usually starts in early infancy; it is characterized by pruritus, eczematous lesions, xerosis, and lichenification (Figure III.18). Research has shown that the factors influencing AD is a complex combination of genetic predisposition, immune responses, epithelial barrier dysfunction, infectious agents, and environmental factors (Nichols & Cook-Bolden, 2009).

AD is the first disease to present in a series of allergic diseases such as food allergy, asthma, and allergic rhinitis that provokes the "atopic march" theory; this suggests that early or severe AD and cutaneous sensitization to environmental allergens may lead to successive allergic diseases at other epithelial barrier surfaces (e.g., gastrointestinal or respiratory tract; Kim, 2013).

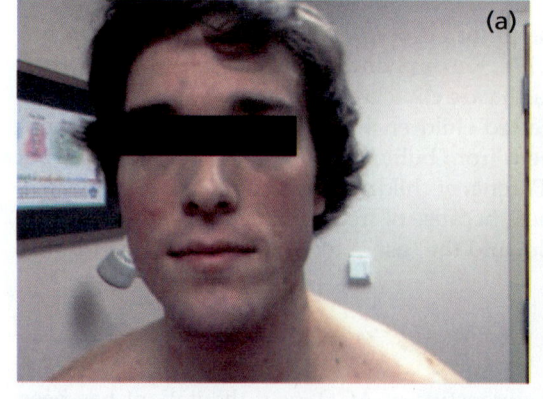

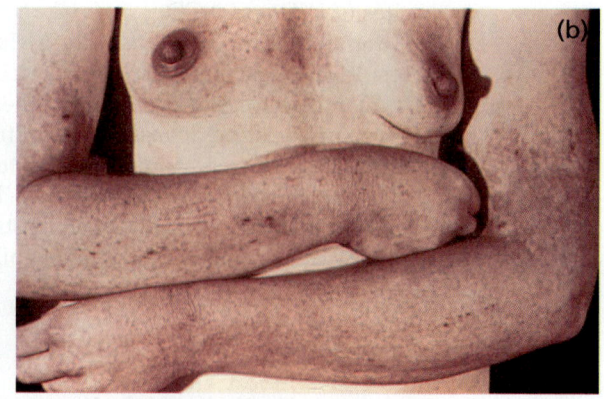

FIGURE III.18 Examples of AD on the **(a)** face and **(b)** arms/trunk
(b) Courtesy of Centers for Disease Control and Prevention

## EPIDEMIOLOGY

The prevalence rate for AD in the United States is 10% to 12% in children and 0.9% in adults; there has been an increase in physician office visits over the past 15 years (Kim, 2013). The onset of AD occurs in 45% of children by the age of 6 months, in 60% of children by age 1 year, and in 85% of children by age 5 years. Females show a slightly higher occurrence of AD than males (4:1). Black and Asian patients visit providers more often than White patients for the treatment of AD. The annual cost to the health care system as a result of AD alone is significant, estimated at between $0.9 and $3.8 billion (Fleischer, 2008; Kim, 2013).

## PATHOLOGY/HISTOLOGY

Two main theories have been proposed regarding the development of inflammation that leads to AD (Fleischer, 2008; Kim, 2013).

1. The first theory suggests a primary immune dysfunction resulting in immunoglobulin E (IgE), that is, sensitization and a secondary epithelial barrier disturbance. In healthy people, there is a balance between important subsets of the T cells. This theory suggests that there is an imbalance in the T-cell subsets in those with AD, which invokes cytokines such as IL-4, IL-5, and IL-13, causing an increase in immunoglobulin E from plasma cells and diminished interferon-gamma levels.
2. The second theory proposes a primary defect in the epithelial barrier leading to secondary immunologic dysregulation and inflammation. This suggests that people develop AD as a result of skin-barrier defects that allow for the entry of antigens, resulting in the production of inflammatory cytokines. Xerosis and ichthyosis are known to be associated signs in many AD patients.

## CLINICAL PRESENTATION

AD is often characterized by hallmark signs and symptoms of pruritus, erythema, dry skin, lichenification, and excoriation, with possible erosions accompanied by exudate, fibrotic papules, and potential for skin infections (Hanna, Moennich, & Jacob, 2009).

Infantile AD presents as generalized xerosis and erythematous scaly plaques affecting the cheeks, forehead, scalp, and extensor extremities. The diaper area is usually spared. As the child ages, AD lesions tend to move to the flexor areas, especially the antecubital and popliteal fossae, and to the creases of the buttocks and thighs. Lichenification and excoriations will appear, secondary to chronic scratching of the affected areas. Other signs of AD include pityriasis alba of the face and Dennie-Morgan lines (Nichols & Cook-Bolden, 2009).

## DIFFERENTIAL DIAGNOSIS

- Contact dermatitis, allergic
- Contact dermatitis, irritant
- Dermatitis herpetiformis
- Dermatophyte infections
- Immunodeficiency
- Impetigo

- Lichen simplex chronicus (LSC)/neurodermatitis (ND)
- Mollusca contagiosa with dermatitis
- Mycosis fungoides
- Nummular dermatitis
- Psoriasis, plaque
- Relative zinc deficiency
- Scabies
- Seborrheic dermatitis
- Tinea corporis

## TREATMENT/MANAGEMENT

There are multiple suspected causes of AD (Kim, 2013), including the following:

- Genetics: A family history of AD is common.
- Infection: The skin of patients with AD is colonized by *Staphylococcus aureus*, which often causes a flare of AD, and *S. aureus* has been suggested as a cause of AD by acting as a superantigen.
- Hygiene: This factor is theorized as a cause for the increase in AD. This theory attributes the rise in AD to reduced exposure to various childhood infections and bacterial endotoxins.
- Climate: AD flares occur in extremes of climate. Extreme heat or cold is poorly tolerated. A dry climate increases xerosis. Sun exposure enhances lesions, whereas sweating intensifies pruritus.
- Food antigens: The role of food antigens in the pathogenesis of AD is debatable regarding both whether diet can prevent AD and whether the withdrawal of foods in persons with established AD can be beneficial. Because the role of food in AD is controversial, most physicians do not recommend dietary changes. However, acute food reactions (urticaria and anaphylaxis) are commonly encountered in children with AD.
- Aeroallergens: A role for aeroallergens and house dust mites has been suggested.
- Tobacco: Exposure to tobacco smoke in childhood is linked to adult-onset AD.

Laboratory testing is usually not needed. However, a swab of infected skin will help define a specific organism or antibiotic sensitivity. A platelet count for thrombocytopenia helps exclude Wiskott-Aldrich syndrome, and testing to rule out other immunodeficiencies may be helpful with potassium hydroxide preparation. Scraping to exclude tinea corporis is occasionally worthwhile (Kim, 2013).

Possible treatment measures include the following:

- Topical emollients
  - Nichols and Cook-Bolden (2009) found that a petroleum-based moisturizer should be applied to the entire body within 3 minutes of bathing each day and applied twice daily if possible.
  - Weston and Howe (2011c) suggested that a topical emollient be used daily after a bath. Patients should use the highest oil content emollient.
- Topical steroids
  - Nichols and Cook-Bolden (2009) recommended that topical steroids be used for AD flares. The topical steroid agent should be used twice daily for 2 weeks only, waiting 2 weeks before initiating treatment again, if necessary.
  - Thomas, Beth-Hextall, Ravenscroft, Charmam, and Williams (2008) stated that there is clear evidence to support the use twice weekly of a potent topical steroid to stabilize AD or eczema to reduce the number of flare ups in adults and children.

- Westin and Howe (2011c) state that topical steroids are the mainstay for AD. A low-potency corticosteroid cream or ointment is effective for patients with mild AD. A medium-potency steroid ointment may be needed if the disease is more severe. Higher potency topical steroids can be used for up to 10 days in some patients with acute flares and then be replaced with a lower potency steroid. For mild hand eczema and dyshidrotic eczema, a moderate to potent topical corticosteroid can control outbreaks.
- Oral steroids
  - Westin and Howe (2011c) concluded that an acute exacerbation of chronic AD, eczema, or dyshidrotic eczema can sometimes benefit from a short course of oral prednisone, but this should be avoided long term.
  - Hanna, Moennich, and Jacob (2009) stated that although systemic steroid therapy is effective, the rapid rate of disease recurrence after stopping the oral steroids and the high risk for potential side effects makes the use of oral steroids impractical.
- Antihistamines
  - Thomas et al. (2008) concluded that there was no evidence that oral antihistamines controlled or prevented AD or eczema flare ups; however, antihistamines can reduce symptoms of pruritus associated with AD and eczema.
  - Hanna et al. (2009) and Westin and Howe (2011c) recommended antihistamines as a therapeutic adjunct in patients with AD to treat both pruritus and eye irritation. The sedating antihistamines appear to be the most effective (diphenhydramine, hydroxyzine, and cyproheptadine). Nonsedating preparations such as fexofenadine or loratadine may occasionally also be useful, especially when there is an urticarial component. Doxepin has potent H1 and H2 blocking properties and is useful when other antihistamines fail.
- Topical tacrolimus (Protopic) or topical pimecrolimus (Elidel)
  - Nichols and Cook-Bolden (2009), Thomas et al. (2008), and Weston and Howe (2011c) suggested that tacrolimus 0.1% is equivalent to a potent cortisone for the treatment of AD. Tacrolimus and pimecrolimus are useful in sensitive areas such as face, skin folds, and perineum.
- Control of dust mites
  - Thomas et al. (2008) and Westin and Howe (2011c) stated that a sleeping environment with minimal dust and upholstery reduces exposure to house dust mites and may potentially reduce the severity of AD and eczema.
- Diet
  - Westin and Howe (2011c) stated that food triggers for AD are eggs, nuts, peanut butter, chocolate, milk, seafood, and soy.
- Probiotics
  - Nichols and Cook-Bolden (2009) reported a significant risk reduction associated with the use of prenatal and postnatal probiotics for primary prevention in pediatric AD and eczema. However, probiotics may help to prevent AD flares, but they were not effective in the treatment of AD.
- Oral antibiotics, antivirals, and antifungals
  - Westin and Howe (2011c) found that topical mupirocin was affective for localized infection of AD, but oral antibiotics were needed for extensive infections. Thomas et al. (2008) concurred that the use of oral antibiotics in the absence of infection would be beneficial.
  - Oral antiviral and antifungal therapies should only be considered if there is a coexisting viral or fungal infection present.
- Herbal therapies
  - Thomas et al. (2008) evaluated multiple trials conducted on the use of Chinese herbs for the treatment of AD. There was little evidence to support their use.

## SPECIAL CONSIDERATIONS

When compared with other childhood dermatologic diseases, AD affects quality of life the most. The possible effects on a child's life include the following (Thomas et al., 2008):

- Sleep disturbance caused by pruritus
- Social stigmatization from peers and their parents
- The need for special clothing and bedding
- Avoidance of activities that cause excessive sweating (sports); avoidance of swimming
- Frequent applications of topical emollients and visits to health care providers
- Loss of school because of AD flares
- For adults, unremitting itching and work loss can cause financial loss (Kim, 2013).

## WHEN TO REFER

Consulting an allergist may be necessary, especially if the patient develops asthma and/or hay fever or an acute reaction to a food. Referral to a dermatologist is warranted for AD if resistant to treatment.

## PATIENT EDUCATION

Advise patients on the following precautions:

- Avoid foods that provoke allergic reactions (hives, anaphylaxis). Common allergic reactions occur with peanuts, eggs, seafood, milk, soy, and chocolate. Applying a barrier of petroleum jelly around the mouth before eating will prevent irritation from tomatoes, oranges, and other acidic foods.
- Avoid activities that cause excessive sweating.
- Avoid soaps, lotions, and topical creams that contain fragrances. Not only could this cause burning to inflamed skin, it could also stimulate an allergic response if patient is sensitive to fragrance.
- Use mild soaps for bathing (Cetaphil or unscented Dove). Cleanse skin gently and do not attempt to exfoliate dry areas. Do not use astringents.
- Dry skin folds well after bathing or swimming to prevent trapped moisture, which can cause increased irritation.

# LICHEN SIMPLEX CHRONICUS/NEURODERMATITIS

## OVERVIEW

Lichen simplex chronicus (LSC) or neurodermatitis (ND) is thickening of the skin that arises secondary to vigorous scratching, rubbing, or picking beyond the normal tolerable pain threshold (Figure III.19). Those with LSC/ND feel pruritus in a specific area of skin (with or without underlying pathology) and cause trauma by scratching to the point of lichenification (Hogan, 2012; James et al., 2006).

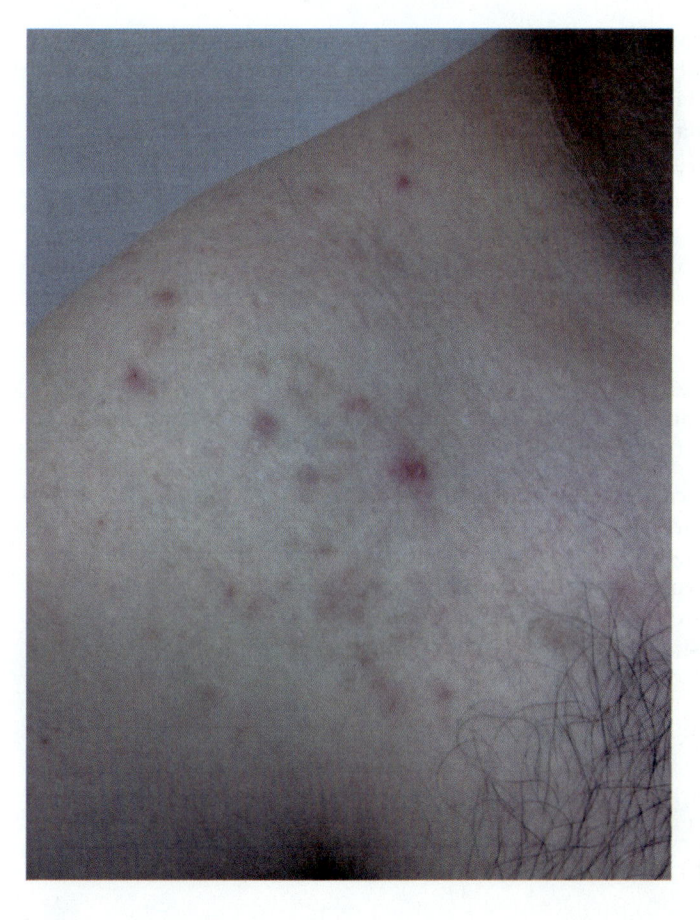

FIGURE III.19  An example of LSC/ND

## EPIDEMIOLOGY

There are no differences reported in the frequency of LSC/ND among races. The appearance of lesions on darker skin may show follicular protrusion and cause secondary pigmentary alterations. LSC/ND is observed more commonly in females than in males in mid to late adulthood. Lichen nuchae is a type of lichen simplex that appears on the mid-posterior neck and is observed almost exclusively in women (Hogan, 2012).

## PATHOLOGY/HISTOLOGY

LSC/ND is found on the skin in areas accessible to scratching. For unknown reasons, those affected feel pruritus, which provokes scratching. There is an association between central and peripheral neural tissue and inflammatory cell products in the sensitivity of pruritus and resultant changes in LSC. Emotional status in affected patients may play a key role in inducing a pruritic sensation, which causes the scratching response. The suspected relationship among LSC/ND, psychic factors, and the severity of pruritus collectively influences the extent and severity of this disorder (Hogan, 2012).

Histologic examination reveals hyperkeratosis, acanthosis, spongiosis, and patches of parakeratosis in the epidermis. Epidermal thickening of all layers is present, with elongation of rete ridges and with pseudoepitheliomatous hyperplasia. Papillary dermal fibrosis with vertical streaking of collagen bundles is characteristic and another finding of LSC that is noted on electron microscopy is frequent collagen fibers attached to and just above the lamina basalis (Hogan, 2012).

## CLINICAL PRESENTATION

Patients with LSC/ND usually describe chronic pruritus in many areas, however, erythema and thickening of the skin is present anywhere on the body that the patient can reach, such as the scalp, nape of neck, extensor forearms and elbows, vulva, scrotum, upper medial thighs, knees, lower legs, and ankles. Areas of atopic dermatitis, irritant or ACD, insect bites, or other past minor skin trauma stimulate pruritus, which intern may cause LSC/ND. Presentation of LSC/ND is likely to have the following characteristics (Hogan, 2012; James et al., 2006):

- Multiple erythematous, scaly, well-demarcated, lichenified, firm, and rough plaques with exaggerated skin lines
- Pigmentary changes (especially hyperpigmentation)
- White scratch marks, erosion, and ulceration from deep scratching
- A cutaneous horn may grow in sites of LSC/ND
- Patients who scratch lesions without conscious effort, especially when discussing their symptoms

## DIFFERENTIAL DIAGNOSIS

- Acanthosis nigricans
- Acne keloidalis nuchae
- Alopecia mucinosa
- Amyloidosis, lichen
- Amyloidosis, macular
- Atopic dermatitis
- Berloque dermatitis
- Contact dermatitis, allergic
- Contact dermatitis, irritant
- Cutaneous T-cell lymphoma
- Dermatitis herpetiformis
- Extramammary Paget disease
- Gastrointestinal disease
- Hematologic disease
- Hyperkeratosis of the nipple and areola
- Lichen nitidus
- Lichen planus
- Lichen striatus
- Neurologic disease
- Nummular dermatitis
- Phytophotodermatitis
- Pretibial myxedema
- Psoriasis, plaque
- Renal disease
- Riehl melanosis
- SD

- Stasis dermatitis
- Tinea cruris

## TREATMENT/MANAGEMENT

The suspected/known causes of LSC/ND are:

- Atopic dermatitis causes increased risk of developing LSC/ND.
- Insect bites, scars (e.g., traumatic, postherpetic/zoster), acne keloidalis nuchae, xerosis, venous insufficiency, and asteatotic eczema cause increased risk of developing LSC/ND.
- Psychological factors, such as anxiety, have been reported to be more prevalent in patients with LSC/ND.
- Lithium has been linked to LSC in one reported case. LSC occurred when lithium was taken and resolved when it was discontinued. Once the lithium was restarted, the LSC returned.
- Long-term exposure to automobile exhaust has been associated with an increase in the frequency of childhood skin diseases, including LSC. (Hogan, 2012)

Perform potassium hydroxide examination and fungal cultures to exclude tinea cruris or candidiasis in patients with genital LSC. Patch testing may help exclude allergic contact dermatitis as an underlying primary dermatosis (e.g., nickel allergy or reaction to topical medication being used to treat LSC). Skin biopsies are advised, especially in elderly patients, to rule out cutaneous T-cell lymphoma (Hogan, 2012).

The goal of therapy is to decrease pruritus, which will decrease lesions. Location and number of lesions and cause of LSC/ND influence treatment options. Habif (2004), Hogan (2012), and James et al. (2006) have recommended the following treatments:

- Topical steroids soften lichenified skin, decrease inflammation, and help control pruritus. High-potency steroid ointments are used to decrease inflammation on large, acute lesions of thick-skinned areas for 3-week courses. Adding occlusion with a mid-potency steroid ointment will increase the steroid potency, promote absorption, and provide protection against scratching. Sensitive areas, such as the vulva, scrotum, axillae, and face should be treated with low-potency topical steroids or topical immunomodulators, such as tacrolimus and pimecrolimus. Nodules on the scalp may benefit from injections of Kenalog at 10 mg/mL to reduce inflammation.
- Oral antianxiety medications and sedation may be useful. Doxepin (Sinequan) and clonazepam (Klonopin) may be appropriate for patients who are anxious.
- Antihistamines such as diphenhydramine (Benadryl) and hydroxyzine (Atarax) are used for pruritus and cause sedation.
- For infected lesions, a topical or oral antibiotic is appropriate.
- Other topical medications to decrease pruritus include doxepin cream and capsaicin cream, although capsaicin may initially cause a burning sensation at the site.
- Other investigational treatments for patients who fail conventional therapy are local botulinum toxin injections and transcutaneous electrical nerve stimulation.

## WHEN TO REFER

Referral to an allergist and/or dermatologist should be considered for resistant cases requiring more aggressive treatments or to facilitate patch testing. Psychiatric care may be necessary for patients with severe anxiety or compulsive scratching (Hogan, 2012).

## PATIENT EDUCATION

Hogan (2012) and James et al. (2006) suggested educating patients about the following concerns:

- LSC/ND worsens or improves depending on the patient's ability to stop scratching. Explain this and disease pathology to patients. Discuss ways to change habitual scratching.
- Extremes of temperature and humidity, psychic stress, and exposure of cutaneous irritants and allergens to vulnerable skin can provoke symptoms.

## CLINICAL PEARLS

- In practice, adding a selective serotonin reuptake inhibitor (SSRI) in the treatment plan for LSC/ND has helped with compulsive behavior of scratching.
- Recommend that patients wear protective clothing (e.g., long sleeves, turtleneck sweaters) if climate allows.

# SEBORRHEIC DERMATITIS

## OVERVIEW

Seborrheic dermatitis (SD) is a disorder that occurs on the sebum-rich areas of the scalp, face, and trunk (Figure III.20). In addition to sebum, SD is linked to *Malassezia*, immunologic abnormalities, and activation of complement. It is commonly aggravated by changes in humidity and temperature, trauma, or emotional stress. The severity varies from mild dandruff to exfoliative erythroderma (Selden, 2013).

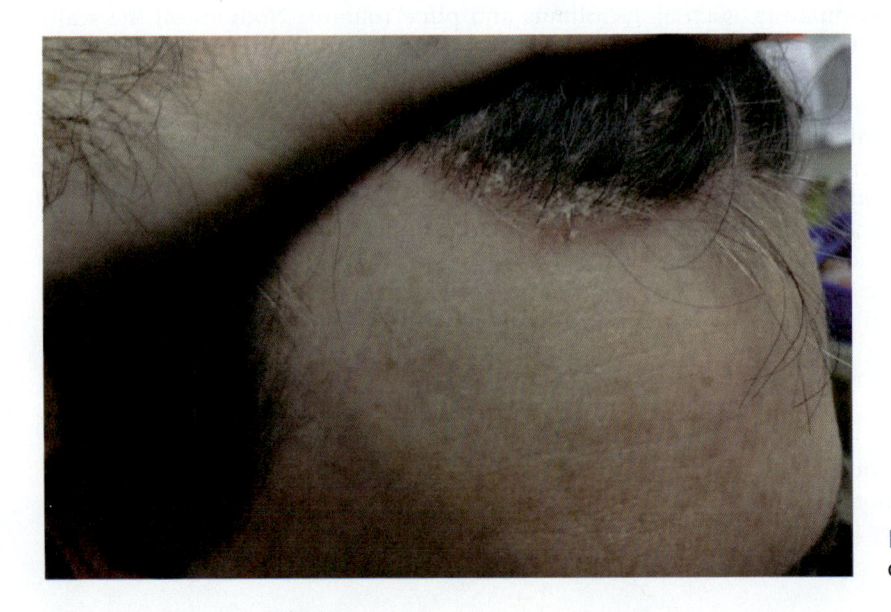

FIGURE III.20 Seborrheic dermatitis

## EPIDEMIOLOGY

The prevalence rate of SD is 3% to 5%, and it occurs worldwide. Dandruff, the mildest form of this dermatitis, is common and present in an estimated 20% of the population. SD occurs in persons of all races, and the condition commonly occurs in infants in the first 3 months of life and in adults at 30 to 60 years of age. In adolescents and adults, it usually presents as scalp scaling or as erythema of the nasolabial fold during times of stress or sleep deprivation. SD of the nasolabial fold tends to affect men more often than women and is often precipitated by stress (Fleischer, 2008; Schwartz, Janusz, & Janniger, 2006; Selden, 2013).

One to three percent of immunocompromised adults are affected with SD. The incidence of SD is high among patients with AIDS, ranging from 30% to 83% (Gupta, Bluhm, Cooper, Summerbell, & Barta, 2003). Patients with Parkinson disease (PD) have worse SD compared with patients without PD (Selden, 2013).

## PATHOLOGY/HISTOLOGY

Despite the commonality of SD, little is known about its etiology. Dermatopathologic findings of SD are inconclusive. Hyperkeratosis, acanthosis, accentuated rete ridges, focal spongiosis, and parakeratosis are characteristic. In contrast, psoriasis is distinguished by regular acanthosis, thinned rete ridges, exocytosis, parakeratosis, and an absence of spongiosis. Neutrophils are often seen in both diseases (Selden, 2013). SD and psoriasis are often mistaken for each other and misdiagnosed.

Several factors are associated with the condition (Gupta et al., 2003; Schwartz et al., 2006; Selden, 2013).

- Hormone levels: This may explain why the condition occurs in infancy, disappears spontaneously, and then reappears during puberty.
- Fungal infections: The growth of *Malassezia* species is found in normal dimorphic human flora. Yeasts of this genus dominate the flora and are found in areas of the body rich in sebaceous lipids (head, trunk, and upper back). The fungal relationship is indicated by the therapeutic response to antifungal agents.
- Nutritional deficits
- Neurogenic factors: There is an association of SD with parkinsonism and other neurogenic conditions, including injuries from cerebrovascular accidents, epilepsy, central nervous system disorders, facial nerve palsy, and syringomyelia induced by neuroleptic drugs.

Skin biopsies may distinguish SD from other similar disorders. SD generally has neutrophils in the scale surface at the margins of follicular ostia. AIDS-associated SD commonly presents as parakeratosis, a few individually necrotic keratinocytes within the epidermis, and plasma cells in the dermis. Yeast cells may be visible within keratinocytes on special stains. If hyphae are present, the diagnosis is dermatomycosis. Shorter hyphae with spores ("spaghetti and meatball" pattern) are present with tinea versicolor (Schwartz et al., 2006).

## CLINICAL PRESENTATION

Adolescent and adult SD usually begins as a mild greasy scale of the scalp and erythema and scaling of the nasolabial folds or the postauricular skin. The scaling is often the result of an oily complexion and occurs in areas of increased sebaceous gland activity (auricles, beard area, eyebrows, trunk flexures, and inframammary areas; Schwartz et al., 2006; Selden, 2013).

Two types of SD occur on the chest (Schwartz et al., 2006).

1. Petaloid type is the most common type and is characterized by small, reddish brown follicular papules with greasy scales that become patches resembling the shape of flower petals.
2. Pityriasiform type is less common and manifests as widespread macules and patches that resemble extensive pityriasis rosea.

In infants, SD may present as a thick, greasy scale of the vertex of the scalp. It is asymptomatic in infants, although older children and adults experience pruritus. The color of the scale varies from off-white to a yellow dermatitis. Generalized SD is uncommon in healthy children and is usually associated with immunodeficiencies (Schwartz et al., 2006).

## DIFFERENTIAL DIAGNOSIS

According to Fleischer (2008) and Selden (2013), the following should be considered in a differential diagnosis of SD:

- Candidiasis, cutaneous
- Contact dermatitis, allergic
- Contact dermatitis, irritant
- Dermatomyositis
- Drug eruptions
- Drug-induced photosensitivity
- Erythrasma
- Extramammary Paget disease
- Gastrointestinal disease
- Glucagonoma syndrome
- Impetigo
- Intertrigo
- Langerhans cell histiocytosis
- LSC
- Lupus erythematosus, acute
- Nummular dermatitis
- Omenn syndrome
- Pemphigus erythematosus
- Pemphigus foliaceus
- Perioral dermatitis
- Pityriasis rosea
- Rosacea
- Tinea capitis
- Tinea corporis
- Tinea cruris
- Tinea versicolor

## TREATMENT/MANAGEMENT

Picardo and Cameli (2008) stated that topical antifungals are well established in the treatment of SD.

- Topical corticosteroids, applied for 1 to 4 weeks, will improve SD and do not cause systemic effects, but relapses occur more frequently than when topical antifungals are used.

- Metronidazole gel is well tolerated and has no side effects.
- Pimecrolimus 1% cream has been shown to improve SD; however, side effects include rosaceiform dermatitis.

Schwartz et al. (2006) recommended conventional treatment for adult SD of the scalp.

- Topical steroids or calcineurin inhibitors therapies can be administered to the scalp by shampoo, topical solutions, lotion, or creams applied to the skin once or twice daily.
- Infants can be treated with low-potency steroids.
- Keratolytics are used to treat scaly build up.
- Antifungal agents attack *Malassezia* associated with SD. Ketoconazole gel mixed equally with desonide cream should be applied daily to facial SD for 2 weeks.
- Shampoos containing selenium sulfide or an azole often are used.
- Ketoconazole shampoo or cream or oral Diflucan and terbinafine can be useful.

Weston and Howe (2011b) concurred with the foregoing recommendations but also recommended anti-inflammatory shampoos (tar, selenium sulfide, and zinc preparations). They also recommended systemic treatments such as ketoconazole or fluconazole. Picardo and Cameli (2008) found limited evidence that oral antifungals were beneficial in the treatment of SD. Selden (2013) recommended early treatment of flares.

Additional strategies that may improve SD include:

- Limiting scratching and excoriations are important in treating scalp SD.
- Topical corticosteroids are used short-term for flares of SD.
- Skin involvement responds to ketoconazole, naftifine, or ciclopirox creams and gels.
- Alternative therapies include calcineurin inhibitors (e.g., pimecrolimus, tacrolimus), sulfur or sulfonamide combinations, or propylene glycol.
- Systemic ketoconazole or fluconazole may help if SD is severe or unresponsive.
- Dandruff responds to frequent shampooing with longer periods of lathering.
- Use of hairspray or hair products should be avoided.
- Shampoos containing salicylic acid, tar, selenium, sulfur, or zinc are effective, and patients can alternate among these daily. Selenium sulfide (2.5%), ketoconazole, and ciclopirox shampoos may help by reducing *Malassezia* yeast scalp reservoirs.
- Overnight occlusion of tar bath, bath oil, or Baker's P&S solution can help soften thick-scaled plaques. Derma-Smoothe F/S oil is helpful in widespread, thick scalp plaques.

## SPECIAL CONSIDERATIONS

Multiple medications may induce SD or cause flares. These medications include auranofin, aurothioglucose, buspirone, chlorpromazine, cimetidine, ethionamide, fluorouracil, gold, griseofulvin, haloperidol, interferon alfa, lithium, methoxsalen, methyldopa, phenothiazines, psoralens, stanozolol, thiothixene, and trioxsalen (Selden, 2013).

## WHEN TO REFER

SD that does not respond to recommended therapies should be referred to dermatology for consideration of a biopsy of the affected area to rule out other etiologies.

## PATIENT EDUCATION

- Good hygiene is recommended to reduce oiliness of the skin. Washing face twice daily and bathing and shampooing hair daily are recommended.
- Shaving beards or trimming facial hair and keeping scalp hair short can help promote the treatment of SD.

# STASIS DERMATITIS

## OVERVIEW

*Stasis dermatitis* is an inflammatory skin disease that occurs on the lower extremities and is usually the earliest sign of chronic venous insufficiency with venous hypertension (Figure III.21). Stasis dermatitis typically affects middle-aged (after age 50) and elderly patients, except for those who have acquired venous insufficiency because of surgery, trauma, or thrombosis (Flugman, 2012; Habif, 2004; Weaver & Billings, 2009).

## EPIDEMIOLOGY

Stasis dermatitis affects approximately 6% to 7% of patients aged older than 50 years, which is approximately 15 to 20 million patients in the United States. This finding makes stasis dermatitis twice as prevalent as psoriasis and only slightly less prevalent than SD (Flugman, 2012).

## PATHOLOGY/HISTOLOGY

Stasis dermatitis occurs as a direct result of venous insufficiency. Disrupted function of the one-way valvular system in the deep venous plexus of the legs results in a backflow of blood from the deep venous system to the superficial venous system,

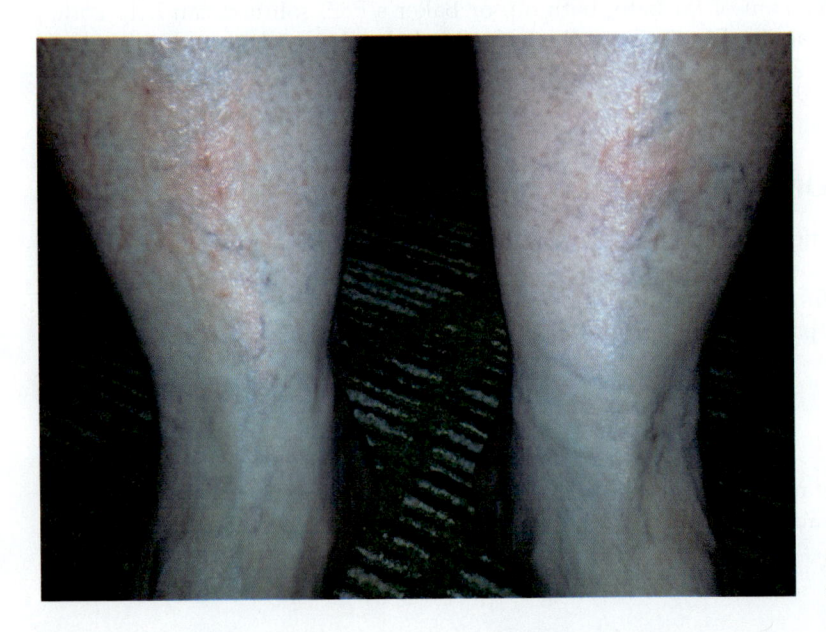

FIGURE III.21 Example of stasis dermatitis

with associated venous hypertension. This valvular dysfunction results in decreased valve competency. Certain events, such as deep venous thrombosis, surgery (e.g., vein stripping, total knee arthroplasty, harvesting of saphenous veins for coronary bypass), or traumatic injury, can severely damage the function of the lower-extremity venous system (Flugman, 2012; Habif, 2004).

Skin biopsies are rarely indicated. Acute lesions may show a superficial, perivascular lymphocytic infiltrate, epidermal spongiosis, serous exudate, scale, and crust. Chronic lesions show epidermal acanthosis with hyperkeratosis. The dermis is characterized by deep dermal aggregates of siderophages as a result of uptake of hemosiderin from degraded erythrocytes. Dermal capillaries are dilated, and long-standing lesions show intimal thickening of small arterioles and venules along with dermal fibrosis (Flugman, 2012).

## CLINICAL PRESENTATION

Histories of patients with stasis dermatitis may reveal the following (Flugman, 2012; Weaver & Billings, 2009):

- Pruritus: Insidious onset of pruritus affecting one or both lower extremities is seen.
- Discoloration: Reddish brown skin discoloration is an initial sign of stasis dermatitis and may herald the onset of symptoms.
- Ankle involvement: The medial ankle is most frequently involved, with symptoms progressing to involve the foot and/or calf.
- Edema: Previous history of dependent leg edema is seen.

Stasis dermatitis is worsened by peripheral edema, caused by congestive heart failure, long-standing hypertension with diastolic dysfunction, pregnancy, obesity, and other causes of increased abdominal pressure are often found in patients with stasis dermatitis. Some antihypertensive medications (e.g., amlodipine) may increase leg edema and cause the onset of stasis dermatitis (Flugman, 2012; Weaver & Billings, 2009).

Physical examination in stasis dermatitis patients reveals erythematous, scaling, and eczematous patches on the lower extremity. Secondary infections cause honey-colored crusting caused by bacteria or can produce monomorphous pustules as a result of cutaneous candidiasis. Severe, acute inflammation may result in exudative, weeping patches, and plaques. Underlying fat necrosis (lipodermatosclerosis) may be painful. In advanced cases, the inflammation may encircle the ankle and the dorsal part of the foot and extend to just below the knee; this is sometimes referred to as stocking erythroderma (Flugman, 2012; Habif, 2004; Weaver & Billings, 2009).

In chronic lesions, lichenification and hyperpigmentation may occur as a result of chronic scratching and rubbing. In addition, patients can have skin induration, which may progress to lipodermatosclerosis (with the classic inverted champagne-bottle appearance), the development of violaceous plaques and nodules on the legs and the dorsal part of the feet, and these lesions frequently undergo painful ulceration and can be clinically indistinguishable from classic Kaposi sarcoma. This clinical appearance has led this entity to be called pseudo–Kaposi sarcoma or acroangiodermatitis (Flugman, 2012).

## DIFFERENTIAL DIAGNOSIS

- Atopic dermatitis
- Cellulitis
- Contact dermatitis, allergic

- Contact dermatitis, irritant
- Cutaneous T-cell lymphoma
- Necrobiosis lipoidica
- Nummular dermatitis
- Pigmented purpuric dermatitis
- Pretibial myxedema
- Tinea pedis

## TREATMENT/MANAGEMENT

Blood tests are generally not indicated unless cellulitis and/or sepsis is suspected or if stasis dermatitis is a result of venous thrombosis, in which case a thorough hematologic workup to rule out underlying hypercoagulability states is warranted. Radiologic and Doppler studies are recommended in patients with acute new-onset stasis dermatitis, in young patients, and if deep venous thrombosis is suspected or if there is severe valve damage because of past thrombosis (Flugman, 2012).

Treatment of stasis dermatitis includes the following:

- Compression is recommended by use of specialized stockings that deliver a controlled pressure gradient (measured in mm Hg) to the affected leg. Compression stockings should be applied early in the morning, before the patient gets out of bed when leg edema is minimal. Also used for compression are elastic wraps, compression (Unna) boots, and more sophisticated devices, such as end-diastolic compression boots. Most of these modalities are applied in a physician's office or wound care center. Frequent leg elevation is also recommended.
- Weeping lesions can be treated with wet to damp gauze dressings soaked with water or with a drying agent, such as aluminum acetate. Topical corticosteroids (triamcinolone 0.1% ointment) are frequently used to reduce inflammation and itching in acute flares. Topical steroids increase the risk for infection in patients with stasis dermatitis. Open wounds should be treated with a topical antibiotic, such as bacitracin or Polysporin. Obvious superficial impetiginization should be treated with topical mupirocin or a systemic antibiotic with activity against *Staphylococcus* and *Streptococcus* species (e.g., dicloxacillin, cephalexin, cefadroxil, levofloxacin). If infection is suspected, culture with sensitivity testing is valuable to aid in appropriate antibiotic therapy and to rule out methicillin-resistant *Staphylococcus aureus* infection.
- The nonsteroidal calcineurin inhibitors tacrolimus and pimecrolimus have been shown to be effective in many steroid-responsive dermatoses and do not carry the risk of skin atrophy or tachyphylaxis.
- Patients with chronic, calm stasis dermatitis can be treated with bland topical emollients to maximize epidermal moisture. Plain white petrolatum is an effective and inexpensive occlusive moisturizer. (Flugman, 2012)

## SPECIAL CONSIDERATIONS

Patients who are immunocompromised or have diabetes may need long-term antibiotic treatment when infectious stasis dermatitis is present.

## WHEN TO REFER

Referrals to a dermatologist are usually all that is required in management of stasis dermatitis; however, patients who have underlying vascular disorders will need referral to a vascular specialist, or a hematologist may be required for deep vein thrombosis–related congenital or acquired hypercoagulable states (Flugman, 2012).

## PATIENT EDUCATION

Flugman (2012) and Habif (2004) recommend:

- Counseling patients regarding the use of compression therapy is vital to the successful management of stasis dermatitis. Demonstrate stocking application and address any patient concerns.
- Recommend frequent leg elevation to reduce leg edema. Increased leg edema will cause compression stockings to be painful, decreasing compliance.

## REFERENCES

Beltrani, V. S. (2003). Occupational dermatoses. *Current Opinion in Allergy Clinical Immunology, 3*, 115–123.

Bourke, J., Coulson, I., & English, J. (2009). *Guidelines for management of contact dermatitis: An update.* Retrieved from http://www.guideline.gov/content.aspx?id=15881&search=contact+dermatitis

Diepgen, T., & Weisshaar, E. (2007). Contact dermatitis: epidemiology and frequent sensitizers to cosmetics. *Journal of the European Academy of Dermatology and Venereology, 21*, 9–13. doi: 10.1111/j.1468-3083.2007.02381.x

Fleischer, A. B. (2008). Diagnosis and management of common dermatoses in children: Atopic, seborrheic, and contact dermatosis. *Clinical Pediatrics, 47*(4), 332–346.

Flugman, S. L. (2012). *Stasis dermatitis.* Retrieved from http://emedicine.medscape.com/article/1084813-overview

Gupta, A. K., Bluhm, R., Cooper, E. A., Summerbell, R. C., & Barta, R. (2003). Seborrheic dermatitis. *Dermatology Clinic, 21*, 401–412.

Habif, T. P. (2004). *Clinical dermatology: A color guide to diagnosis and therapy* (4th ed.). Philadelphia, PA: Mosby.

Hanna, D. M., Moennich, J., & Jacob, S. E. (2009). A practical management of atopic dermatitis—Palliative care to contact dermatitis. *Journal of the Dermatology Nurses' Association, 1*(2), 97–105.

Herro, E. M., & Jacob, S. E. (2011). Allergic contact dermatitis in children. *Journal of the Dermatology Nurses; Association, 3*(3), 142–147.

Hill, M. J. (2003). *Dermatologic nursing essentials: A core curriculum* (2nd ed.). Pitman, NJ: Dermatology Nurses Association.

Hogan, D. (2012). *Lichen simplex chronicus.* Retrieved from http://emedicine.medscape.com/article/1123423

James, W. D., Berger, T. G., & Elston, D. M. (2006). *Andrews' diseases of the skin: Clinical dermatology* (10th ed.). Philadelphia, PA: Elsevier/Saunders.

Kim, B. S. (2013). *Atopic dermatitis.* Retrieved from http://emedicine.medscape.com/article/1049085-overview

Koch, P. (2001). Occupational contact dermatitis. Recognition and management. *American Journal of Clinical Dermatology, 2*(6), 353–365.

Militello, G., Jacob, S. E., & Crawford, G. H. (2006). Allergic contact dermatitis in children. *Current Opinion in Pediatrics, 18*, 385–390.

Nichols, K. M., & Cook-Bolden, E. F. (2009). Allergic skin disease: Major highlights and recent advances. *Medical Clinics of North America, 93*, 1211–1224.

Nijhawen, R. I., Matiz, C., & Jacob, S. E. (2009). Contact dermatitis: From the basics to allergodromes. *Pediatric Annals, 38*(2), 99–108.

Picardo, M., & Cameli, N. (2008). Seborrheic dermatitis. In H. Williams, M. Bigby, T. Diepgen, A. Herxheimer, L. Naldi, & B. Rzany (Eds.), *Evidence-based dermatology* (2nd ed., pp. 164–167). Malden, MA: Blackwell.

Schwartz, R. A., Janusz, C. A., & Janniger, C. K. (2006). Seborrheic dermatitis: An overview. *American Family Physician, 74*(1), 125–130.

Selden, S. T. (2013). *Seborrheic dermatitis*. Retrieved from http://emedicine.medscape.com/article/1108313-overview#aw2aab6b2b2

Thomas, K., Beth-Hextall, F., Ravenscroft, J., Charmam, C., & Williams, H. (2008). Atopic eczema. In H. Williams, M. Bigby, T. Diepgen, A. Herxhiemer, L. Naldi, & B. Rzany (Eds.), *Evidence-based dermatology* (2nd ed., pp. 128–158). Malden, MA: Blackwell.

Van Coevorden, A. M., Diepgen, T., & Coenraads, P. (2008). Hand eczema. In H. Williams, M. Bigby, T. Diepgen, A. Herxheimer, L. Naldi, & B. Rzany (Eds.), *Evidence-based dermatology* (2nd ed., pp. 117–127). Maldem, MA: Blackwell.

Weaver, J., & Billings, S. D. (2009). Initial presentation of stasis dermatitis mimicking solitary lesions: A previously unrecognized clinical scenario. *Journal of the American Academy of Dermatology, 61*(6), 1028–1032.

Weston, W. L., & Howe, W. (2011a). *Overview of dermatitis*. Retrieved from http://uptodate.com/contents/overview-of-dermatitis

Weston, W. L., & Howe, W. (2011b). *Patient Information: Seborrheic dermatitis (including dandruff and cradle cap)*. Retrieved from http://uptodate.com/contents/patients-information-seborrheic-dermatitis-including-dandruff-and-cradle-cap

Weston, W. L., & Howe, W. (2011c). *Treatment of atopic dermatitis (eczema)*. Retrieved from http://www.uptodate.com/contents/treatment-of-atopic-dermatitis-eczema

Yang, Y., & Zirwas, M. (2009). Hand dermatitis in primary care: A nurse practitioner's role in management. *Journal of the American Academy of Nurse Practitioners, 21*, 671–676.

# Erythema Multiforme

## OVERVIEW

*Erythema multiforme* (EM) is an acute, immune-mediated condition characterized by the appearance of unique target-like lesions on the skin (Figure III.22). These lesions may be accompanied by erosions or bullae involving the oral, genital, and/or oral mucosa. *EM major* is the term used to describe EM with mucosal involvement, and *EM minor* refers to EM without mucosal involvement (Wetter, 2012a).

## EPIDEMIOLOGY

The precise incidence of EM in the United States is unknown; however, approximately 1% of dermatologic outpatient visits are for EM (Plaza, 2013). EM most commonly occurs in adults between the ages of 20 and 40 years and affects males slightly more than females (male-to-female ratio of 3:2 to 2:1; Wetter, 2012a). Before the human immunodeficiency virus (HIV) endemic among young men, females were affected more than males (Plaza, 2013).

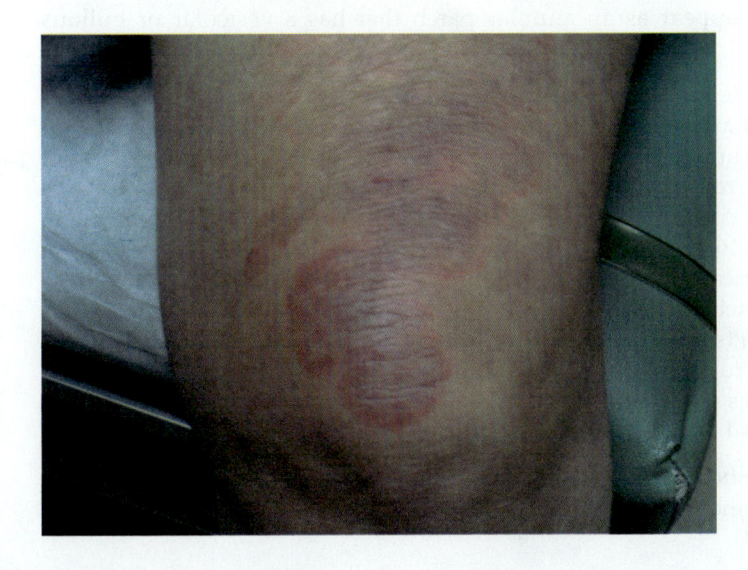

FIGURE III.22   Erythema multiforme
Courtesy of Nancy Seal, FNP

The following medical conditions put people in a higher risk category for developing EM (Plaza, 2013):

- HIV infection
- Corticosteroid exposure
- Bone marrow transplant
- Systemic lupus erythematosus
- Graft-versus-host disease
- Inflammatory bowel disease
- Individuals undergoing radiation, chemotherapy, or neurosurgery for brain tumors
- Infections (viral, bacterial, and fungal; most common in approximately 90% of occurrences, with herpes simplex virus [HSV] being the most frequent precipitator)
- Certain drugs and medications (e.g., nonsteroidal anti-inflammatory drugs, sulfonamides, antiepileptics, and antibiotics)
- Malignancy
- Autoimmune diseases
- Immunizations
- Radiation
- Sarcoidosis
- Menstruation
- Mycoplasma pneumonia infection in children

Early in the disease process, the epidermis becomes infiltrated with CD8 T lymphocytes and macrophages, and the dermis displays a slight influx of CD4 lymphocytes. These immunologically active cells are low in number and do not directly cause epithelial cell death, but they do release diffusible cytokines, which start the inflammatory reaction and resultant cell death of epithelial cells. Findings of immunohistochemical analysis have also shown lesion blister fluid to contain tumor necrosis factor, an essential proinflammatory cytokine (Plaza, 2013).

## CLINICAL PRESENTATION

EM lesions may present as two types (Ghislain & Roujeau, 2008; Patel & Patel, 2009):

1. *Iris type* (target lesions) have an annular patch with a cyanotic center (Figure III.22). Typically, these lesions look like a bull's eye.
2. *Vesiculobullous* types appear as an annular patch that has a vesicular or bullous center (Figure III.23). The hands and feet are the most commonly affected areas.

EM occurs in a wide spectrum of severity. EM minor signifies a localized eruption of the skin with little, if any, mucosal involvement. Lesions remain in a fixed location for 1 week and then begin to heal. Because this condition may be related to a persistent antigenic stimulus, recurrences may appear up to twice a year. Prodromal symptoms in persons with EM minor consist of a mild, nonspecific upper respiratory tract infection. The sudden onset of a nonpruritic rash usually occurs 3 days after prodrome, starting on the extremities symmetrically, with centripetal dispersion. In EM major, 50% of patients have prodromes that include moderate fever, malaise, cough, sore throat, vomiting, chest pain, and diarrhea (secondary to gastrointestinal tract ulceration) that can last up to 2 weeks before skin eruption occurs. The lesions begin on the acral areas and spread in the same presentations as EM minor (James, Berger, & Elston, 2006; Plaza, 2013).

Prominent mucosal involvement can occur with EM major (Plaza, 2013).

- Erosions of the oral mucosa affect eating, drinking, or opening the mouth.
- Conjunctival involvement may cause lacrimation, photophobia, burning eyes, or visual impairment.

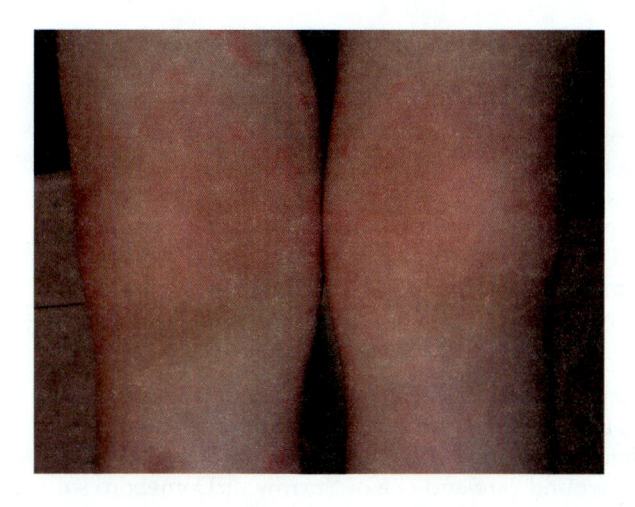

FIGURE III.23  Example of erythema multiforme
Courtesy of Nancy Seal, FNP

- Genital lesions are painful, making it difficult to urinate.
- Shortness of breath or difficulty breathing may occur because of tracheobronchial epithelial involvement.

## DIFFERENTIAL DIAGNOSIS

- Acute febrile neutrophilic dermatosis
- Acute hemorrhagic edema of infancy
- Behçet disease
- Bullous pemphigoid
- Contact dermatitis, allergic
- Contact dermatitis, irritant
- Drug eruptions
- Pemphigus, paraneoplastic
- Polymorphous light eruption
- Rowell syndrome
- Staphylococcal scalded skin syndrome
- Stevens-Johnson syndrome and toxic epidermal necrolysis
- Sweet syndrome
- Urticarial vasculitis

## TREATMENT/MANAGEMENT

EM is usually diagnosed clinically, so no specific laboratory tests are indicated. Cultures are recommended in severe cases and should be obtained from blood, sputum, and mucosal lesions. If there are specific respiratory signs and symptoms, a chest x-ray may be needed; otherwise, imaging studies are usually not necessary. Blood urea nitrogen and creatinine tests are indicated to screen for renal involvement and dehydration in severe cases requiring hospitalization. When laboratory testing is performed, results are as follows (Plaza, 2013):

- Complete blood cell count with differential will reveal moderate leukocytosis with atypical lymphocytes and lymphopenia, possibly because of the depletion of CD4 lymphocytes (90% of patients). An eosinophil count greater than 1,000/mm$^3$ may also be seen. The presence of neutropenia indicates a poor prognosis. A severely

elevated total white blood cell count indicates infection. Mild anemia may be present, and thrombocytopenia is found in 15% of patients.
- Electrolyte values may be abnormal with severe skin and mucous membrane involvement because of fluid losses.
- Erythrocyte sedimentation rate may be elevated, but this is a nonspecific finding. Mildly elevated liver transaminase levels may be found with hepatic involvement.
- Specific HSV antigens have been detected within keratinocytes by immunofluorescence study. The HSV DNA has been identified primarily within the keratinocytes by polymerase chain reaction amplification.
- Direct immunofluorescence staining and examination may also identify an alternative diagnosis (e.g., pemphigoid, immunoglobulin A [IgA] linear dermatosis).

For all types of EM, treatment is usually symptomatic, including oral antihistamines, analgesics, local skin care, and relieving mouthwashes (e.g., oral rinsing with warm saline or a solution of diphenhydramine, lidocaine, and bismuth subsalicylate). For more difficult cases, thorough wound care and use of Burrow or Domeboro solution dressings may be necessary (Plaza, 2013). Treatment for EM includes the following:

- Corticosteroids
    - Ghislain and Roujeau (2008) reported that corticosteroids appear to be of little use. However, Patel and Patel (2009) advocated treatment of EM with steroid use for symptom management only. James, Berger, and Elston (2006) stated that steroids can be used; however, if EM is initially caused by HSV, then reactivation of HSV may occur. Wetter (2012b) concurred that topical steroids may be effective for symptomatic relief of EM symptoms such as pruritis. Oral steroids are recommended of there is severe mucosal involvement.
- Antibiotics
    - Ghislain and Roujeau (2008) and Patel and Patel (2009) reported that the use of antibiotics is favorable only if *Mycoplasma pneumonia* infection is suspected.
- Antivirals
    - Ghislain and Roujeau (2008) reported that the initiation of acyclovir in treatment of full-blown postherpetic EM was of no benefit.
    - James et al. (2006) stated that the treatment of EM is determined by cause and extent. EM is usually caused by HSV, and the use of antiviral medication is appropriate.
    - Patel and Patel (2009) reported that the use of acyclovir is warranted until the cause of EM can be confirmed. Acyclovir can also be used prophylactically to prevent recurrent EM.
    - Wetter (2012b) stated that in patients with HSV-induced EM, treatment with oral antivirals in the acute setting does not alter the course of EM and is not indicated. However, for patients with HSV-induced EM that recurs more than six times per year or patients who have fewer but disabling episodes, it is recommended that antivirals be used on a continuous basis (Grade 1B).
    - Plaza (2013) stated that the suppression of HSV can prevent HSV-associated EM, but antiviral treatment started after the eruption of EM has no effect on the course of EM.
- Other
    - After cultures are done, treat infections accordingly. The use of liquid antiseptics, such as 0.05% chlorhexidine, when bathing helps prevent infection. Topical treatment can be applied with a gauze dressing or a hydrocolloid (Plaza, 2013).
    - Local supportive care for eye involvement is important and includes topical lubricants for dry eyes, sweeping of conjunctival fornices, and removal of fresh adhesions (Plaza, 2013).
    - Antihistamines are used for pruritus (Wetter, 2012b).

## SPECIAL CONSIDERATIONS

Advanced age, visceral involvement, increased serum urea nitrogen level, and previous bone marrow transplantation are poor prognostic factors. Two additional unusual clinical forms of EM have been described by Plaza (2013):

- Continuous EM demonstrates a persistent course with overlapping attacks and may be associated with systemic administration of glucocorticoids.
- Persistent EM has a protracted clinical course over months, is commonly associated with atypical skin lesions, and is resistant to standard treatment. It has been associated with inflammatory bowel disease, occult renal carcinoma, persistent or reactivated Epstein-Barr virus infection, and HSV infection.

## WHEN TO REFER

Consultation with the following specialists is recommended (Plaza, 2013):

- Dermatologist: For diagnosis and management of EM
- Internal medicine specialist or a pediatric specialist: For evaluation of the underlying causes of disorders and systemic sequelae
- Ophthalmologist: For consultation in the management of ocular involvement
- Infectious disease specialist: For evaluation of difficult infections and treatment recommendations
- Respiratory therapist: For tracheobronchial involvement
- Physical or occupational therapist
- Psychologists, psychiatrists, or social workers as needed

## PATIENT EDUCATION

Educate patients with EM about recommended symptomatic treatment and assure patients that the disease is usually self-limited. In addition, advise patients to avoid identified triggers for EM, which may cause recurrence (Plaza, 2013).

## CLINICAL PEARLS

- Erythema multiforme: ICD-9, 695.10; ICD-10, L51.9
- EM is usually diagnosed clinically by history and physical examination.
- Typical lesions are erythematous macules, papules, and characteristic target or "iris" lesions.
- EM is symmetrically distributed on palms, soles, dorsum of the hands, and extensor surfaces of extremities and face.
- Management of EM involves determining the etiology, treating the causative infection, or discontinuing the responsible drug.
- Complications are rare.
- Recurrent cases often are secondary to HSV infection. (Marat, 2013)

# REFERENCES

Ghislain, P. D., & Roujeau, J. C. (2008). Erythema multiforme. In H. Williams, M. Bigby, T. Diepgen, A. Herxheimer, L. Naldi, & B. Rzany (Eds.), *Evidence-based dermatology* (2nd ed., pp. 608–611). Malden, MA: Blackwell.

James, W. D., Berger, T. G., & Elston, D. M. (2006). *Andrews' diseases of the skin: Clinical dermatology* (10th ed.). Philadelphia, PA: Elsevier/Saunders.

Marat, J. P. (2013). *Erythema multiforme—Causes, symptoms, diagnosis, treatment, and ongoing care.* Retrieved from http://health.tipsdiscover.com/erythema-multiforme-causes-symptoms-diagnosis-treatment-and-ongoing-care

Patel, N. N., & Patel, D. N. (2009). Erythema multiforme syndrome. *American Journal of Medicine, 122*(7), 623–625.

Plaza, J. A. (2013). *Erythema multiforme.* Retrieved from http://emedicine.medscape.com/article/1122915-overview

Wetter, D. A. (2012a). *Pathogenesis, clinical features, and diagnosis of erythema multiforme.* Retrieved from http://uptodate.com/contents/pathogenesis-clinical-features-and-diagnosis-of-erythema-multiforme

Wetter, D. A. (2012b). *Treatment of erythema multiforme.* Retrieved from http://www.uptodate.com/contents/treatment-of-erythema-multiforme

# Erythema Nodosum

## OVERVIEW

Erythema nodosum (EN) is the most commonly diagnosed form of inflammatory panniculitis, which is characterized by an acute, nodular, erythematous eruption that usually affects the extensor parts of the lower legs (Figure III.24). EN is suspected to represent a delayed hypersensitivity response to an antigenic provocation (Gilchrist & Patterson, 2011). The acute process typically lasts 3 to 6 weeks. A chronic or recurrent form can also occur (Gilchrist & Patterson, 2011), but it is rare (Habif, 2004; Hebel, 2012; James, Berger, & Elston, 2006; Shojania, 2012).

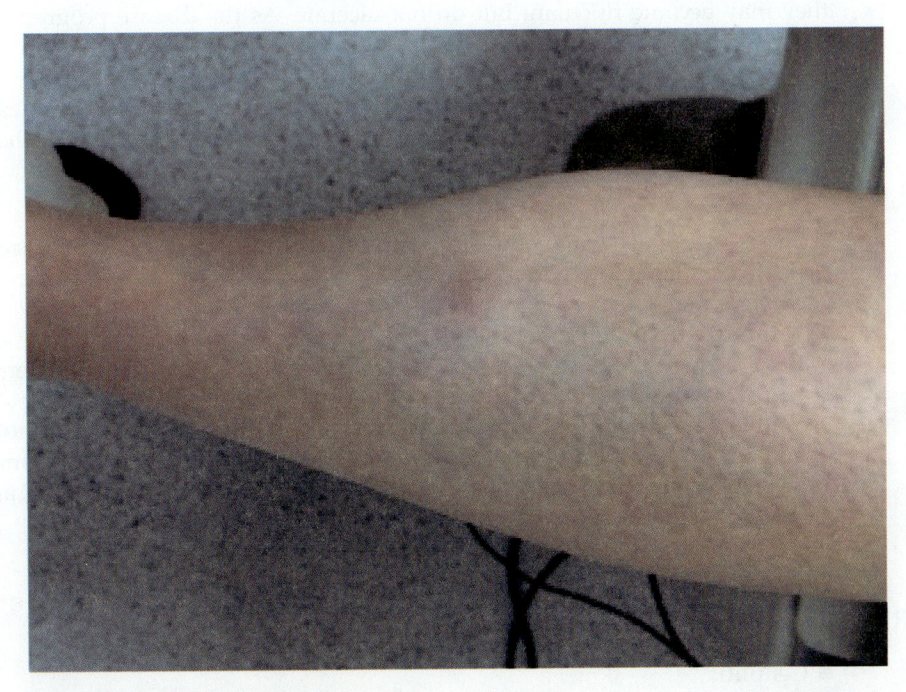

**FIGURE III.24** Erythema nodosum
Courtesy of Nancy Seal, FNP

## EPIDEMIOLOGY

In the United States, age and gender distributions of EN vary according to etiology and geographic location. The annual incidence of EN is approximately 1 to 5 in 100,000 persons, most often women aged 15 to 40 years, with a male-to-female ratio of one to four. EN is most common in adults aged 18 to 34, although children and the elderly can be affected (Hebel, 2012; Shojania, 2012).

## PATHOLOGY/HISTOLOGY

The classic features of EN on histopathology include a thickened septal panniculitis with mild superficial and deep perivascular inflammatory lymphocytic infiltrate. As lesions grow, periseptal fibrosis, giant cells, and granulation tissue appear. Miescher granulomas are a trademark feature of EN. Small, well-defined nodular aggregates of histiocytes around a central stellate cleft are scattered throughout the lesions. A lymphohistiocytic infiltrate is noted in the septum and in small- and medium-sized vessels (Hebel, 2012; James et al., 2006).

## CLINICAL PRESENTATION

The eruptive phase of EN starts with flulike symptoms of fever, generalized aching, and arthralgia followed by a painful rash within 2 days. Infection-induced EN heals usually within 6 to 8 weeks, but active disease can last up to 4 or 5 months (Habif, 2004; Hebel, 2012; James et al., 2006).

Individual lesions last 1 to 2 weeks, but sometimes new lesions will continue to occur for 3 to 6 weeks. Lesions begin as red tender nodules measuring 2 to 6 cm with poorly defined borders, then lesions become tense, hard, and painful; the second week, they may become fluctuant but do not ulcerate. As the disease progresses, the tender lesion size varies from 3 to 20 cm (Wolff, Johnson, & Saavedra, 2013). Aching and swelling of lower extremities may persist for weeks. Lesions change color in the second week from bright red to bluish or livid. As the color is absorbed, the color slowly fades to a yellowish hue, resembling a bruise (Habif, 2004; Hebel, 2012; James et al., 2006; Shojania, 2012).

Other associated symptoms of EN include the following (Habif, 2004; Hebel, 2012):

- Hilar adenopathy may develop as part of the hypersensitivity reaction of EN. Bilateral hilar lymphadenopathy is associated with sarcoidosis, whereas unilateral changes may occur with infections and malignancy.
- Arthralgia occurs in more than half of patients affected with EN and begins during the eruptive phase or precedes the eruption by 2 to 4 weeks. Erythema, swelling, tenderness, and stiffness occur over the joint with occasional morning stiffness. Any joint can be affected, but the ankles, knees, and wrist are most common. Erythema and edema resolves within a few weeks, but joint pain and stiffness may last up to 6 months. No joint damage occurs with EN. Synovial fluid is acellular, and the rheumatoid factor is negative.

## DIFFERENTIAL DIAGNOSIS

- Cellulitis
- Erysipelas
- Erythema induratum (nodular vasculitis)

- Infected insect bites
- Minor trauma
- Other forms of panniculitis
- Superficial and deep thrombophlebitis
- Urticaria, acute

## TREATMENT/MANAGEMENT

The most common causes of EN are streptococcal infection in children and adults and adult sarcoidosis. The causes reported most often in the literature are as follows (Habif, 2004; Hebel, 2012; James et al., 2006; Shojania, 2012):

- Bacterial infections
  - Streptococcal infections
  - Tuberculosis, especially in developing countries
  - *Yersinia enterocolitica,* a gram-negative bacillus that causes acute diarrhea and abdominal pain; most common in France and Finland
  - Mycoplasma pneumoniae infection
  - Lymphogranuloma venereum
  - *Salmonella* infection
  - Campylobacter infection
- Fungal infections
  - Coccidioidomycosis (San Joaquin Valley fever) is the most common cause of EN in the American Southwest. EN develops after the primary fungal infection (which may be asymptomatic or involve symptoms of upper respiratory infection).
  - Histoplasmosis
  - Blastomycosis
- Drugs
  - Sulfonamides and halide agents
  - Gold, sulfonylureas, and oral contraceptives
  - Penicillins, bromides, and iodides (Gilchrist & Patterson, 2011)
  - Opiates (Gilchrist & Patterson, 2011)
- Enteropathies
  - Ulcerative colitis and Crohn's disease may trigger EN.
- Hodgkin disease and lymphoma
  - EN may precede the diagnosis of non-Hodgkin lymphoma by months.
  - EN may precede the onset of acute myelogenous leukemia.
- Sarcoidosis
  - The most common skin manifestation of sarcoidosis is EN. A characteristic form of acute sarcoidosis involves the association of EN, hilar lymphadenopathy, fever, arthritis, and uveitis, which has been termed Löfgren syndrome.
- Behçet disease
  - This can cause mucocutaneous and gastrointestinal findings identical to Crohn's disease.
- Pregnancy
  - Some patients develop EN during pregnancy, most frequently during the second trimester.

The following diagnostic studies may be helpful (Hebel, 2012; Shojania, 2012):

- Perform a throat culture to exclude Group A beta-hemolytic streptococcal infection.
- Perform an antistreptolysin titer. The results will be elevated in some patients with streptococcal disease, but normal values do not exclude streptococcal infection.

- Order complete blood count and differential.
- Order liver enzymes (aspartate aminotransferase, alanine aminotransferase, alkaline phosphatase), checking bilirubin and albumin levels.
- Order erythrocyte sedimentation rates; these are often high.
- Order stool examination. Along with the appropriate history of gastrointestinal complaints, a stool examination can exclude infection by *Yersinia, Salmonella*, and *Campylobacter* organisms.
- Order blood cultures.
- Order chest radiographs as part of the initial workup to exclude sarcoidosis and tuberculosis and to document hilar adenopathy.
- Perform intradermal skin tests to exclude tuberculosis and coccidioidomycosis.
- Because the diagnosis of EN often is clinical, perform a biopsy for diagnostically difficult cases. Deep skin incisional biopsies are required to adequately sample the subcutaneous tissue. The specimen should be obtained from the center of a well-developed lesion, and it is vital that it includes subcutaneous fat (Gilchrist & Patterson, 2011).

The management of EN involves three elements: (1) identification and treatment of the trigger, (2) rest and elevation of the affected extremity, and (3) specific anti-inflammatory medications (e.g., acetyl salicylic acid, ibuprofen, naproxen, indomethacin). EN will resolve without treatment, but symptomatic relief can be given using nonsteroidal anti-inflammatory drugs, cool wet compresses, elevation, and bed rest. Corticosteroids are effective but seldom necessary in self-limited disease. Potassium iodide may relieve lesional tenderness, arthralgia, and fever. Colchicine has shown efficacy. After treatment has stopped, recurrences of EN are common, and underlying infectious diseases may be exacerbated (Hebel, 2012; James et al., 2006).

## SPECIAL CONSIDERATIONS

Treatment of children may be difficult because bed rest is recommended.

## WHEN TO REFER

Dermatologist and internist involvement is warranted for evaluation of the underlying cause of EN (Hebel, 2012).

## PATIENT EDUCATION

If pain and swelling are present, the patient's ability to walk may be limited. Bed rest and restriction of physical activities are encouraged during the active phase.

## CLINICAL PEARLS

- EN: ICD-9, 695.2; ICD-10, L52
- Nonskin findings may include fever, malaise, diarrhea, headache, conjunctivitis, and cough (Gilchrist & Patterson, 2011).
- Ankle edema and leg pain are common (Gilchrist & Patterson, 2011).
- Firm supportive stockings should be prescribed (Goodheart, 2011).

# REFERENCES

Gilchrist, H., & Patterson, J. (2011). Panniculitis. In J. E. Fitzpatrick & J. G. Morelli (Eds.), *Dermatology secrets plus* (4th ed., p. 135). Philadelphia, PA: Elsevier/Saunders.

Goodheart, H. (2011). *Goodheart's same-site differential diagnosis: A rapid method of diagnosing and treating common skin disorders.* Philadelphia, PA: Lippincott Williams & Wilkins.

Habif, T. P. (2004). *Clinical dermatology: A color guide to diagnosis and therapy* (4th ed.). Philadelphia, PA: Mosby.

Hebel, J. L. (2012). *Erythema nodosum.* Retrieved from http://emedicine.medscape.com/article/1081633-overview

James, W. D., Berger, T. G., & Elston, D. M. (2006). *Andrews' diseases of the skin: Clinical dermatology* (10th ed.). Philadelphia, PA: Elsevier/Saunders.

Shojania, K. G. (2012). *Erythema nodosum.* Retrieved from http://www.uptodate.com/contents/erythema-nodosum

Wolff, K., Johnson, R., & Saavedra, A. (2013). *Fitzpatrick's color atlas and synopsis of clinical dermatology* (7th ed.). Philadelphia, PA: McGraw-Hill Medical.

# Granuloma Annulare

## OVERVIEW

*Granuloma annulare* (GA) is a self-limited benign inflammatory skin condition that is fairly common and occurs in all age groups, although it is rare in infancy (Figure III.25; Brodell, 2012; Cyr, 2006; Ghadially, 2012). The disease typically occurs in children and young adults (Wolff, Johnson, & Saavedra, 2013).

## EPIDEMIOLOGY

The frequency of GA in the general population is unknown. GA does not favor a particular race, ethnic group, or geographic area. Females are affected by GA twice as often as males, with a ratio of 2.5 to 1.0 (Brodell, 2012). Localized GA is the most

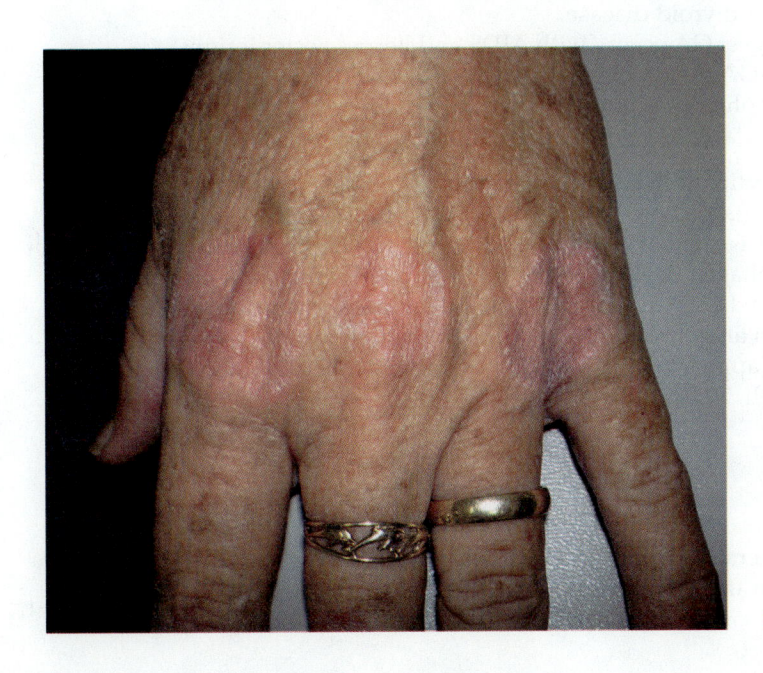

**FIGURE III.25** Granuloma annulare

common type of GA and is most frequently seen in children and adults younger than age 30. Generalized variant GA affects 9% to 15% of patients with GA, with equal distribution between sexes, occurring in patients younger than 10 years and in patients aged 30 to 60 years. Perforating GA has a prevalence of 5% among GA subtypes and most often affects children. Subcutaneous GA can occur in adults; however, it predominantly affects healthy children, typically those aged 2 to 10 years (Cyr, 2006; Ghadially, 2012).

## PATHOLOGY/HISTOLOGY

The pathogenetic mechanisms of GA are poorly understood, with a vast majority of GA cases occurring in patients who are otherwise healthy. There is a large range of predisposing events and associated diseases that can initiate a GA reaction (Brodell, 2012; Cyr, 2006; Ghadially, 2012).

- It has been speculated that GA is associated with tuberculosis, insect bites, trauma, sun exposure, thyroiditis, vaccinations, and viral infections, including HIV, Epstein-Barr virus, hepatitis B virus, hepatitis C virus, and herpes zoster virus; however, these etiologic factors have not been researched. GA also has a tendency to occur on sun-exposed areas and photodamaged skin.
- GA has been observed in identical twins and siblings in several generations, along with an association of GA with human leukocyte antigen (HLA) phenotypes, suggesting that genetics plays a role in the development of GA.
- Some research has cited chronic stress as a trigger of GA.
- Photosensitive GA has been associated with HIV infection.
- A few cases of GA have been reported in association with gold therapy and treatment with the following medications: allopurinol, diclofenac, quinidine, calcitonin, amlodipine, angiotensin-converting enzyme inhibitors, daclizumab, and calcium channel blockers.
- GA has been associated mainly with type 1 diabetes mellitus and rarely with type 2 diabetes mellitus and thyroid disease.
- Limited reports suggest GA occurs with AIDS and herpes zoster lesions.
- Lesions that mimic GA or are histologically confirmed as GA have occurred with various types of lymphoma, leukemia, and solid tumors (e.g., breast, cervical, colon, lung, prostate, testicular, and thyroid tumors).

A lymphohistiocytic infiltrate, degeneration of collagen, and mucin deposition are characteristic histopathologic features of GA. These features are present as an interstitial pattern that is characterized by histiocytes embedded in basophilic mucin infiltrating between collagen bundles in the mid to upper dermis or a palisading pattern that is characterized by lymphohistiocytic inflammatory infiltrates that palisade around foci of collagen and elastin degeneration in the mid to upper dermis. Areas of collagen degeneration appear as eosinophilic fibrillar material separated by basophilic mucin deposits (Brodell, 2012).

## CLINICAL PRESENTATION

Both localized and generalized GA lesions usually present as asymptomatic cutaneous lesions. GA is worse in the summer and will be stable for months, then may rapidly enlarge over the course of weeks (Ghadially, 2012).

The following clinical variants are recognized (Brodell, 2012; Cyr, 2006; Ghadially, 2012):

1. *Localized GA:* This is the most common form. Localized GA frequently occurs on the feet, ankles, lower limbs, hands, fingers, and wrists and will present with groups of 1- to 2-mm papules that range in color from flesh-toned to erythematous, often in an annular arrangement that can be up to 5 cm in diameter. Centers of lesions may be slightly hyperpigmented and depressed with raised borders, which may be solid or composed of numerous dermal papules.
2. *Generalized GA:* This form occurs predominantly in adults. The entire body can be involved. Patients with generalized GA may present with multiple 1- to 2-mm papules or nodules that range in color from flesh-toned to erythematous. Lesions may merge into annular plaques measuring 3 to 6 cm in diameter and may enlarge centrifugally over weeks to months.
3. *Subcutaneous GA:* This form occurs predominantly in children and occurs on the shins, ankles, dorsal feet and hands, buttocks, scalp, and eyelids. Patients present with a firm, nontender, flesh-colored or pinkish nodule without overlying epidermal alteration.
4. *Perforating GA:* This form is rare and usually present on the dorsal hands and fingers but can be generalized on the trunk and extremities. Patients with perforating GA present with multiple grouped 1- to 4-mm papules that range in color from flesh-toned to erythematous. Papules can merge to form annular plaques and may evolve into yellowish pustular lesions that will have a clear or creamy discharge, which then forms an umbilicating, crusting, or scaling area that heals, leaving atrophic hypopigmented or hyperpigmented scars. Larger and more ulcerated plaques are common in middle-aged and elderly patients.
5. *Arcuate Dermal Erythema:* This is a rare form of GA that manifests as infiltrated erythematous patches that may form large, hyperpigmented rings with central clearing.

## DIFFERENTIAL DIAGNOSIS

- Annular elastolytic giant cell granuloma
- Annular lichen planus
- Erythema annulare centrifugum
- Erythema elevatum diutinum
- Erythema migrans of Lyme disease
- Interstitial granulomatous dermatitis
- Lichen planus
- Nodular tertiary syphilis
- Nummular eczema
- Pityriasis rosea
- Rheumatoid nodules
- Sarcoidosis
- Subcutaneous cutaneous lupus erythematous
- Tinea corporis
- Urticaria

## TREATMENT/MANAGEMENT

Laboratory studies do not add to the diagnosis of GA. With negative history and physical examination findings, no additional workup is necessary, unless a thorough history is not available or systemic disease is present. A biopsy is useful for atypical presentations or when the diagnosis is in question. To rule out fungal infection, a potassium hydroxide preparation or fungal culture should be performed. Imaging studies are not generally necessary unless the evaluation of atypical subcutaneous lesions are needed (Brodell, 2012; Ghadially, 2012).

Many cases of GA resolve spontaneously within a few years, and treatment is indicated only for patients who have symptomatic lesions or cosmetic concerns. Treatments of GA include the following (Brodell, 2012; Cyr, 2006; Ghadially, 2012):

- Localized GA is often asymptomatic and resolves without treatment. However, localized lesions can be treated with very-high-potency topical corticosteroids with or without occlusion for 2 to 4 weeks, as well as with intralesional corticosteroid injection of 0.1 mL with 2.5 to 10.0 mg/mL triamcinolone acetonide, given with a 30-gauge needle into the elevated border. Treatment with cryotherapy using liquid nitrogen or nitrous oxide as refrigerants can also be used. Other potential treatments in both localized and generalized GA involve tacrolimus and pimecrolimus and imiquimod cream.
- Generalized GA tends to be more persistent and unsightly. Treatment is unfortunately difficult and ineffective. Although the treatment of choice is uncertain, research supports the use of isotretinoin or phototherapy with oral psoralen and ultraviolet-A (PUVA) as first-line options. There has also been some efficacy with dapsone, systemic steroids, pentoxifylline, hydroxychloroquine, cyclosporine, fumaric esters, interferon-gamma, potassium iodide, nicotinamide, etanercept, infliximab, adalimumab, and efalizumab for the treatment of generalized GA.

## SPECIAL CONSIDERATIONS

The appearance of GA can resemble a tinea infection and can cause social stigma because of fear of contagion.

## WHEN TO REFER

Dermatology referral is warranted if conventional treatment of GA is ineffective.

## PATIENT EDUCATION

Patients and families should be reassured about the typically benign nature and course of GA.

## CLINICAL PEARLS

- Granuloma annulare: ICD-9, 695.89; ICD-10, L92.0
- If generalized GA is diagnosed, diabetes mellitus should be ruled out (Fitzpatrick & Morelli, 2011; Wolff et al., 2013).
- GA resolves within 2 years in 75% of patients (Wolff et al., 2013).
- On occasion, GA will present as subcutaneous nodules similar to rheumatoid nodules (Goodheart, 2011).

# REFERENCES

Brodell, R. (2012). *Granuloma annulare*. Retrieved from http://www.uptodate.com/contents/granuloma-annulare

Cyr, P. R. (2006). Diagnosis and management of granuloma annulare. *American Family Physician, 74*(10), 1729–1734.

Fitzpatrick, J. E., & Morelli, J. G. (2011). *Dermatology secrets plus* (4th ed.). Philadelphia, PA: Elsevier/Saunders.

Ghadially, R. (2012). *Granuloma annular*. Retrieved from http://emedicine.medscape.com/article/1123031-overview

Goodheart, H. (2011). *Goodheart's same-site differential diagnosis: A rapid method of diagnosing and treating common skin disorders.* Philadelphia, PA: Lippincott Williams & Wilkins.

Wolff, K., Johnson, R., & Saavedra, A. (2013). *Fitzpatrick's color atlas and synopsis of clinical dermatology* (7th ed.). Philadelphia, PA: McGraw-Hill Medical.

# Herpes Simplex Virus

*Herpes simplex virus* (HSV) is a human pathogenic DNA virus that causes a variety of disease presentations, ranging from a localized skin and mucous membrane lesion to severe distributed infections (e.g., neonatal herpes simplex, eczema herpeticum, and herpetic meningoencephalitis). In localized infections, vesicles are grouped primarily around the lips and nostrils, on the mouth and face, and on the genitals. The vesicles may rupture and ulcerate, and may be painful or itch (Mahler, 2008).

## HERPES SIMPLEX VIRUS TYPE 1

### OVERVIEW

*Herpes simplex virus type 1* (HSV-1) infections are frequently asymptomatic but can produce a variety of signs and symptoms (Figure III.26). Contact with herpetic lesions or oral secretions can cause an infection with HSV-1. The viral titer is 100 to 1,000 times greater when lesions are present; as a result, transmission is much more likely when the patient has lesions (Klein, 2012).

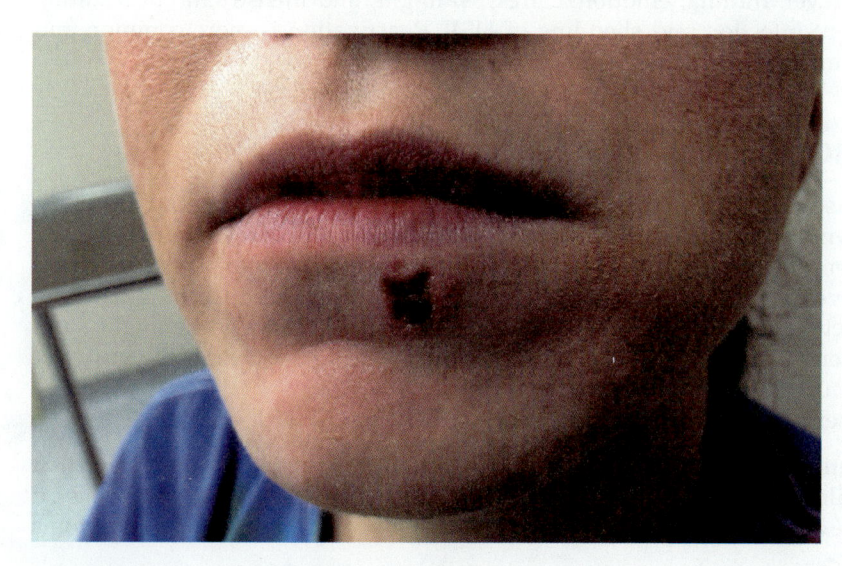

**FIGURE III.26** A herpes simplex virus type 1 infection, commonly known as a cold sore

HSV-1 infections are oral lesions that are also called *cold sores*. HSV-1 can occur in other areas such as the genitalia, liver, lung, eye, and central nervous system. These infections can be severe, especially if the patient is immunosuppressed (Klein, 2012).

## EPIDEMIOLOGY

Worldwide, more than 90% of people are seropositive for HSV-1 by the fourth decade of life, especially those of lower socioeconomic groups. This pattern was also present in the United States during the 1940s and 1950s; however, the prevalence rates for people from industrialized countries and middle-class societies have been declining (Klein, 2012).

HSV-1 is frequently acquired as a child because of contact with infected individuals. Antibodies to HSV-1 start in childhood and increase with age and relate to socioeconomic status, race, and cultural group. By the third decade of life, approximately half of all those in higher socioeconomic classes and three-fourths of individuals in lower socioeconomic classes are seropositive for HSV-1 (Salvaggio, 2012).

## PATHOLOGY/HISTOLOGY

HSV-1 infects mucosal surfaces that are susceptible (broken skin areas); the virus enters the epidermis, the dermis, and the sensory and autonomic nerve endings. HSV-1 usually occurs suddenly when a person is ill, in the form of multiple grouped vesicular papules with an inflammatory, erythematous base. Initial infection is associated with symptoms such as fever and malaise (Klein, 2012).

HSV (both types 1 and 2) is part of the family *Herpesviridae* and to the subfamily *Alphaherpesvirinae*. It is a double-stranded DNA virus characterized by the following specific biological properties (Salvaggio, 2012):

- Neurovirulence: The ability to invade and duplicate in the nervous system
- Latency: The creation and preservation of dormant infection in nerve cell ganglia proximal to the site of infection
    - In orofacial HSV infections, the trigeminal ganglia are most commonly involved, whereas in genital HSV infection, the sacral nerve root ganglia (S2–S5) are involved.
- Reactivation: The reactivation and replication of dormant HSV
    - The area supplied by the ganglia affected can be triggered by various stressors (e.g., fever, trauma, emotional stress, sunlight, and menstruation), resulting in recurrent infection and shedding of HSV. Reactivation is more common and severe in immunocompromised individuals.

## CLINICAL PRESENTATION

HSV-1 can cause rare cases of encephalitis with high rates of morbidity and mortality. This clinical syndrome is often characterized by the rapid onset of fever, headache, seizures, focal neurologic signs, and impaired consciousness. Multiple other neurologic syndromes have been linked to infection with HSV, including aseptic meningitis, autonomic dysfunction, transverse myelitis, benign recurrent lymphocytic meningitis, and Bell' palsy (Klein, 2012). Infected saliva from an adult or another child is the source of HSV-1. The incubation period is 4 to 7 days.

The presentations for HSV-1 are as follows (Salvaggio, 2012):

- Acute herpetic gingivostomatitis: This is a manifestation of initial HSV-1 infection that occurs in children aged 6 months to 5 years. Adults can be affected as well; however, it is less severe and is often associated with a posterior pharyngitis. Clinical symptoms for herpetic gingivostomatitis include sudden onset, high temperature (102°F–104°F), anorexia, listlessness, gingivitis (the most striking feature, with moderately swollen, erythematous, friable gums), vesicular lesions (these develop on the oral mucosa, tongue, and lips and later rupture and merge, leaving ulcerated plaques), tender regional lymphadenopathy, and perioral skin involvement as a result of contamination with infected saliva. Acute herpetic gingivostomatitis lasts 5 to 7 days, with symptoms lasting approximately 2 weeks. Viral shedding from patient's saliva may continue for more than 3 weeks.

- Acute herpetic pharyngotonsillitis: This is an oropharyngeal HSV-1 infection in adults. Fever, malaise, headache, and sore throat are presenting features. The vesicles rupture and form ulcerative erosions with grayish exudate on the tonsils and the posterior pharynx. Associated oral and labial lesions occur in fewer than 10% of patients.
- Herpes labialis: This is the most common appearance of recurrent HSV-1 infection. Prodrome consists of pain, burning, and tingling followed by the development of erythematous papules that quickly evolve into tiny vesicles that become pustular and ulcerate. Recurrences manifest twice yearly (most common) to monthly. Viral shedding occurs within 24 hours of onset of illness and lasts for 1 week.

## DIFFERENTIAL DIAGNOSIS

- Aphthous ulcers
- Bacterial pharyngitis
- Enteroviruses (herpangina)
- Epstein-Barr virus
- Hand–foot–mouth disease
- Steven–Johnson syndrome
- Syphilis

## TREATMENT/MANAGEMENT

The diagnosis of HSV infection can be made using a variety of techniques, including viral culture, serology, immunofluorescence, or a bedside Tzanck prep.

According to Klein (2012), randomized trials of patients with sporadic recurrences of HSV-1 infection showed that antiviral therapy with topical creams or ointments are of uncertain benefit. Most of these topical applications are based on acyclovir or related compounds (e.g., penciclovir) as the active component. The choice of oral agents includes acyclovir (200–400 mg five times daily), famciclovir (750 mg twice daily for 1 day or 1,500 mg as a single dose), or valacyclovir (2 g twice daily for 1 day). Single-day dosing with either famciclovir or valacyclovir is more convenient and less costly. Salvaggio (2012) states that it is important to recognize HSV infections in immunocompromised patients and the diagnosis of HSV encephalitis because this requires high-dose intravenous acyclovir, often started as a precaution.

## SPECIAL CONSIDERATIONS

HSV-1 infections can be more severe and have increased frequency of recurrences in the following patients (Klein, 2012):

- Immunocompromised hosts (e.g., those with HIV infection or transplant patients)
- Burn patients and patients who have other skin disorders because of decreased skin integrity

- Children (primary HSV-1 oral infection usually presents as gingivostomatitis, which can decrease nutritional intake)

## WHEN TO REFER

Consultation with a dermatologist is warranted for unusual presentations of HSV, and consultation with an infectious disease specialists is needed for immunocompromised patients (Salvaggio, 2012).

## PATIENT EDUCATION

No cure exists for HSV infection, and recurrences may be sporadic. Cold sores spread from person to person by close personal contact, such as kissing. Cold sores are caused by HSV-1 and are closely related to the virus that causes genital herpes (HSV-2). Both of these herpes simplex viruses can affect the mouth or genitals and can be spread via oral sex (Mayo Clinic, 2012).

To prevent the spread of HSV-1 to other people or self-inoculation, use the following precautions (Mayo Clinic, 2012):

- Avoid close contact with others when vesicles are present.
- Protect the eyes and genital areas because they are susceptible to spread of the virus.
- Do not share utensils, towels, or lip balms.
- Wash hands frequently.

### CLINICAL PEARLS

- Herpes simplex virus type 1: ICD-9, 054; ICD-10, B00
- The majority of herpes infections are transmitted by persons who shed the virus but are asymptomatic (Habif, Campbell, Chapman, Dinulos, & Zug, 2011).
- Intermittent asymptomatic viral shedding is the major reason herpes continues to spread (Habif et al., &2011).

## HERPES SIMPLEX VIRUS TYPE 2

### OVERVIEW

Genital herpes simplex virus (*herpes simplex virus type 2*; HSV-2) is a recurrent lifelong viral infection with the overwhelming majority of people unaware they have disease. In 2000, 1.6 million new cases were estimated, with more than 50 million persons believed to be infected in the United States (Grimshaw-Mulcahy, 2007).

### EPIDEMIOLOGY

HSV-2 infections are a major global public health problem. HSV-2 occurs in at least 50 million people in the United States alone (Albrecht, 2013). Recently, in the United States, surveys revealed a seropositive of HSV-2 antibodies in 45% of Blacks, 22% of Mexican Americans, and 17% of Whites. Seropositivity of HSV-2 antibodies is more common in women (25%) than men (17%). HSV-2 genital infections in children can be acquired perinatally from vaginal delivery by an infected mother or can be an indication of sexual abuse (Salvaggio, 2012).

## PATHOLOGY/HISTOLOGY

As noted earlier, HSV (both types 1 and 2) is part of the family *Herpesviridae* and the subfamily *Alphaherpesvirinae*. It is a double-stranded DNA virus characterized by the following specific biological properties (Salvaggio, 2012):

- Neurovirulence: The ability to invade and duplicate in the nervous system
- Latency: The creation and preservation of dormant infection in nerve cell ganglia proximal to the site of infection
    - In orofacial HSV infections, the trigeminal ganglia are most commonly involved, whereas in genital HSV infection, the sacral nerve root ganglia (S2–S5) are involved.
- Reactivation: The reactivation and replication of dormant HSV
    - The area supplied by the ganglia affected can be triggered by various stressors (e.g., fever, trauma, emotional stress, sunlight, and menstruation), resulting in recurrent infection and shedding of HSV. Reactivation is more common and severe in immunocompromised individuals.

## CLINICAL PRESENTATION

A diagnosis of HSV-2 should be confirmed with laboratory testing using the following techniques: viral culture, polymerase chain reaction (PCR), direct fluorescence antibody, and type-specific serologic tests. Cell culture and PCR-based testing are the preferred tests for a patient presenting with active lesions (Albrecht, 2013).

HSV-1 and HSV-2 can cause genital herpes infections. The clinical symptoms and course of genital herpes caused by both types are impossible to distinguish, but recurrences are more common with HSV-2. Preexisting antibodies to HSV-1 have an enhancing effect on severity of symptoms caused by HSV-2. Previous oro-labial HSV-1 infection protects against genital HSV-1 but not HSV-2 (Salvaggio, 2012).

The severity and frequency of recurrence of the disease depend on numerous factors: virus type, previous immunity to autologous or heterologous virus, gender, and immune status of the patient. Symptoms are usually more severe in women than men (Salvaggio, 2012).

In both genders, the ulcerative lesions persist from 4 to 15 days until encrusting and re-epithelialization occur. New lesions can occur during the course of the illness for up to 10 days in 75% of patients. The median duration of viral shedding is about 12 days. Clinical features are as follows (Salvaggio, 2012):

- In women, herpetic vesicles appear on the external genitalia, labia majora, labia minora, vaginal vestibule, and introitus. In moist areas, the vesicles rupture, leaving tender ulcers. The vaginal mucosa is inflamed and edematous. Cervicitis is present in 70% to 90% of cases and is characterized by ulcerative or necrotic cervical mucosa. Dysuria is associated with urethritis, and HSV can be isolated in the urine. HSV-1 infection causes urethritis more often than does HSV-2 infection.
- In men, herpetic vesicles appear in the glans penis, the prepuce, the shaft of the penis, and sometimes on the scrotum, thighs, and buttocks. In dry areas, the lesions progress to pustules and then encrust. Herpetic urethritis occurs in one third of affected men and is characterized by severe dysuria and mucoid discharge.

- The perianal area and rectum may be involved in persons who engage in anal intercourse, resulting in herpetic proctitis.

## DIFFERENTIAL DIAGNOSIS

- Behçet disease
- Candidiasis
- Drug eruptions
- Gonococcal erosion
- Syphilis and chancroid
- Trauma

## TREATMENT/MANAGEMENT

According to Grimshaw-Mulcahy (2007), for the initial outbreak of genital herpes, acyclovir 400 mg three times daily for 7 to 10 days, famciclovir 250 mg three times daily for 7 to 10 days, or valacyclovir 1 g twice daily for 7 to 10 days can be used. For recurrent or episodic occurrences, acyclovir 400 mg three times daily or 800 mg twice daily for 5 days or 800 mg three times daily for 2 days; famciclovir 125 mg twice daily for 5 days or 1,000 mg twice daily for 1 day; or valacyclovir 500 mg for 3 days or 1 g each day for 5 days.

## SPECIAL CONSIDERATIONS

Pregnant women may experience an increase in the number of recurrences in the course of pregnancy. Primary infections can have severe consequences for mother and infant; therefore identifying women at risk for a primary infection is vital. Infection in the third trimester of pregnancy is associated with neonatal HSV infections, intrauterine growth retardation, and prematurity (Salvaggio, 2012).

Neonatal HSV infection is caused by contact with the mother during vaginal delivery. The risk of transmission from a mother with an active primary infection is approximately 50%. Therefore, cesarean delivery is recommended. However, presence of active genital lesions is not a good indicator of HSV viral shedding. The American College of Obstetricians and Gynecologists recommends that suppressive antiviral therapy be given in the last 4 weeks of pregnancy to all women with a history of recurrent genital HSV. HSV-infected neonates and infants (aged < 6 weeks) have a high frequency of visceral and central nervous system infections. Without therapy, the mortality rate is 65%, and there is a high risk of neurologic complications. The disease may be confined to the skin, eyes, or oral areas, or it may manifest as encephalitis or disseminated visceral disease involving the lungs, liver, heart, adrenals, and skin (Salvaggio, 2012).

## WHEN TO REFER

Referral is warranted for the following extragenital complications, which may occur in a minority of patients with HSV-2 (Albrecht, 2013).

- Meningitis
- Proctitis
- Urinary bladder retention caused by sacral autonomic nervous system dysfunction and distant skin lesions

## PATIENT EDUCATION

Patients with HSV-2 need to be counseled that recurrence is expected. The frequency of recurrence depends on the severity and duration of the initial episode. After resolution of the primary HSV-2 infection, asymptomatic viral shedding occurs in both men and women, even in the absence of viral lesions (Albrecht, 2013). Genital herpes is contagious; those with active disease should avoid any sexual contact. The use of a condom does not prevent the spread of disease because not all sores are covered by the condom. Asymptomatic viral shedding may occur in 1% to 2% of infected immunocompromised persons and may be as high as 6% in the first few months after acquisition of the infection (Salvaggio, 2012).

### CLINICAL PEARLS

- Herpes simples virus type 2: ICD-9, 054; ICD-10, A60
- Genital herpes is a lifetime infection, and recurrences are the norm (Wolff, Johnson, & Saaverda, 2013)
- Chronic antiviral suppressive therapy reduces viral shedding

## HERPETIC WHITLOW

### OVERVIEW

*Herpetic whitlow* is an HSV infection of the fingers that can occur as a complication of primary oral or genital herpes by inoculation of the virus through a break in the skin barrier (Figure III.27). When the nail and cuticle are involved, it can be mistaken as a bacterial infection and inappropriately subjected to incision and drainage (Salvaggio, 2012).

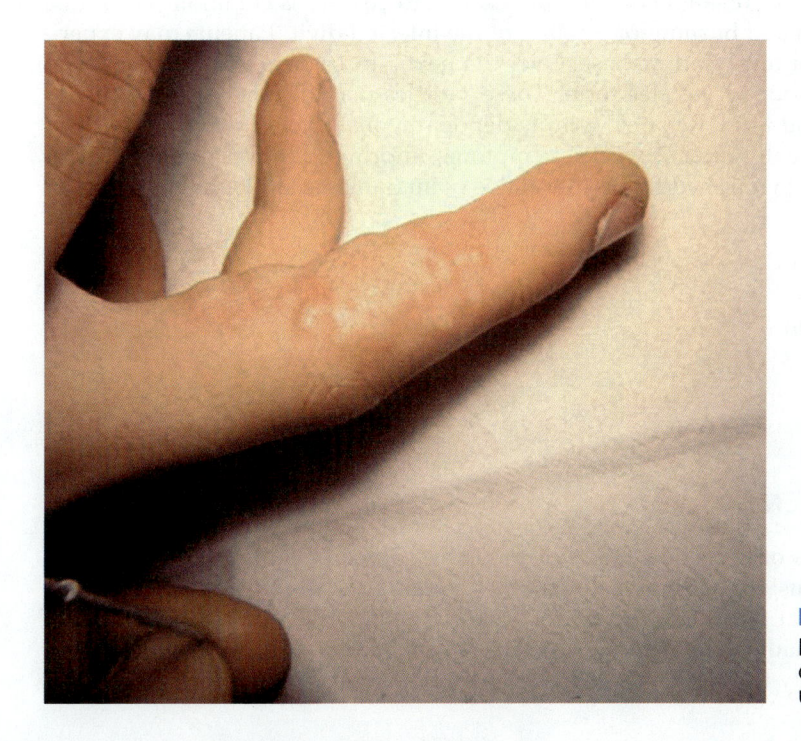

**FIGURE III.27** An example of herpetic whitlow
Courtesy of Dr. Thomas Sellers, Emory University

Herpetic whitlow is a painful infection of the hand involving one or more fingers. HSV-1 is the cause in 60% of cases of herpetic whitlow, and HSV-2 causes the other 40% (Omori, 2012).

## EPIDEMIOLOGY

In the United States, the annual incidence of herpetic whitlow is estimated at 2.4 to 5.0 cases per 100,000 people. Mortality related to herpetic whitlow is rare; however, morbidity is related primarily to bacterial super infection or to iatrogenic complications because of inappropriate incision and drainage (Omori, 2012).

Females are twice as likely as males to be affected by herpetic whitlow. In adults, 55% of cases occur between the ages of 20 and 40. Toddlers and preschool children who suck their thumb or fingers are at risk for herpetic whitlow if they have herpes labialis or herpetic gingivostomatitis (James, Berger, &Elston, 2006; Omori, 2012).

## PATHOLOGY/HISTOLOGY

Herpetic whitlow is transmitted by viral transmission through exposure to infected body fluids via a break in the skin, most commonly a torn cuticle. The virus then invades the cells of the dermis and subcutaneous tissue and then enters cutaneous nerve endings and migrates to the peripheral ganglia and Schwann cells, where it lies dormant. The primary infection usually has the worst symptoms, and recurrences are milder and shorter in duration. Herpetic whitlow in children is usually from HSV-1, whereas HSV-2 infection from genital herpes is the most frequent cause in the general adult population (Omori, 2012).

## CLINICAL PRESENTATION

After the initial exposure, an incubation period of 2 to 20 days is common. The initial symptoms are pain and burning or tingling of the infected digit. Patients may experience a prodrome of fever and malaise. Over the next 7 to 10 days, erythema, edema, and 1- to 3-mm grouped vesicles form. These vesicles may ulcerate or rupture and usually contain clear fluid. Regional lymphadenopathy may occur in epitrochlear and axillary nodes. Usually after 2 weeks, symptoms improve, and vesicles crust over and heal. The risk of viral shedding is low at this point (James et al., 2006; Omori, 2012).

## DIFFERENTIAL DIAGNOSIS

- Bacterial infection
- Cellulitis
- Felon
- Paronychia

## TREATMENT/MANAGEMENT

A clinical diagnosis of herpetic whitlow is made based on appearance and history. In children, a recent history of gingivostomatitis is common, whereas in adults, the presence of occupational risk factors or recent oral or genital HSV is common. Definitive diagnosis can be made by using the Tzanck test, viral cultures, serum antibody titers, fluorescent antibody testing, or DNA hybridization. Patients with frequent recurrent infections may have immunodeficiency; consider HIV testing for these patients (James et al., 2006; Omori, 2012).

Herpetic whitlow resolves without treatment, and any treatment is given for symptom relief. In primary infections, topical acyclovir 5% has shown efficacy in shortening duration of symptoms and viral shedding. Oral acyclovir in doses of 800 mg twice daily initiated at the first sign of symptoms may prevent recurrences. Famciclovir or valacyclovir may also be used. Use antibiotic treatment if bacterial infection is suspected (Omori, 2012).

## SPECIAL CONSIDERATIONS

Immunocompromised persons who are at increased risk for herpetic whitlow, frequent recurrences, and potential complications include the following (James et al., 2006; Omori, 2012):

- Health care workers are at risk because of exposure to infected patients.
- Patients with other herpetic lesions are at risk for self-inoculation.

## WHEN TO REFER

Herpetic whitlow that is recurrent and not responsive to treatment should be referred to a dermatologist.

## PATIENT EDUCATION

Advise patients that reoccurrences will occur and take precautions to prevent spreading herpetic whitlow to other parts of the body and to other individuals. Also advise patients who have HSV in other areas to use precaution to prevent infecting fingers. Health care workers should use gloves, practice strict hand washing, and follow universal fluid precautions (Omori, 2012).

### CLINICAL PEARLS

- Herpetic whitlow can resemble a group of warts or bacterial infection (Habif et al., 2011).
- Herpetic whitlow is caused by direct exposure of herpes simplex virus to the fingertips (Goodheart, 2011).
- Gloves have significantly decreased the occupational hazard of the disease for dental and medical workers (Goodheart, 2011).
- Both HSV-1 and HSV-2 cause herpetic whitlow.

# DERMATITIS HERPETIFORMIS

## OVERVIEW

*Dermatitis herpetiformis* (DH) is an autoimmune blistering disorder that is caused by a gluten-sensitive enteropathy (GSE). DH is characterized by grouped excoriations caused by severe pruritus; erythematous, urticarial plaques; and papules with vesicles.

The areas commonly affected with lesions are the extensor surfaces of the elbows, knees, buttocks, and back. DH is a lifelong disease, although periods of exacerbation and remission are common (James et al., 2006).

## EPIDEMIOLOGY

Research has shown a DH prevalence of 11.2 cases per 100,000 persons in the United States. Internationally, the prevalence of DH has been reported as high as 10 cases per 100,000 people. DH occurs more often in persons of northern European ancestry and is rare in Asians and persons of African descent. DH is most common in Ireland and Sweden. In the United States, males are affected slightly more often than females (1.4:1), and internationally the male-to-female ratio is higher (2:1). Although any age can be affected, the average onset is age 20 to 40 years. DH is rare in children (James et al., 2006; Miller, 2011).

## PATHOLOGY/HISTOLOGY

DH is caused by the accumulation of immunoglobulin A (IgA) in the papillary dermis, which triggers an immunologic surge, resulting in neutrophil recruitment and complement activation. This causes an immunity reaction that stimulates gut mucosa when dietary intake of gluten occurs. Theories suggest that a genetic predisposition for gluten sensitivity, in combination with a diet high in gluten, leads to the formation of IgA antibodies to gluten-tissue transglutaminase (t-TG), which is found in the intestines. These antibodies cross-react with epidermal transglutaminase (e-TG). eTG is highly homologous with t-TG. Serum studies from patients with gluten-sensitive enteropathy contain IgA antibodies to both skin and gut types. Deposition of IgA and e-TG complexes in the papillary dermis causes the lesions of DH (James et al., 2006; Miller, 2011).

## CLINICAL PRESENTATION

Patients typically present with complaints of intermittent pruritic eruption typically on the extensor surfaces of the arms, knees, and buttocks; however, it may become generalized. Patients report small vesicles initially, but these may appear as excoriations by the time of presentation to the physician. The skin eruption will worsen with dietary intake of gluten. Gastrointestinal symptoms are not reported in subjective findings (Miller, 2011).

DH rarely occurs on the posterior (nuchal) scalp, face, or the oral mucosa; males have more oral and genital involvement than females. The eruption is intensely pruritic; patients often present with erosions and crusts instead of vesicles because the vesicles have ruptured as a result of excoriation (James et al., 2006; Miller, 2011).

## DIFFERENTIAL DIAGNOSIS

- Bullous pemphigoid
- Erythema multiforme
- Linear IgA dermatosis
- Neurotic excoriations
- Scabies
- Transient acantholytic dermatosis

## TREATMENT/MANAGEMENT

The diagnosis of DH is made on the basis of skin biopsy results. Treatment of DH includes (James et al., 2006; Miller, 2011):

- Avoidance of gluten by consuming a gluten-free diet and pharmacotherapy. Improvement of skin disease with a gluten-free diet may take several months. Foods that contain gluten are wheat, barley, and rye, which are normally consumed on a daily basis.
- Dapsone (diaminodiphenylsulfone) and sulfapyridine are the primary medications used to treat DH. The exact mechanism of action is unknown but it is speculated to be related to inhibition of neutrophil migration and function. There is a symptomatic improvement within hours after starting dapsone treatment. Patients should be evaluated for the adverse effects of dapsone, primarily hemolytic anemia (monitor for GDPD deficiency), methemoglobinemia, agranulocytosis, and neuropathy.
- Other treatments for DH include colchicine, cyclosporine, azathioprine, and prednisone. Ultraviolet light may provide some relief of symptoms. Cyclosporine should be used with caution in patients with DH because of a potential increase in the risk of developing intestinal lymphomas.
- Nonsteroidal anti-inflammatory drugs may exacerbate DH.
- Iodides may provoke or aggravate DH.

## SPECIAL CONSIDERATIONS

Those with DH will experience pain, severe pruritus, and insomnia. Some may develop secondary bacterial infections. Patients will be unable to work, go to school, or engage in normal activities while affected. Following a gluten-free diet can also be difficult (Miller, 2011).

## WHEN TO REFER

Consultation with a gastroenterologist for evaluation and management regarding GSE is recommended. Consult with a dietitian regarding a gluten-free diet (Miller, 2011).

## PATIENT EDUCATION

Educate patients regarding a gluten-free diet as well as the adverse effects and complications of dapsone.

## CLINICAL PEARLS

- Dermatitis herpetiformis: ICD-9, 694.0; ICD-10, L13.0
- Intense pruritus nonresponsive to steroids is suggestive of DH or scabies (Habif et al., 2011).
- According to Habif et al. (2011), immunofluorescence confirms the diagnosis of DH.
- Bullae formation is rare in this disease.
- This disease is related to gluten sensitivity (Wolff et al., 2013).
- DH is a lifelong disease with brief remissions (Fitzpatrick & Morelli, 2011).

# HERPES ZOSTER

## OVERVIEW

*Herpes zoster* (shingles) is a cutaneous viral infection caused by the reactivation of varicella-zoster virus (VZV; Figure III.28), a herpes virus that also causes varicella (chickenpox). The response to varicella and herpes zoster depends on an individual's immune status; those with no previous exposure to VZV, most commonly children, develop varicella, whereas those with previous exposure to varicella develop a localized recurrence, zoster (Jacobsen & Hull, 2013; James et al., 2006; Janniger, 2013).

The incidence of zoster appears to be dependent with the host's ability to mount a cellular immune response. However, many patients with zoster will have normal immunity. In these patients, zoster is assumed to occur when VZV antibody titers and cellular immunity decrease to levels that will no longer completely prevent viral invasion (Albrecht, 2013; Jacobsen & Hull, 2013; Janniger, 2013).

Zoster most often occurs from a failure of the immune system to contain latent VZV replication; other factors, such as radiation, trauma, medications, other infections, and stress, can also potentially trigger zoster. It is unclear why existing varicella antibodies and cell-mediated immune mechanisms do not prevent recurrent overt disease, as is the case with other viral illnesses (Centers for Disease Control and Prevention, 2012a; James et al., 2006; Janniger, 2013).

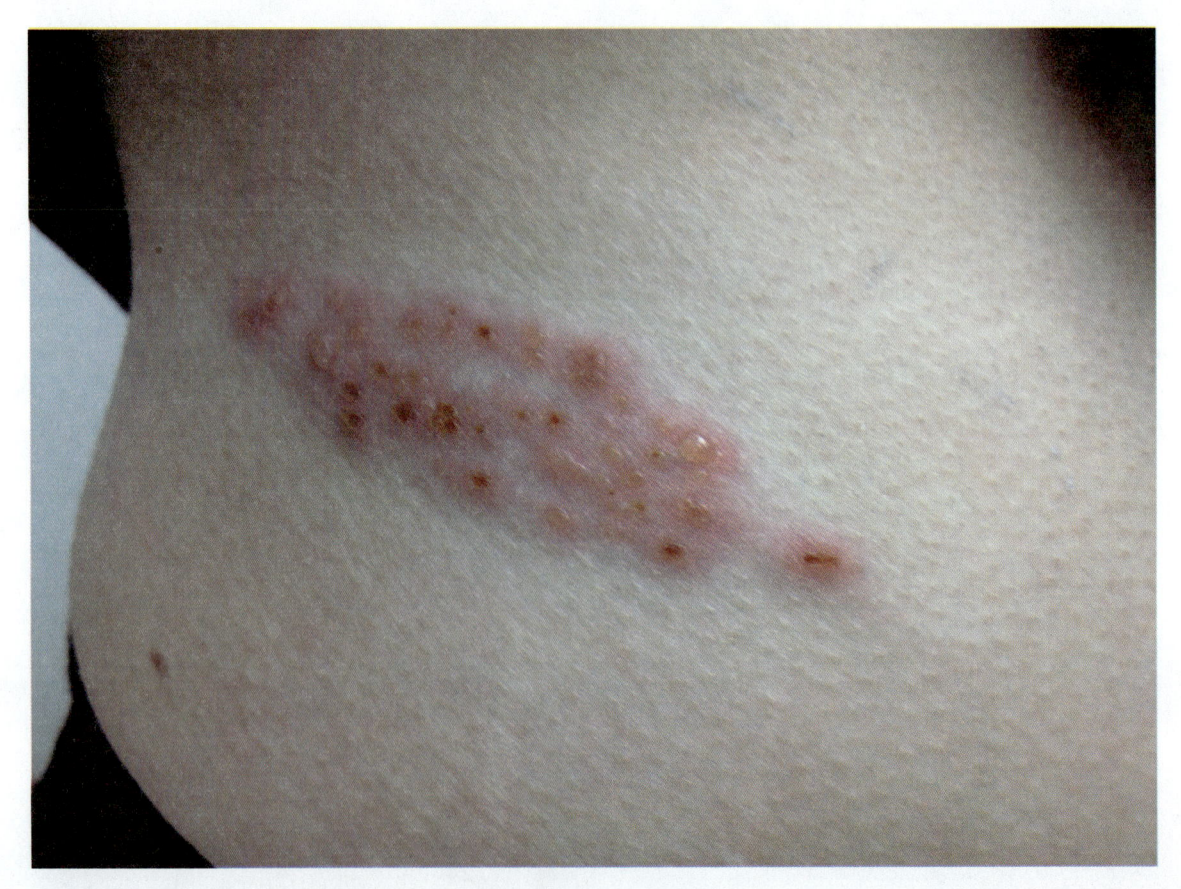

FIGURE III.28  Example of herpes zoster infection

## EPIDEMIOLOGY

Persons who have had previous infections with VZV (either by natural infection or varicella vaccination) may develop shingles. Approximately 99.5% of people born in the United States who are age 40 and older have had varicella. An estimated 500,000 to 1 million episodes of zoster occur annually in the United States. In 2000, the incidence of herpes zoster was approximately 4 per 1,000 in the U.S. population. The lifetime incident rate of developing herpes zoster is 10% to 20% (Centers for Disease Control and Prevention, 2012b; Jacobsen & Hull, 2013; Janniger, 2013).

## PATHOLOGY/HISTOLOGY

VZV infection gives rise to two distinct syndromes. The primary infection, chickenpox, is a contagious and usually benign febrile illness. After this infection resolves, viral particles remain in the dorsal root or other sensory ganglia, where they may lay dormant for years to decades. When host immunologic mechanisms suppressing replication of the virus fail to contain the virus, VZV reactivates (Janniger, 2013).

Once VZV is activated at the spinal root or cranial nerve neurons, an inflammatory response occurs that includes the leptomeninges. This inflammation in the dorsal root ganglion can be accompanied by hemorrhagic necrosis of the nerve cell, which results in neuronal loss and fibrosis. The frequency of dermatologic involvement correlates with the centripetal distribution of the primary varicella lesions. This pattern suggests that the latency may be from nearby spread of the virus during varicella from infected skin cells to sensory nerve endings, with successive ascent to the ganglia. Instead, the ganglia may become infected hematogenously during the viremic phase of varicella, and the frequency of the dermatome involvement in herpes zoster may reflect the ganglia most often exposed to reactivating stimuli (James et al., 2006; Janniger, 2013).

The appearance of the cutaneous rash as a result of zoster coincides with a profound VZV-specific T-cell proliferation. Production of interferon alfa appears with the resolution of zoster. In immunocompetent patients, specific antibodies (immunoglobulins G, M, and A [IgG, IgM, and IgA, respectively]) appear more rapidly and reach higher titers during reactivation (herpes zoster) than during the primary infection. The patient has a long-lasting, enhanced, cell-mediated immunity response to VZV (James et al., 2006; Janniger, 2013).

## CLINICAL PRESENTATION

The presenting clinical manifestations of zoster are usually characterized by rash and acute neuritis. The rash starts as erythematous papules, which rapidly transforms into vesicles or bullae. Within a few days, these vesicular lesions become more pustular or may hemorrhage. In healthy individuals, the lesions crust by 7 to 10 days and are no longer considered contagious. The development of new lesions more than a week after initial presentation should raise concern of underlying immunodeficiency. Scarring and hypopigmentation or hyperpigmentation can last months to years after the infection has cleared (Albrecht, 2013; Jacobsen & Hull, 2013; James et al., 2006; Janniger, 2013).

Zoster usually affects one dermatome, but the two or three neighboring dermatomes may also be affected. The thoracic and lumbar areas are the most common sites for zoster. The following are signs and symptoms (Jacobsen & Hull, 2013; Janniger, 2013):

- Scattered erythema can occur, with possible induration in the dermatome involved.
- Regional lymphadenopathy can occur.

- Grouped herpetiform vesicles can appear on an erythematous base.
- Pain in the dermatomal area of involvement can arise. It may be mild or change in character and intensity with the onset of other symptoms. Many patients describe the pain as burning, throbbing, or stabbing in nature.
- Vesicles initially are clear but eventually cloud, rupture, crust, and involute, a process that is accelerated by treatment.
- The remaining erythematous plaques follow a slow resolution. However, the pain may persist. This is called postherpetic neuralgia (PHN), which is usually confined to the area of original dermatomal involvement; can persist for weeks, months, or years; and is often severe.

## DIFFERENTIAL DIAGNOSIS

In addition to the differential diagnosis, other conditions that should be considered include the following (Janniger, 2013):

- Abscess
- Acne keloidalisnuchae
- Acneiform eruptions
- Angina
- Aphthous stomatitis
- Atopic dermatitis
- Atypical measles
- Back pain
- Bell's palsy
- Candidiasis, mucosal
- Cellulitis
- Cholecystitis and biliary colic
- Conjunctivitis
- Contact dermatitis, allergic
- Contact dermatitis, irritant
- Contact stomatitis
- Corneal ulceration and ulcerative keratitis
- Cowpox infection, human
- Coxsackievirus infection
- Cystitis
- Dental infection or abscess
- Ecthyma
- Eczema
- Erysipelas
- Erysipeloid
- Folliculitis
- Furunculosis
- Herpangina
- Herpes simplex
- Insect bites
- Jellyfish stings
- Leptomeningitis
- Lichen striatus
- Malignant and nonmalignant pain syndromes
- Ménière disease

- Myelitis
- Renal calculi
- Spinal nerve compression
- Stroke
- Superficial pyoderma
- Syphilis
- Trigeminal neuralgia
- Varicella
- Vestibular neuronitis

## TREATMENT/MANAGEMENT

Diagnosis of herpes zoster is usually based on history and clinical examination. Systemic manifestations are uncommon and usually confined to patients in whom the immune system has been compromised (James et al., 2006; Janniger, 2013).

For most patients, confirming the diagnosis with laboratory testing has no benefit. In some patient populations, however, the appearance of herpes zoster can be unusual and may require additional testing, such as the following (Jacobsen & Hull, 2013; James et al., 2006; Janniger, 2013):

- A malignancy workup may be called for because zoster has been considered a herald of other occult disease. Patients with malignancies, especially Hodgkin disease and leukemia, are five times more likely to develop herpes zoster than are their age-matched peers. Approximately 3% of pediatric zoster cases occur in children with malignancies. A malignancy workup is not indicated in an otherwise healthy child who has herpes zoster, however.
- The Tzanck smear is simple and inexpensive. It is used to test for VZV and other herpes viruses. The Tzanck smear confirms that the lesion is herpetic but does not differentiate the herpes viruses.
- When acute diagnostic confirmation is desired, modern tests, such as direct fluorescent antibody (DFA) testing or PCR (if available), are preferred to the Tzanck smear. DFA testing of vesicular fluid or a corneal lesion can yield the VZV antigen. Both DFA and PCR have greater sensitivity and specificity than the Tzanck smear and allow differentiation between HSV and VZV infections.
- Herpes zoster is seen approximately seven times more frequently in patients with HIV infection; therefore, when clinically indicated, an HIV test should be ordered.

Treatment recommendations for VZV are as follows:

- Antivirals
  - According to Jacobsen and Hull (2013) and Janniger (2013), many studies have found acyclovir and its derivatives (valacyclovir, famciclovir, and penciclovir) to be safe and effective in treating active disease and preventing PHN. Acyclovir is dosed at 800 mg five times per day for 7 to 10 days; valacyclovir is dosed at 1,000 mg three times daily for 7 days; and famciclovir is dosed at 500 mg three times daily for 7 days.
  - Albrecht (2013) and Dworkin et al. (2007) recommended the use of acyclovir, valacyclovir, or famciclovir for patients 50 years of age or older with uncomplicated herpes zoster who present within 72 hours of clinical symptoms (Grade 2C). The benefit of antiviral therapy in younger patients is not as clear, although the risk of adverse events is low. Valacyclovir (1,000 mg three times per day for 7 days) was preferred over the others.

- Steroids
    - Albrecht (2013) does not recommend the routine use of steroids with antivirals because steroids do not decrease the risk of PHN (Grade 1B).
    - Dworkin et al. (2007) recommend the use of steroids as soon as possible after diagnosis for patients with moderately severe pain and no contraindications.
    - Janniger (2013) recommends a large dose (40–60 mg every morning) given as soon as possible and continued for 1 week, followed by a quick taper over 2 weeks. In view of the potential adverse effects of and contraindications to corticosteroid use, it has been suggested that these agents be limited to cases of moderate to severe zoster pain or cases in which significant neurologic symptoms (e.g., facial paralysis) or central nervous system involvement is present and when the use of corticosteroids is not otherwise contraindicated.
- Gabapentin
    - Dworkin et al. (2007) states that gabapentin and pregabalin can both be used and that, if used in the first 2 weeks of rash onset, they can provide the greatest benefit of treatment for pain.
- Therapeutic Interventions
    - Jacobsen and Hull (2013) and Janniger (2013) recommend nonsteroidal anti-inflammatory drugs; wet dressings with 5% aluminum acetate (Burow solution), applied for 30 to 60 minutes four to six times daily; and lotions (such as calamine).
    - Most patients with acute herpes zoster experience pain. Efforts should be made to reduce patients' pain and suffering, even if opioid therapy is required. Nonpharmacologic modalities that may be used for acute zoster-associated pain include sympathetic, intrathecal, and epidural nerve blocks and percutaneous electrical nerve stimulation.

## SPECIAL CONSIDERATIONS

Immunocompromised patients, such as transplant patients and HIV-infected individuals with advanced disease, are at increased risk for developing complicated herpes zoster infections (Albrecht, 2013). In immunocompromised persons, zoster may disseminate, causing generalized skin lesions and central nervous system, pulmonary, and hepatic involvement (Centers for Disease Control and Prevention, 2012a). Herpes zoster is rare in children and young adults, except in younger patients with AIDS, lymphoma, other malignancies, and other immune deficiencies and in patients who have received bone marrow or kidney transplants. Fewer than 10% of zoster patients are younger than 20 years, and only 5% are younger than 15 years. Although zoster is primarily a disease of adults, it has been noted as early as the first week of life, occurring in infants born to mothers who had primary VZV infection (chickenpox) during pregnancy (Albrecht, 2013).

Pain is the most common symptom of zoster. Approximately 75% of patients have prodromal pain in the dermatome where the rash will appear. Prodromal pain may be constant or intermittent and can precede the rash by days or weeks. As noted earlier, most patients describe the pain as a deep burning, throbbing, or stabbing sensation. Some patients complain of the pain only when the area is lightly touched (allodynia; Albrecht, 2013).

PHN is the most common complication of herpes zoster. It is a chronic pain in the area where the herpes zoster occurred and can last for weeks, months, or even years. Older adults are at higher risk for PHN that lasts longer and is more painful (Centers for Disease Control and Prevention, 2012b; Jacobsen & Hull, 2013; James et al., 2006). Other complications of herpes zoster include the following (Centers for Disease Control and Prevention, 2012b):

- Ophthalmic involvement with acute or chronic ocular sequelae (herpes zoster ophthalmicus) can occur.
- Bacterial superinfection of the lesions, usually caused by *Streptococcus aureus* or group A beta-hemolytic *Streptococcus*, is a possibility.
- Cranial and peripheral nerve palsies can occur.
- Visceral involvement, such as meningoencephalitis, pneumonitis, hepatitis, and acute retinal necrosis can occur.
- Zoster can be a presenting symptom of hyperparathyroidism, and it occurs twice as often (frequency, 3.7%) among patients older than 40 years with hypercalcemia as it does among age-matched cohorts of patients who have normal calcium levels.

Approximately 1% to 4% of people with herpes zoster get hospitalized for complications. Older adults and people with compromised or suppressed immune systems are more likely to get hospitalized. In fact, about 30% of all people hospitalized with herpes zoster are those with compromised or suppressed immune systems. Approximately 25% of patients with HIV and 7% to 9% of those receiving renal transplantation or cardiac transplantation experience a bout of zoster.

## WHEN TO REFER

The following situations warrant quick referral to ophthalmology; neurology; or an ear, nose, and throat specialist (Albrecht, 2013; Jacobsen & Hull, 2013):

- Herpes zoster ophthalmicus is a serious sight-threatening condition. The frontal branch with the first division of the trigeminal nerve is the most frequently involved. Clinicians should also be aware that vesicular lesions on the nose are associated with a high risk of herpes zoster ophthalmicus (Hutchinson sign). Early diagnosis is critical to prevent progressive corneal involvement and potential loss of vision. Zoster has been implicated as the leading causative pathogen of acute retinal necrosis and has been described in patients with a history of herpes encephalitis.
- Herpes zoster oticus (Ramsay Hunt syndrome) typically includes a triad of ipsilateral facial paralysis, ear pain, and vesicles in the auditory canal and auricle. Taste perception, hearing, and lacrimation are affected in selected patients. Ramsey–Hunt syndrome is generally considered a polycranial neuropathy with frequent involvement of cranial nerves V, IX, and X. Vestibular disturbances (vertigo) are also frequently reported.
- Other referable conditions:
  - Aseptic meningitis
  - Peripheral motor neuropathy
  - Myelitis
  - Encephalitis
  - Guillain-Barré syndrome
  - Stroke syndrome (secondary to infection of the cerebral arteries)
  - Bacterial infections

## PATIENT EDUCATION

Careful explanation of the disease, including risk of viral transmission to individuals who have not had chickenpox, and the proposed treatment plan are essential for adherence to therapy (Dworkin et al., 2007). People with active herpes zoster lesions should avoid contact with the following susceptible people (Centers for Disease Control and Prevention, 2012b):

- Pregnant women
- Those who have never had chickenpox or the varicella vaccine
- All premature infants born to susceptible mothers
- Infants born at less than 28 weeks gestation or weighing less than 1,000 grams
- People of all ages who have compromised or suppressed immune systems, such as those with cancer (especially leukemia and lymphoma) or HIV infection; those who have undergone bone marrow or solid organ transplantation; and those taking immunosuppressive medications, including steroids, chemotherapy, or transplant-related immunosuppressive medications

In 2006, the herpes zoster vaccine (Zostavax), was approved by the Food and Drug Administration for prevention of zoster in adults aged 60 and older. Since then, this vaccine has also been approved for individuals aged 50 and older if other comorbidities exist (Jacobsen & Hull, 2013).

## CLINICAL PEARLS

- Herpes zoster: ICD-9, 0.53; ICD-10, B02
- Herpes zoster is most common on the trunk, followed by the head (Fitzpatrick & Morelli, 2011).
- Five percent of patients with herpes zoster will have a recurrence (Fitzpatrick & Morelli, 2011).
- If not treated with antivirals, up to 50% of patients will develop ocular complications (Habif et al., 2011).
- PHN causes great morbidity (Wolff et al., 2013).
- If gabapentin is taken with valacyclovir within 72 hours of disease, it may significantly reduce the pain associated with herpes zoster (Goodheart, 2011).

# VARICELLA

## OVERVIEW

Varicella is an acute infectious disease caused by VZV. VZV is a DNA virus, a member of the herpesvirus group, and has the ability to remain in the sensory nerve ganglia as a latent infection after the primary infection has resolved (Bechtel, 2012; Centers for Disease Control and Prevention, 2012a; James et al., 2006).

## ETIOLOGY

The infectious particles of VZV are cell-free virus particles derived from skin lesions or the respiratory tract. Transmission occurs mainly through respiratory droplets that contain the virus, making the disease highly contagious even before the rash appears. Direct person-to-person contact with lesions also spreads the virus. Papules and vesicles, but not the crusts, have high populations of the virus. In addition, maternal varicella with viremia can spread to the fetus transplacentally. This leads to neonatal varicella. Risk factors for severe varicella in the neonate are as follows: A neonate's first month of life is a susceptible period for severe varicella, especially if the mother is seronegative. Delivery of an infant before 28 weeks gestation also renders a baby susceptible because transplacental transfer of immunoglobulin G (IgG) antibodies occurs after this time.

Risk factors for severe varicella in children, adolescents, and adults are as follows:

- Steroid therapy: High doses (i.e., doses equivalent to 1–2 mg/kg/day of prednisolone) for 2 weeks or more are definite risk factors for severe disease. Even short-term therapy at these doses immediately preceding or during the incubation period of varicella can cause severe or fatal varicella.
- Malignancy: All children with cancer have an increased risk for severe varicella. The risk is highest for children with leukemia. Almost 30% of patients who are immunocompromised and who have leukemia have visceral dissemination of varicella; 7% may die.
- Other immunocompromised states (e.g., antimalignancy drugs, HIV, or other congenital or acquired immunodeficient conditions): Defects of cellular but not humoral immunodeficiency are believed to render a person susceptible to severe varicella.
- Pregnancy: Pregnant women have high risk of severe varicella particularly the complication of varicella-induced pneumonia.

## EPIDEMIOLOGY

Before the varicella vaccine was available in the United States, the disease affected about 4 million children per year, caused approximately 100 deaths in children annually, and cost an estimated $400 million in medical costs and lost wages each year. In 1995, the varicella vaccine became available, and the disease was significantly decreased (Figure III.29). National seroprevalence data for 1988 through 1994 indicated that by age 40, 99.6% people were immune to varicella (Bechtel, 2012).

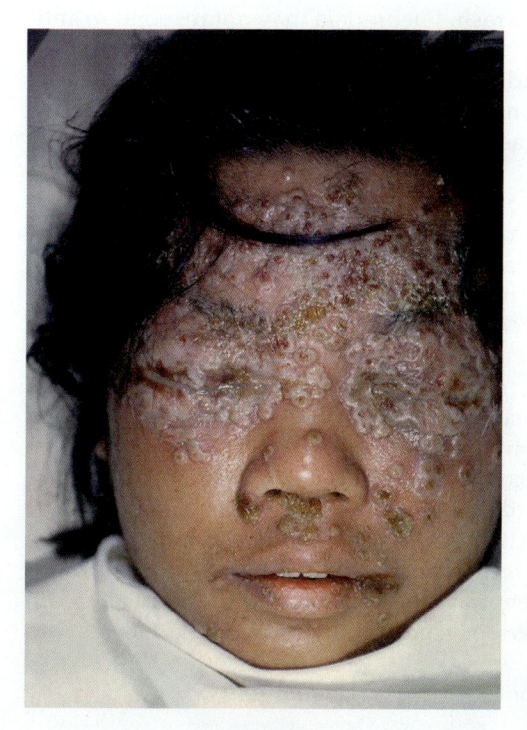

FIGURE III.29 Although the introduction of the varicella vaccine in 1995 has greatly reduced the incidence of the disease, some individuals do have skin reactions to the vaccine.
Courtesy of Allen W. Mathies, MDCDC

## PATHOLOGY/HISTOLOGY

VZV enters through the respiratory tract and conjunctiva. The virus replicates in the nasopharynx and in regional lymph nodes. A primary viremia occurs 4 to 6 days after infection and spreads the virus to other organs, such as the liver, spleen, and sensory ganglia. The virus continues to replicate and a secondary viremia occurs in which a skin rash appears. VZV can be cultured from an infected person 5 days before and 2 days after the rash is visible (Centers for Disease Control and Prevention, 2012a; James et al., 2006).

## CLINICAL PRESENTATION

The incubation period is 14 to 16 days after exposure, with a range of 10 to 21 days. In adults, a prodrome may occur 1 or 2 days before the outbreak with fever and malaise (Bechtel, 2012; Centers for Disease Control and Prevention, 2012a; James et al., 2006).

The pruritic rash is generalized and progresses rapidly from macules to papules to 1- to 4-mm vesicular lesions before crusting. The rash usually appears first on the head, then the trunk, and then the extremities. Most of the rash is concentrated onto the trunk. Lesions can also occur on mucous membranes of the oropharynx, respiratory tract, vagina, conjunctiva, and the cornea. The vesicles are superficial, delicate, and contain a clear fluid with an erythematous base and may rupture or become purulent before they dry and crust. Groups of lesions appear over several days, with lesions present in several stages of development (Bechtel, 2012; Centers for Disease Control and Prevention, 2012a; James et al., 2006).

Healthy children may have mild fever, achiness, and itchiness for 2 to 3 days. However, adults usually have more symptoms and have a higher occurrence of complications (Centers for Disease Control and Prevention, 2012a; James et al., 2006).

Complications of varicella include:

- Viral pneumonia primarily occurs in older children and adults. Respiratory symptoms usually appear 3 to 4 days after the rash. Pneumonia may not respond to antiviral therapy and can lead to death.
- Varicella causes increased risk for secondary bacterial infection. Symptoms of a bacterial infection are not recognized during the first few days because of the active varicella infection. Complications such as cellulitis, impetigo, septicemia, and other serious infections can occur.
- The most common infectious organisms are Group A streptococci and *S. aureus*. Varicella places the patient at high risk for acquiring invasive Group A streptococcal disease, which may cause toxic shock syndrome. Group A streptococci may also cause necrotizing fasciitis, bacteremia, osteomyelitis, pyomyositis, gangrene, subgaleal abscess, arthritis, and meningitis in patients with varicella.
- Acute postinfectious cerebellar ataxia is the most common neurologic complication and has a sudden onset that usually occurs 2 to 3 weeks after the onset of varicella. Symptoms may range from mild unsteadiness to complete inability to stand and walk, with accompanying incoordination and dysarthria. This condition may persist for 2 months. The prognosis for total recovery is good, but a few patients may have residual ataxia, incoordination, or dysarthria.
- Encephalitis occurs in 1.7 patients per 100,000 cases of varicella among otherwise healthy children aged 1 to 14 years. A few days after rash onset, lethargy, drowsiness, and confusion can occur. Children may have seizures, and encephalitis can rapidly progress to deep coma. This serious complication of varicella has a 5% to 20% mortality rate.

- Other neurologic complications include aseptic meningitis, myelitis (including Guillain-Barré syndrome), polyradiculitis, and meningoencephalitis.
- Approximately 5% of children with varicella develop otitis media.
- Hepatitis may occur with varicella but resolves when rash clears. Liver involvement is independent of the severity of skin and systemic manifestations.
- Retinitis and optic neuritis are rare complications of varicella in children who are immunocompetent.
- Other reported complications include glomerulonephritis, hemorrhagic varicella, thrombocytopenia, myocarditis, appendicitis, pancreatitis, Henoch-Schonleinpurpura, orchitis, iritis, and keratitis. (Bechtel, 2012)

## DIFFERENTIAL DIAGNOSIS

Conditions and differential diagnoses is that should be considered in the diagnosis of pediatric varicella include the following (Bechtel, 2012):

- Contact dermatitis
- Dermatitis herpetiformis
- Drug reactions
- Eczema herpeticum
- Encephalitis
- Enteroviralinfections
- Henoch-Schonleinpurpura
- Herpes simplex virus infection
- Herpes zoster
- Impetigo
- Insect bites
- Measles
- Meningococcemia (can be confused with hemorrhagic varicella)
- Other common viral exanthems (e.g., coxsackievirus, echovirus)
- Papularurticaria
- Pediatrics, hand–foot–mouth disease
- Scabies
- Smallpox (no cases since 1949; virus officially eradicated in 1996)
- Stevens–Johnson syndrome
- Toxic shock syndrome
- Urticaria

## TREATMENT/MANAGEMENT

Imaging and laboratory testing is usually not needed in VZV unless secondary complications occur or if confirmation of disease is needed. A Tzanck smear is done by scraping the base of the lesions and then staining the scrapings to show multinucleated giant cells. Multinucleated giant cells suggest a herpes virus infection but are not specific for VZV. Polymerase chain reaction is the method of choice for diagnosis of varicella (Bechtel, 2012; Centers for Disease Control and Prevention, 2012a).

Treatment approaches include symptom management antiviral therapy, administration of varicella-zoster immune globulin, and management of secondary bacterial infection. Other treatments are as follows:

- Pruritus can be controlled with cool compresses, regular bathing with oatmeal or cornstarch, topical calamine lotion, and antihistamines.

- Acetaminophen is recommended for fever reduction.
- The routine use of acyclovir in healthy children is not universally recommended. Intravenous acyclovir is recommended only for the treatment of varicella in immunocompromised children or in healthy children with varicella pneumonia or encephalitis. (Bechtel, 2012)

## SPECIAL CONSIDERATIONS

The risks of complications from varicella include the following (Bechtel, 2012; Centers for Disease Control and Prevention, 2012a):

- Immunocompromised individuals have a high risk of severe disease. These people may have multiple organ system involvement, and the disease may become fulminant and hemorrhagic. The most frequent complications in this group are pneumonia and encephalitis.
- The onset of maternal varicella from 5 days before to 2 days after delivery may result in overwhelming infection of the neonate and a fatality rate as high as 30%. This is the result of fetal exposure to the varicella virus without the benefit of passive maternal antibody.
- High doses of steroids (i.e., doses equivalent to 1 to 2 mg/kg/day of prednisolone) immediately preceding or during the incubation period of varicella can cause severe or fatal varicella.
- All children with cancer have an increased risk for severe varicella. The risk is highest for children with leukemia.
- Defects of cellular but not humoral immunodeficiency are believed to render a person susceptible to severe varicella.

  Pregnant women have high risk of severe varicella, especially varicella pneumonia.

## WHEN TO REFER

Patients with varicella may require hospitalization if these symptoms develop (Bechtel, 2012).

- Abnormal erythema, swelling, or pain over an area of the rash
- Refusal or inability to drink fluids
- Signs of dehydration, such as scanty and yellow-colored urine, increasing drowsiness, dry mouth and lips, excessive thirst, or lethargy
- Confusion, irritability, drowsiness, or difficulty waking
- Inability to walk or unusual weakness
- Complaints of severe headache, stiff neck, and/or back pain
- Frequent vomiting
- Difficulty breathing, chest pain, wheezing, fast breathing, or severe cough
- Fever persisting more than 4 days or fever that returns after varicella has resolved

## PATIENT EDUCATION

Parents should be instructed to bathe the affected child regularly to reduce itching and prevent secondary infection. To prevent scratching, the child's fingernails should be kept short, mittens or socks may be worn on the hands at night, and medication for itching can be given as needed. Aspirin-containing medications should not be used (Bechtel, 2012).

Those affected with VZV should avoid nonimmune pregnant women, unimmunized young infants, and others with immunodeficiencies or who are taking prednisone long term. Children with chickenpox may not return to school or day care until all lesions are crusted over (Bechtel, 2012).

## CLINICAL PEARLS

- Varicella: ICD-9, 052; ICD-10, B01
- Varicella is the primary infection with VZV (Brice, 2011).
- In varicella, lesions are present at different stages, and the majority are located on the trunk (Habif et al., &2011).
- Varicella is a highly contagious disease.
- Primary disease is symptomatic (Wolff et al., 2013).
- Adults with primary infection can develop the complications of pneumonia and encephalitis (Wolff et al., 2013).

## REFERENCES

Albrecht, M. A. (2013). *Epidemiology, clinical manifestations, and diagnosis of genital herpes simplex virus infection*. Retrieved from http://www.uptodate.com/contents/epidemiology-clinical-manifestations-and-diagnosis-of-genital-herpes-simplex-virus-infection

Bechtel, K. A. (2012, December 28). *Pediatric chickenpox*. Retrieved from http://emedicine.medscape.com/article/969773-overview

Brice, S. (2011). Bullous viral eruptions. In J. Fitzpatrick & J. Morelli. *Dermatology secrets plus* (4th ed.). Philadelphia, PA: Elsevier/Saunders.

Centers for Disease Control and Prevention. (2012a). *Varicella. epidemiology and prevention of vaccine-preventable diseases. The pink book—Course textbook* (12th ed.). Retrieved from http://www.cdc.gov/vaccines/pubs/pinkbook/varicella.html

Centers for Disease Control and Prevention. (2012b). *Shingles clinical overview—Herpes zoster*. Retrieved from http://www.cdc.gov/shingles/hcp/clinical-overview.html

Dworkin, R. H., Johnson, R. W., Breuer, J., Gnann, J. W., Backonja, M., Betts, R. F., ... Whitley, R. J. (2007). *Recommendations for the management of herpes zoster*. Retrieved from http://guideline.gov/content.aspx?id=10222&search=herpes+zoster

Fitzpatrick, J. E., & Morelli, J. G. (2011). *Dermatology secrets plus* (4th ed.). Philadelphia, PA: Elsevier/Saunders.

Goodheart, H. (2011). *Goodheart's same-site differential diagnosis: A rapid method of diagnosing and treating common skin disorders*. Philadelphia, PA: Lippincott Williams & Wilkins.

Grimshaw-Mulcahy, L. J. (2007). Now I know my STDs. *Journal for Nurse Practitioners*, 641–649.

Habif, T., Campbell, J., Chapman, M., Dinulos, J., & Zug, K. (2011). *Skin disease diagnosis and treatment* (3rd ed.). Philadelphia, PA: Elsevier/Saunders.

Jacobsen, E., & Hull, C. E. (2013). Herpes zoster infection. *Clinician Reviews*, 42–49.

James, W. D., Berger, T. G., & Elston, D. M. (2006). *Andrews' diseases of the skin: Clinical dermatology* (10th ed.). Philadelphia, PA: Elsevier/Saunders.

Janniger, C. K. (2013, February 26). *Herpes zoster*. Retrieved from http://emedicine.medscape.com/article/1132465-overview

Klein, R. S. (2012). *Clinical manifestations and diagnosis of herpes simplex virus type 1 infection*. Retrieved from http://www.uptodate.com/contents/clinical-manifestations-and-diagnosis-of-herpes-simplex-virus-type-1-infection

Mahler, V. (2008). Herpes simplex. In H. Williams, M. Bigby, T. Diepgen, A. Herxheimer, L. Naldi, & B. Rzany (Eds.), *Evidence-based dermatology* (2nd ed., pp. 428–437). Malden, MA: Blackwell.

Mayo Clinic. (2012). *Cold sore*. Retrieved from http://www.mayoclinic/health/cold-sore/DS00358

Miller, J. L. (2011, April 13). *Dermatitis herpetiformis*. Retrieved from http://emedicine.medscape.com/article/1062640-overview

Omori, M. S. (2012, May 23). *Herpetic whitlow*. Retrieved from http://emedicine.medscape.com/article/788056-overview

Salvaggio, M. R. (2012, January 5). *Herpes simplex*. Retrieved from http://emedicine.medscape.com/article/218580-overview

Wolff, K., Johnson, R., & Saavedra, A. (2013). *Fitzpatrick's color atlas and synopsis of clinical dermatology* (7th ed.). Philadelphia, PA: McGraw-Hill Medical.

# Impetigo

Impetigo is an acute, contagious Gram-positive bacterial infection of the upper layers of the epidermis (Figure III.30). Impetigo arises near the site of *Staphylococcus aureus* colonization, for example, in the nares (Wolff, Johnson, & Saavedra, 2013). Impetigo affects children most often, usually those living in warm, moist climates. Impetigo accounts for 50% to 60% of all bacterial skin infections. Impetigo is a result of a disruption of the environmental factors that protect the skin (Feaster & Singer, 2010).

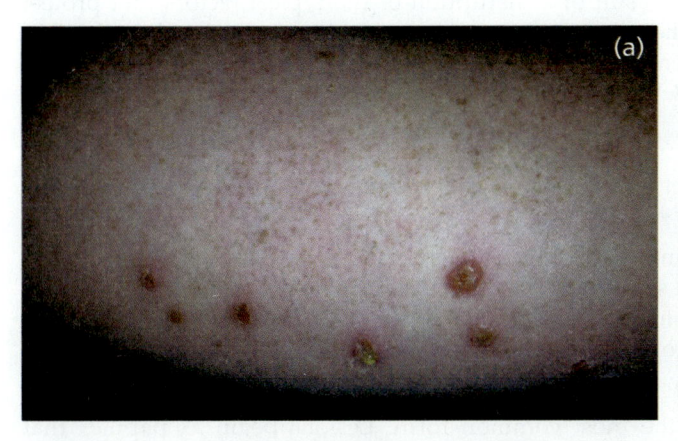

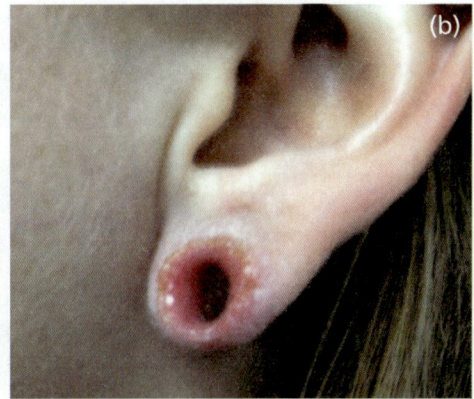

FIGURE III.30  Examples of impetigo on a child's **(a)** arm and **(b)** ear

## EPIDEMIOLOGY

Impetigo is responsible for 10% of dermatology conditions that are seen in pediatric clinics. This condition occurs more in the southeastern United States because impetigo thrives on hot, humid climates (Lewis, 2013).

Impetigo can affect people of all races. Overall, the incidence of impetigo in males and females is equal. The infection affects individuals of all ages but most frequently occurs in children 2 to 5 years of age. Day-care centers, nurseries, and grade schools are significant sources for the spread of impetigo. Bullous impetigo is most common in newborns and infants (Lewis, 2013).

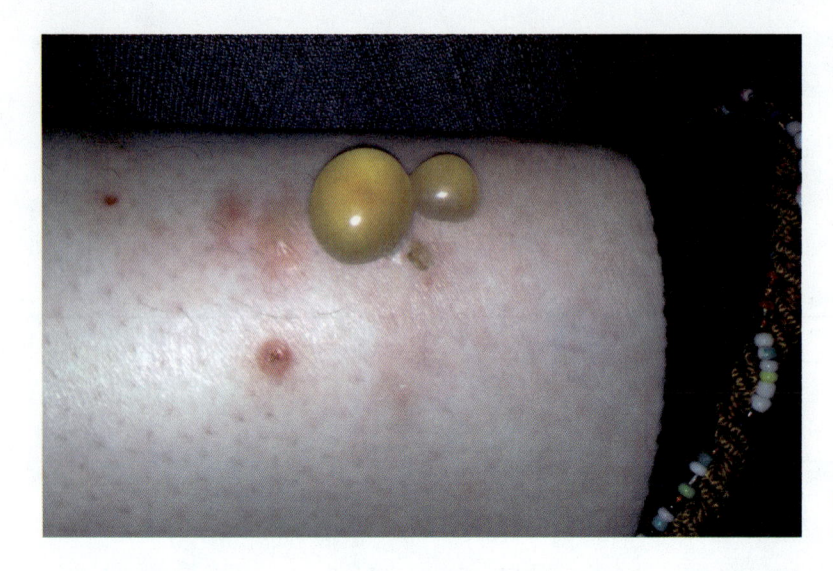

FIGURE III.31  Bullous impetigo

## PATHOLOGY/HISTOLOGY

The principal pathogen of impetigo is *S. aureus*; however, beta-hemolytic streptococci infection can also occur, either alone or in combination with *S. aureus* (Baddour, 2012; Morelli, 2011). Impetigo is a result of a disruption of the typical factors that protect the skin against invasion. The primary cause of impetigo involves a break in the skin caused by trauma or as a secondary cause resulting from another etiology (i.e., dermatitis, herpes zoster; Feaster & Singer, 2010; Lewis, 2013).

## CLINICAL PRESENTATION

Impetigo can be classified into two categories: primary impetigo (direct invasion of bacteria to normal skin) and secondary impetigo (infection at the site of minor trauma or underlying skin conditions such as eczema; Baddour, 2012). Variants of impetigo include nonbullous impetigo, bullous impetigo, and ecthyma (Baddour, 2012; Lewis, 2013; Popovich & McAlhany, 2008):

- Nonbullous impetigo is the most common form. Lesions begin as papules that progress to vesicles surrounded by erythema, then they become pustules that enlarge and break down to form thick, adherent, honey-colored crust. This process usually occurs over about 1 week. Lesions generally involve the face and extremities. Multiple lesions tend to be well localized and regional lymphadenopathy may occur.
- Bullous impetigo (Figure III.31) is a form of impetigo seen in young children in which vesicles enlarge to form flaccid bullae (2–5 mm) with clear yellow fluid, which later becomes darker and more turbid; ruptured bullae leave a thin brown crust. Usually there are fewer lesions than in nonbullous impetigo, and the trunk is more frequently involved.
- Ecthyma is an ulcerative form of impetigo in which lesions extend through the epidermis and deep into the dermis. They consist of "punched-out" ulcers covered with yellow crust surrounded by raised violaceous margins.

# DIFFERENTIAL DIAGNOSIS

Alternative diagnostic possibilities to consider are as follows (Lewis, 2013):

- Atopic dermatitis in emergency medicine
- Bullous—fixed drug reaction
- Bullous lupus erythematosus
- Bullous pemphigoid reactions
- Bullous scabies
- Burns, chemical
- Candidiasis in emergency medicine
- Contact dermatitis
- Cutaneous candidiasis
- Dermatitis herpetiformis
- Dermatophytic infections
- Discoid lupus erythematosus
- Erysipelas
- Follicular mucinosis
- Herpes simplex virus infection
- Herpetic impetigo
- Inflammatory dermatophytosis
- Insect bites
- Kerion
- Linear immunoglobulin A bullous dermatosis
- Pediculosis (lice)
- Pemphigus vulgaris (rare in children)
- Scabies
- Staphylococcal scalded skin syndrome in emergency medicine
- Sweet syndrome (acute febrile neutrophilic dermatosis)
- Tinea
- Varicella-zoster virus

# TREATMENT/MANAGEMENT

The diagnosis of impetigo is made on the bases of clinical characteristics. Cultures of pus or bullae fluid may be warranted in patients who fail to respond to treatment with antibiotics to rule out methicillin-resistant *S. aureus* (MRSA). Serologic testing for streptococcal antibodies is not useful for the diagnosis of impetigo but can be helpful in impetigo with associated poststreptococcal glomerulonephritis (Baddour, 2012).

Treatments for impetigo include the following:

- Topical antibiotics: Baddour (2012), Feaster and Singer (2010), Koning et al. (2009), and Popovich and McAlhany (2008) have recommended that topical therapy be administered if there are a limited number of lesions without bullae. The topical drug of choice is mupirocin three times per day (Grade 1A) for 10 days. Reasonable alternatives include fusidic acid, retapamulin, and tetracycline. An alternative to topical antibiotics is hydrogen peroxide cream.
- Oral antibiotics: Baddour (2012), Koning et al. (2009), and Popovich and McAlhany (2008) recommend that oral antibiotics be used for impetigo when the lesions are bullous and when it is unfeasible to use a topical preparation because of extent or location of lesions. Recommended antibiotics include doxycycline, Keflex, or clindamycin (Grade 1B). Macrolides are not adequate because of increased resistance

among *Streptococcus pyogenes* and *S. aureus*. Bactrim DS is active against MRSA but does not have activity against *streptococci*. Seven days of treatment are usually effective but follow-up is recommended.

Follow-up in 1 week is important to ensure complete clearing of lesions. If the lesions have not improved, bacterial culture and sensitivity should be done (Lewis, 2013).

## SPECIAL CONSIDERATIONS

- Impetigo is the most common bacterial skin infection in children (Habif, Campbell, Chapman, Dinulos, & Zug, 2011).
- While collecting a superficial bacterial culture keep in mind that a higher concentration of bacteria may be found at the area of maximal inflammation (Spates, 2011).
- Systemic symptoms of impetigo are infrequent (Habif et al., 2011).
- Children (especially aged 2–4 years) may experience the rare complication of post-streptococcal glomerulonephritis 1 to 5 weeks after impetigo infection (Habif et al., 2011).

## WHEN TO REFER

The age of the patient and the extent of the impetigo determine the need for consultation. Newborns with bullous impetigo may require a consult with a neonatologist. Recurrent impetigo is uncommon and should be evaluated by dermatology or infectious disease. If signs of acute glomerulonephritis develop, consult a nephrologist (Lewis, 2013).

## PATIENT EDUCATION

Parental education is important in the prevention and successful treatment of impetigo. Promote good hand washing with antibacterial soap, and keep fingernails trimmed. Nasal *S. aureus* has been implicated in recurrent impetigo, so parents should consistently encourage the use of tissues. Children infected with impetigo should not bathe together, share towels, or have skin-to-skin contact (Popovich & McAlhany, 2008).

Instruct patients to avoid contact with newborn babies, the elderly, and pregnant women, especially if MRSA is involved. Patients should be discouraged from visiting hospitals or nursing homes until the infection is resolved (Zajac & Jacobson, 2009).

## CLINICAL PEARLS

- Impetigo: ICD-9, 686.80; ICD-10, B08.0
- The majority of cutaneous erosions with honey-colored crusts are not impetigo (Wolff et al., 2013).
- Impetigo is typically asymptomatic and painless (Habif et al., 2011).
- If infectious skin lesions do not improve with treatment for *S. aureus*, diagnosis of MRSA must be considered (Goodheart, 2011).

# REFERENCES

Baddour, L. M. (2012). *Impetigo*. Retrieved from http://www.uptodate.com/contents/impetigo

Feaster, T., & Singer, J. I. (2010). Topical therapies for impetigo. *Pediatric Emergency Care, 26*(3), 222–231.

Goodheart, H. (2011). *Goodheart's same-site differential diagnosis: A rapid method of diagnosing and treating common skin disorders*. Philadelphia, PA: Lippincott Williams & Wilkins.

Habif, T., Campbell, J., Chapman, M., Dinulos, J., & Zug, K. (2011). *Skin disease diagnosis and treatment* (3rd ed.). Philadelphia, PA: Elsevier/Saunders.

Koning, S., Verhagen, A. P., Van Suijiekom-Smit, L., Morris, A. D., Butler, C., & Van der Wouden, J. C. (2009). *Interventions for impetigo*. Retrieved from Cochrane Database of Systemic Reviews (00075320-100000000-02329)

Lewis, L. S. (2013, March 20). *Impetigo*. Retrieved from http://emedicine.medscape.com/article/965254-overview

Morelli, J. G. (2011). Pediatric dermatology. In J. E. Fitzpatrick & J. G. Morelli (4th ed.). *Dermatology secrets plus* (pp. 404–408). Philadelphia, PA: Elsevier/Saunders.

Popovich, D., & McAlhany, A. (2008). Accurately diagnosing commonly misdiagnosed circular rashes. *Dermatology Nursing, 20*(4), 294–300.

Spates, T. (2011). Diagnostic techniques. In J. E. Fitzpatrick & J. G. Morelli (4th ed.). *Dermatology secrets plus* (pp. 22–27). Philadelphia, PA: Elsevier/Saunders.

Wolff, K., Johnson, R., & Saavedra, A. (2013). *Fitzpatrick's color atlas and synopsis of clinical dermatology* (7th ed.). Philadelphia, PA: McGraw-Hill Medical.

Zajac, L., & Jacobson, A. (2009, July). Impetigo: Taking on a common skin infection. *Clinical Advisor*. Retrieved from http://www.clinicaladvisor.com/impetigo-taking-on-a-common-skin-infection/article/139474

# Insect Bites

## SCABIES

### OVERVIEW

Human *scabies* is a contagious disease caused by the mite *Sarcoptes scabiei* (Figure III.32). Also known as the itch mite, it is an oval-shaped, ventrally flattened mite with dorsal spines. The fertilized female burrows into the stratum corneum and deposits her eggs. Scabies spreads where there is frequent personal contact and sharing of personal items. Sensitization begins about 2 to 4 weeks after onset of infection (Andrews, McCarthy, Carapetis, & Currie, 2009; Habif, 2004; James, Berger, & Elston, 2006).

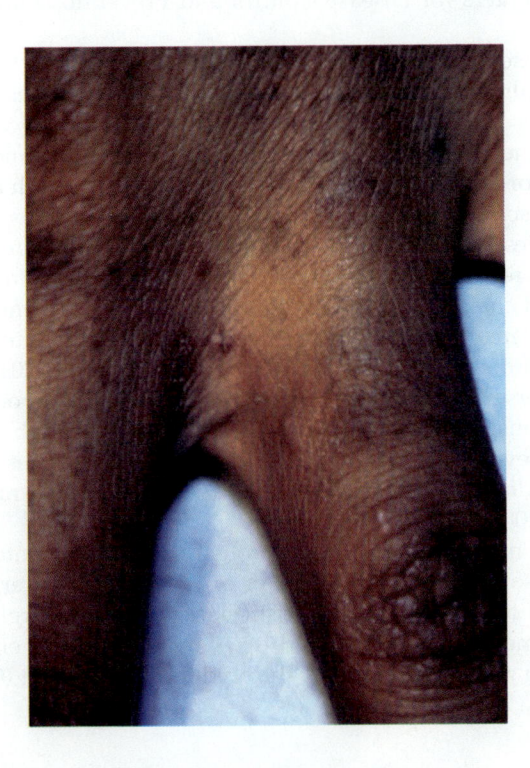

**FIGURE III.32** Scabies
Courtesy of J. Pledger, Centers for Disease Control (CDC)

## EPIDEMIOLOGY

Each year about 300 million cases of scabies occur worldwide, affecting people of all races and social classes. In developed countries, scabies epidemics are common in institutional settings, such as prisons; long-term care facilities, such as nursing homes; hospitals; and child care facilities (Centers for Disease Control and Prevention, 2010; Cordoro, 2012).

## PATHOLOGY/HISTOLOGY

Transmission of scabies occurs with prolonged contact with an infected individual. Scabies mites can live for 3 days away from human skin, so objects (bedding, clothing) can also be a source of transmission (Cordoro, 2012; Goldstein & Goldstein, 2011).

The mites live for 30 days within the human epidermis. After mating, the male mite dies, and the female mite burrows into the superficial skin layers and lays approximately 60 to 90 eggs, of which only 10% will mature. The ova take 10 days to progress through larval and nymph stages before becoming mature adult mites. Mites travel through the superficial layers of skin by secreting proteases that degrade the stratum corneum. They feed on dissolved tissue but do not ingest blood. Scybala (feces) are left behind as they travel through the epidermis, creating linear lesions clinically recognized as burrows. An affected individual harbors a variable number of living mites, typically less than 100 and usually no more than 10 to 15. The incubation period before onset of symptoms is dependent on whether the infestation is a new exposure or a relapse/reinfestation. Once initial infestation occurs, a delayed type IV hypersensitivity reaction to the mites, eggs, or scybala develops over the next 4 to 6 weeks. However, previously infested individuals may have symptoms within hours of reexposure. The intense pruritus caused by a hypersensitivity reaction is the clinical hallmark of the disease (Centers for Disease Control and Prevention, 2010; Cordoro, 2012; Habif, 2004).

In immunocompromised hosts, the weak immune response fails to control the disease and results in a fulminant hyperinfestation termed *crusted scabies*. Crusted scabies usually infects those with immunodeficiency disorders or a compromised ability to mount an immune response secondary to drug therapy. A modified host response may be a key factor in patients with malnutrition. Patients with motor nerve impairments are unable to scratch in response to the pruritus. The number of mites in a patient with crusted scabies can exceed 1 million. In these cases, the mite can survive off the host for up to 7 days, feeding on the sloughed skin in the local environment such as bed sheets, clothing, and chair covers. Failure to implement environmental control measures in this situation may result in relapse and reinfestation after successful treatment of the host (Centers for Disease Control and Prevention, 2010; Cordoro, 2012; Habif, 2004). A hypersensitivity reaction rather than a foreign-body response is responsible for the lesions, which may delay the diagnosis of scabies. Elevated immunoglobulin E titers develop in some patients infested with scabies, along with eosinophilia, and an immediate-type hypersensitivity reaction to an extract prepared from female mites (Habif, 2004; James et al., 2006).

Positive diagnosis is made only by the demonstration of the mite under the microscope. A burrow is sought, and the position of the mite is determined. The majority of mites are found on the hands and wrist (Figure III.33). A surgical blade or sterile needle is used to remove the parasite. A drop of mineral or immersion oil can be placed on the lesion then gently scrape away the epidermis beneath it (Goldstein & Goldstein, 2011; James et al., 2006).

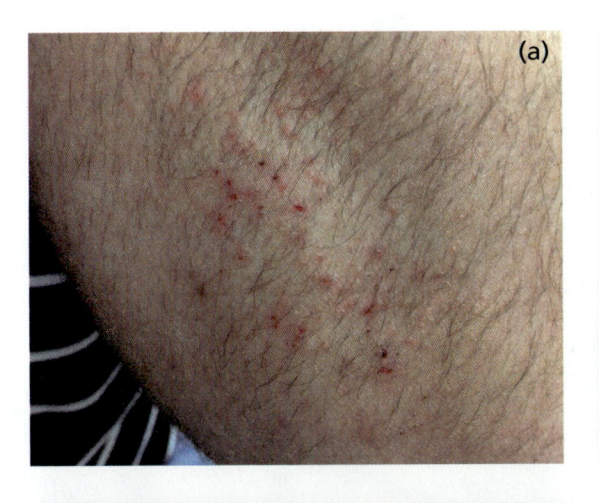

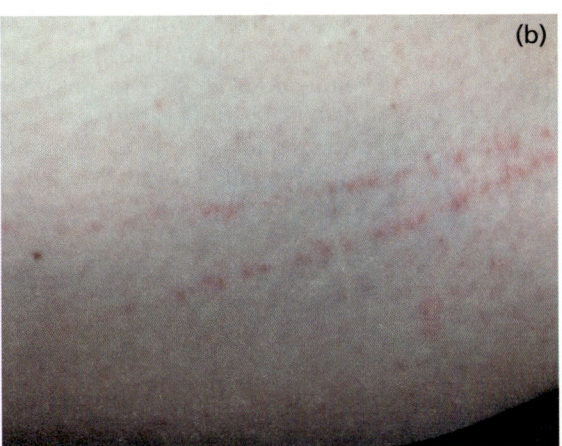

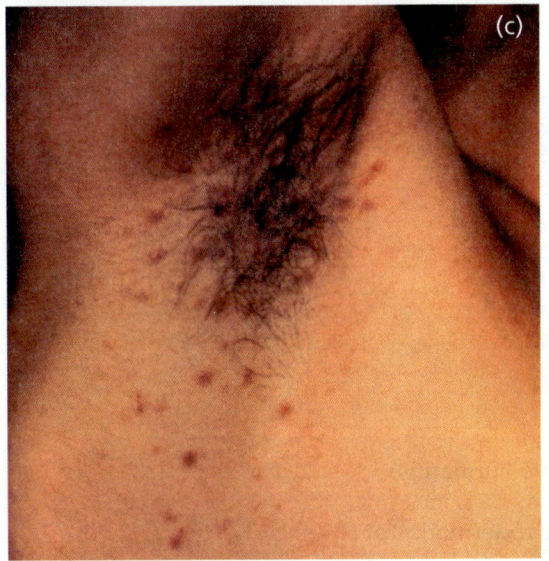

FIGURE III.33 (a and b) Scabies are often found on the arm. (c) Scabies in the axilla
Courtesy of Susan Lindsley, CDC

The histologic features of scabies are specific. If a burrow is excised, mites, larvae, ova, and feces may be seen within the stratum corneum. A superficial and deep dermal infiltrate comprised of lymphocytes, histiocytes, mast cells, and eosinophils is characteristic. Biopsy of older lesions is nondiagnostic, demonstrating only excoriation and scale crusts (Cordoro, 2012).

## CLINICAL PRESENTATION

Scabies is characterized by pruritic papular lesions, excoriation, and burrows. Sites of preference include the finger webs, wrists, axillae, areola, umbilicus, lower abdomen, genitals, and buttocks. In adults the scalp and face are spared, but in infants lesions are commonly present over the entire cutaneous surface. The burrows appear as slightly elevated, grayish, tortuous lines in the skin. A vesicle or pustule containing the mite may be present in the end of the burrow, especially in infants and children (Andrews et al., 2009; Centers for Disease Control and Prevention, 2010; Habif, 2004; James et al., 2006).

After initial contact (2–4 weeks) the parasites burrow into the skin without causing pruritus or discomfort. Severe itching begins with sensitization of the host. In reinfections, itching begins within days and the reaction may be clinically more intense. The itching is worse at night. In women, itching of the nipples associated with pruritic papular eruption is characteristic. In men, itchy papules on the scrotum and penis are equally typical. When more than one member of a family has pruritus, a suspicion of scabies should be present (Centers for Disease Control and Prevention, 2010; Habif, 2004; James et al., 2006).

The eruption varies depending on the length of infestation, previous sensitization, and previous treatment. It also varies with climate and the host's immunologic status. Lichenification, impetigo, and furunculosis may be present. Bullous lesions may contain eosinophils, resembling bullous pemphigoid. Dull red nodules (3–5 mm) may appear during active phase of scabies. They may or may not itch and persist on the scrotum, penis, and vulva; these are termed nodular scabies (James et al., 2006).

## DIFFERENTIAL DIAGNOSIS

- Acropustulosis of infancy
- Asteatotic eczema
- Atopic dermatitis
- Bedbug bites
- Bullous pemphigoid
- Chickenpox
- Contact dermatitis, allergic
- Contact dermatitis, irritant
- Dermatitis artifacta
- Dermatitis herpetiformis
- Dyshidrotic eczema
- Eosinophilic pustular folliculitis
- Erythroderma (generalized exfoliative dermatitis)
- Folliculitis
- Gianotti-Crosti syndrome (papularacrodermatitis of childhood)
- Id reaction (autoeczematization)
- Kyrle disease
- Langerhans cell histiocytosis
- Lice
- Lichen planus
- Neurotic excoriations
- Other insect bites
- Papular urticaria
- Parapsoriasis
- Prurigo nodularis
- Psoriasis, guttate
- Psoriasis, pustular
- Renal disease
- Seabathereruption
- Syphilis
- Urticaria, cholinergic
- Vesicular palmoplantar eczema

## TREATMENT/MANAGEMENT

Treatment for scabies requires a scabicidal agent, an anti-itch agent, and an appropriate antimicrobial agent if secondarily infection is present. Patients with crusted scabies should have excess scale removed to allow for penetration of the topical scabicidal agent and decrease further infestation. To remove excess scale, soak in warm water and apply a keratolytic agent such as 5% salicylic acid in petrolatum or Lac-Hydrin cream. Avoid salicylic acid if large body areas are involved. The scales can be removed with a tongue blade or similar nonsharp instrument (Cordoro, 2012).

Permethrin 5% cream (Elimite) is the most widely used medication for scabies. It is a synthetic pyrethroid that is lethal to mites and has low toxicity for humans. Lindane is also effective, with a low incidence of adverse effects when used properly. Internationally, benzyl benzonate and 10% sulfur in white petrolatum are also used to treat scabies. The topical medication should be rubbed into the skin from the neck to the feet, especially in the skin creases, perianal areas, umbilicus, and free nail edge and folds. It is washed off 8 to 10 hours later (Calianno, 2013; Centers for Disease Control and Prevention, 2010; Goldstein & Goldstein, 2011; Habif, 2004; James et al., 2006).

Ivermectin has been used for scabies and is supplied in 3- and 6-mg pills. It is given in a dose of 200 µg/kg. Although oral treatment is convenient, usually topical therapy is used in conjunction with oral therapy, especially in the crusted type of scabies (Andrews et al., 2009; Centers for Disease Control and Prevention, 2010; Goldstein & Goldstein, 2011; Habif, 2004; James et al., 2006).

## SPECIAL CONSIDERATIONS

As noted earlier, crusted scabies (Norwegian, or hyperkeratotic, scabies) is found in immunocompromised patients, including those with neurologic disorders, Down syndrome, organ transplants, graft-versus-host disease, adult T-cell leukemia, leprosy, and AIDS. In these patients, the infestation assumes a heavily scaling and crusted appearance. These populations present with clinically atypical lesions and often are misdiagnosed, thus delaying treatment and elevating the risk of local epidemics (Centers for Disease Control and Prevention, 2010; Cordoro, 2012; Goldstein & Goldstein, 2011; Habif, 2004; James et al., 2006).

Infants will have widespread involvement. Infants are often affected on the face and the scalp, which is rare for adults. Vesicles are common on the palms and the soles of the feet, making them a highly characteristic sign of scabies in infants. Nodules may be present in the axillae and diaper area. Elderly patients have few cutaneous lesions other than excoriation, dry skin, and scaling, but they experience intense itching (Habif, 2004).

## WHEN TO REFER

The intense itching of scabies leads to scratching that can lead to secondary bacterial infections, such as *Staphylococcus aureus* or beta-hemolytic streptococci. Occasionally the bacterial skin infection can lead to an inflammation of the kidneys called poststreptococcal glomerulonephritis. Referral to nephrology should be considered (Centers for Disease Control and Prevention, 2010; Cordoro, 2012).

## PATIENT EDUCATION

The following should be explained when educating patients on scabies (Centers for Disease Control and Prevention, 2010; Cordoro, 2012):

- The importance of compliance and complete eradication of scabies.
- All close contacts should be treated for scabies. All carpets and furniture should be vacuumed and vacuum bags disposed. Pets do not require treatment.
- All bedding and clothing should be washed in hot water and dried using hot dryer cycles or dry cleaned. If items cannot be laundered or dry cleaned, place them in an air tight plastic bag for a week.
- Patients treated may return to day care, school, or work the day after treatment.

## CLINICAL PEARLS

- To aid in identification of burrows, add a drop of gentian violet to the infested area, then remove with alcohol.
- The burrows will retain the ink (James et al., 2006).

# LICE

## OVERVIEW

Pediculosis is not reported often because of the social embarrassment associated with the diagnosis and the assumption that lice are related to poor personal hygiene. This stigma aids the spread of infestation. Affected families are reluctant to share information with their neighbors and when children are treated, it tends to be on an individual basis, not school or community wide to totally eradicate the lice (Goldstein & Goldstein, 2013; Guenther, 2012; Habif, 2004).

## EPIDEMIOLOGY

In the United States, pediculosis has become more common over the past 30 years, which makes the diagnosis and treatment of lice a common task in general primary practice, with more than 12 million Americans infested each year (Guenther, 2012; Habif, 2004).

Head lice infestation is more common in the warmer months, whereas pubic lice occurs more in the cooler months. Head lice infestation is most common in urban areas and is seen in all socioeconomic groups. Head lice infestation occur more in school-age children (10%–40% in U. S. schools), typically in late summer and autumn. Body lice infestation mainly affects the homeless, whereas pubic lice generally are transmitted as a sexually transmitted infection (STI). Lice infestation occurs in all races, but in North America, the incidence of head lice is lower in African Americans than in other racial groups (Goldstein & Goldstein, 2013; Guenther, 2012).

Girls are at higher risk for head lice infestation because of social behavior (e.g., social acceptance of close physical contact; sharing hats, combs, and hair ties). Children aged 3 to 11 years are usually infested with head lice because of close contact in classrooms and day-care facilities. Head lice are much less common after puberty (Guenther, 2012).

## PATHOLOGY/HISTOLOGY

Human lice (*Pediculus humanus* and *Pediculus pubis*) are found in all countries and climates. They belong to the phylum *Arthropoda*, the class *Insecta*, the order *Phthiraptera*, and the suborder *Anoplura* (known as the sucking lice). The size and shape of their claws conform to the texture and shape of the hair or clothing fibers they grasp (Goldstein & Goldstein, 2013; Guenther, 2012).

Body lice infest clothing, laying their eggs on fibers in the fabric seams. Head and pubic lice infest hair, laying their eggs at the base of hair fibers (Guenther, 2012; Habif, 2004; James et al., 2006). Histology is not needed for diagnosis. Examination of a bite reveals intradermal hemorrhage and a deep, wedge-shaped infiltrate with many eosinophils and lymphocytes (Guenther, 2012).

## CLINICAL PRESENTATION

There are three types of human lice: the head louse, *Pediculus humanus capitis* (also known as *Pediculus humanus*); the body louse, *Pediculus humanus corporis*; and the crab louse, *Pthirus pubis* (Guenther, 2012; Habif, 2004; James et al., 2006):

- The head louse, *P. humanus capitis*, causes symptoms of scalp pruritus, postcervical lymphadenopathy, and impetigo. The scalp may have excoriations, evidence of louse feces, nits, and active lice. Lice are typically present in the retroauricular scalp. For the diagnosis of *P. capitis*, the use of a louse comb will provide better direct visual examination of the scalp. Bite reactions manifested as pruritic papules and/or wheals may be present. The hair of patients who are heavily infested is frequently matted with exudates, predisposing the area to fungal infection. Numerous lice and nits are found under the matted hair. Nits are difficult to separate from the hair. A definitive diagnosis can be made by using a Wood's light. A Wood's light can be used to illuminate the live nits, which will fluoresce white, and the empty nits, which will appear gray. Eggs rely on body warmth to incubate, so nits are attached to the hair shafts just above the level of the scalp.
- *P. humanus corporis*, the body louse, warrants a physical examination. Physical examination findings include multiple lesions from bites. Uninfected bites present as erythematous papules, 2 to 4 mm in diameter, with an erythematous base. Bites can appear anywhere on the body but are seen most frequently on the axillae, groin, and trunk (i.e., areas most often covered by clothing). Body lice tend to avoid the scalp, except at the margins. Maculae cerulea are blue–gray macules, which are actually a discoloration of the skin caused by the insect's bite. This is indicative of lice infestation. Enzymes in the louse saliva cause the breakdown of human bilirubin to biliverdin, which changes the skin color associated with maculae cerulea. Patients who have had a chronic infestation can develop a condition termed *vagabond skin*. The skin becomes thickened and hyperpigmented after years of bites and recurrent scratching and excoriations.
- Crab louse, *P. pubis*, is also referred to as pubic lice. Pubic lice and nits are visible in the pubic hair. Pubic lice are less mobile so they are easily seen when attached to the hair on the skin surface. The eyebrows and eyelashes are also common sites of infestation. In children, this infestation is usually acquired from an infested parent and is rarely attributed to sexual abuse; however, *P. pubis* infestation can be acquired secondary to sexual abuse, so the child should be examined thoroughly. Excoriations are common. Inguinal lymphadenopathy and axillary lymphadenopathy may be noted with pubic lice infestation.

## DIFFERENTIAL DIAGNOSIS

Differential diagnosis of head lice infestation includes:

- Dandruff
- Dermatophyte infection
- Dried hairspray/gel
- Hair shaft abnormalities (i.e., monilethrix, trichorrhexis nodosa)
- Piedra (black piedra from *Piedraia hortae*, white piedra from *Trichosporon asahii*, and other species of *Trichosporon*) (Guenther, 2012)

Differential diagnosis of body lice infestation includes:

- Acne
- Delusions of parasitosis
- Folliculitis
- Impetigo
- Other insect bites
- Postinflammatory hyperpigmentation
- Scabies
- Xerosis with excoriations (Guenther, 2012)

Differential diagnosis of pubic lice infestation includes:

- Conjunctivitis (if eyelash involvement)
- Contact dermatitis
- Delusions of parasitosis
- Dermatophyte infection
- Folliculitis (Guenther, 2012)

## TREATMENT/MANAGEMENT

Treatment of pediculosis has two components: medication and environmental changes. Multiple topical pediculicidal agents are available for treatment of head and pubic lice. Pyrethrin shampoos and permethrin 1% rinse are available over the counter; permethrin 5%, malathion, lindane, ivermectin topical, and spinosad are prescribed agents. These products are applied topically as directed and then washed off. This application can be repeated in 7 to 10 days. All close contacts should be treated. In addition to medical therapies, other therapies include the following (Goldstein & Goldstein, 2013; Guenther, 2012; Habif, 2004; James et al., 2006):

- Using a fine-tooth comb can aid in the removal of nits. Metal nit combs (e.g., LiceMeister) are effective and can be purchased over the Internet.
- Soaking the hair in a solution of equal parts water and white vinegar and then wrapping the hair in a towel for at least 15 to 20 minutes will help with removal of nits. Commercial products available include an 8% formic acid preparation (GenDerm Step 2) and an enzymatic nit remover (Clear).
- Occlusive therapy techniques that have not been scientifically proven are vinegar, mayonnaise, petroleum jelly, olive oil, butter, isopropyl alcohol, and water submersion as long as 6 hours.
- Any item that the infested child or parent has come into contact with should be considered infested. It is recommended that contact items (e.g., towels, pillowcases, sheets, hats, toys) be laundered in hot water, followed by machine drying using the

hottest cycle. Items that are not machine washable may be placed in a dryer at high heat for 30 minutes, or dry cleaning may be an effective alternative. Items that cannot be laundered can be placed in a sealed plastic bag for 1 to 2 weeks, which will effectively kill lice and their eggs. Vacuuming selected areas of the home, such as the couch used by infested patients, is recommended.
- Combs and hair brushes should be thrown away or can be treated by soaking for 5 to 10 minutes in very hot water (>131°F, or 55°C) or treated with pediculicides.
- Chemical insecticide sprays used in the home environment have not been shown to be effective.
- The same pediculicides used for head louse infestation can be used for pediculicides in other body areas such as pubic lice or body louse infestation. *P. pubis* infestations of the eyelashes are treated with occlusive therapies. Petrolatum (twice daily for 7–10 days) is often used as an asphyxiant for eyelash infestation. Remove dead lice with tweezers. Mercuric oxide ointment is also useful in the treatment of eyelash infestation and fluorescein dye strips, which are used in the diagnosis of corneal abrasions, may be used in combination with white petrolatum for 3 days.
- Topical agents should be applied to the seams of clothing. Data suggest that permethrin spray is also effective against infestation.

## SPECIAL CONSIDERATIONS

Infestation with *P. pubis* is considered an STI, and 30% of these patients have an additional STI. Therefore, it is recommended that these patients be screened for other STIs (Guenther, 2012; James et al., 2006).

# STINGS

## OVERVIEW

Insects make up the most diverse and largest group in the animal kingdom and include many species. Insects represent more than 50% of all living organisms and could represent more than 90% of all differing life forms on Earth. Therefore, contact with insects cannot be prevented. Exposures to insect bites or stings can result in a serious emergency (Burns, 2013).

## EPIDEMIOLOGY

In the United States, the American Association of Poison Control Centers reported 42,620 cases of exposures to insects in 2007, with more than 200 cases resulting in moderate or major reactions (Burns, 2013).

Mortality from insect bites occurs from hypersensitivity reactions or from complications resulting from infections. The U.S. Centers for Disease Control and Prevention estimates that approximately 100 deaths annually are from insect venom anaphylaxis (Centers for Disease Control and Prevention, 2010). Risk factors for increased severity of reaction include older age, cardiovascular disease or mast cell disorder, concomitant treatment with beta-adrenergic blockage or angiotensin-converting enzyme inhibitors, previous severe reactions, and the type of insect (honeybees presenting the highest risk; Burns, 2013).

## PATHOLOGY/HISTOLOGY

Mouth parts of biting insects can be classified into three major groups: piercing, sponging, and biting. There is a large diversity in the morphology of these groups. Insect saliva will inhibit coagulation, increase blood flow to the bite, or anesthetize the bite area. Most localized reactions are caused by the immune response of the victim to the insect secretions. Usually insect bites result in superficial puncture wounds to the skin but this is not always the case; a horsefly bite, for example, causes a deep, painful wound (Burns, 2013).

## CLINICAL PRESENTATION

When patient history is limited, diagnosis of an insect bite can be difficult because the initial response may be limited to erythema, local pain, pruritus, or edema. Wheals and urticaria may also occur. This can be confusing for the provider because multiple other dermatologic conditions produce the same presentations (Burns, 2013; Castellis, 2012).

Patients usually do not seek treatment unless a severe reaction occurs. Reactions to bites can be delayed because the host is unaware or because the saliva of some insects contains an anesthetic secreted to allow uninterrupted bloodfeeding. Patients at risk include the following:

- Homeless persons
- Patients with impairment from mental illness
- Those who are exposed to pets or outside animals (Burns, 2013)

Bedbug bites are painless because the insect injects salivary proteins that contain anesthetic and an anticoagulant. Bedbugs cannot bite through clothing, plastic, or paper. Therefore, the most commonly affected areas are the exposed skin and areas that can be reached through open sleeves or clothing. The bite reaction is often delayed and can occur up to 2 weeks after an exposure. Patients will present with pruritic erythematous papules, macules, urticarial, and possibly bullae and bites are often in linear groups of three (Figure III.34a–e) (Calianno, 2013).

Fleas inflict bites that are usually papules arranged in a nonfollicular pattern. Flea bites can induce papular urticarial. Flea allergy may cause respiratory symptoms in humans, particularly in patients allergic to cats. Types of reactions are as follows:

- With a local reaction, patients will have itching, moderate or severe pain, erythema, and tenderness at the site.
- In a systemic or anaphylactic reaction, the symptoms are more severe. Initially, patients will have rash, urticaria, pruritus, and angioedema. Then symptoms can progress to anxiety, weakness, dizziness, gastrointestinal disturbances, urinary incontinence, syncope, hypotension, and shortness of breath. Patients can experience respiratory failure and cardiovascular collapse.
- Delayed reactions may appear 10 to 14 days after a sting. Symptoms of delayed reactions resemble serum sickness and include fever, malaise, headache, urticaria, lymphadenopathy, and polyarthritis. (Burns, 2013; Castellis, 2012)

Insect Bites ■ 209

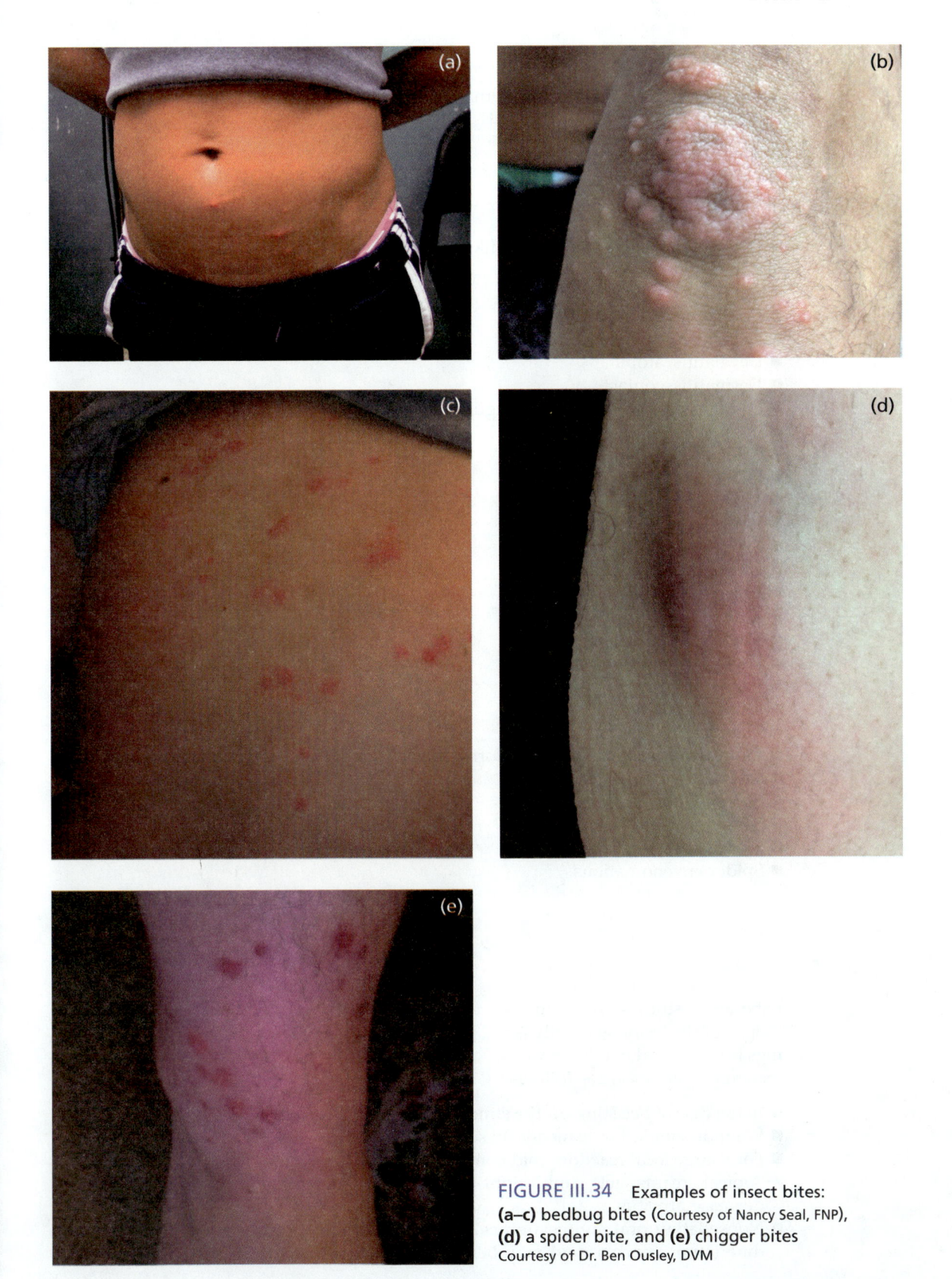

FIGURE III.34  Examples of insect bites: **(a–c)** bedbug bites (Courtesy of Nancy Seal, FNP), **(d)** a spider bite, and **(e)** chigger bites
Courtesy of Dr. Ben Ousley, DVM

## DIFFERENTIAL DIAGNOSIS

Because of the various reactions that stings may cause, the differential diagnosis is quite large (Burns, 2013):

- Acute coronary syndrome
- Anaphylaxis
- Arthritis, rheumatoid
- Bites, animal
- Burkitt lymphoma and Burkitt-like lymphoma
- Caterpillar envenomations
- Cat-scratch disease
- Centipede envenomations
- Delusions of parasitosis
- Dermatitis, atopic
- Dermatitis, contact
- Disseminated intravascular coagulation
- Erysipelas
- Folliculitis
- HIV infection and AIDS
- Impetigo
- Lice
- Lymphomatoid papulosis
- Lymphoma, cutaneous T-cell
- Lymphoma, mantle cell
- Millipede envenomations
- Mycosis fungoides
- Pediatrics, anaphylaxis
- Pediculosis
- Pityriasis rosea
- Plant poisoning, resins
- Pityriasis lichenoides et varioliformis acuta (PLEVA)
- Scabies
- Scorpion envenomations
- Serum sickness
- Snake envenomations
- Spider envenomations

## TREATMENT/MANAGEMENT

Laboratory studies are seldom necessary, unless severe reaction or cellulitis occurs. Biopsy of the lesion generally is not necessary. Microscopic examination of skin scrapings is warranted if a diagnosis of scabies or mite infestation are suspected. Treatment recommendations are as follows:

- In the case of bee stings, if the stinger is present in the wound, it should be removed.
- Wounds should be cleaned with soap and water.
- For a large local reaction, cold compresses decrease swelling.
- Topical creams, gels, and lotions such as those containing calamine or pramoxine decrease pruritus.
- Nonsedating oral antihistamines such as cetirizine (10 mg once a day) or loratadine (10 mg once a day) may be helpful for patients with pruritus. The sedating

agent hydroxyzine (10–25 mg every 4–6 hours as needed) may be helpful for controlling pruritus in adults.
- Use of $H_2$-blocking drugs (usually used to reduce gastric acid secretion) may be used concurrently with $H_1$-blocking antihistamines.
- Prescribe epinephrine autoinjector if the patient has had a systemic response to an insect bite.
- Corticosteroids may be used for 3 to 4 days if reaction is moderate to severe.
- Eradication of fleas in homes without an obvious animal vector involves insecticidal dusts or sprays, vacuuming, and cleaning (Burns, 2013; Calianno, 2013; Castellis, 2012)

## SPECIAL CONSIDERATIONS

Castellis (2012) listed the following special considerations:

- Immunocompromised patients, such as those with AIDS, chronic lymphocytic leukemia, histiocytosis-X disorders, and disorders of monocyte function, may develop severe local bite reactions. In such patients, local reactions can progress to become necrotic, or may be accompanied by systemic symptoms, including lymphadenopathy and fever.
- Patients with delusional parasitosis believe they are being bitten by imaginary insects.
- Similarly, amphetamine and cocaine abusers with formication (feeling that ants are crawling on the skin) can present with self-inflicted skin lesions from imaginary infestation.

## WHEN TO REFER

If determining the insect species that caused the reaction is necessary, contacting the health department, agriculture extension, or university entomologist is recommended. If the patient has traveled to a tropical region, consider contacting a tropical medicine specialist or the Centers for Disease Control and Prevention at (877) 394-8747 (Traveler's Health Hotline). A regional poison center may be of assistance in difficult or complicated cases or for general information (Burns, 2013).

## PATIENT EDUCATION

Burns (2013) and Castellis (2012) recommended instructing patients on the following tips:

- Periodically implement pest control measures to eliminate nests and minimize reproduction of biting insects.
- Wear protective clothing (i.e., long pants, long sleeves, footwear, and gloves), especially when outdoors. Most insects are incapable of biting through clothing. Additionally, light-colored, nonfloral clothing appears to be less attractive to many biting insects, including mosquitos.
- Avoid use of heavy perfumes, scented soaps, sprays, or lotions that may attract insects.
- Be aware of surroundings; for example, avoid dense vegetation or animals suspected of carrying fleas, chiggers, or ticks.
- Judicious use of insect repellent can help minimize exposure to insect bites and stings.

- Be aware of the potential for bees or other foraging insects to enter opened soft drink containers that are left idle.
- Consult with a veterinarian if pets or other animals are believed to be the source of the infestation because direct treatment of the pet is required.

## REFERENCES

Andrews, R. M., McCarthy, J., Carapetis, J. R., & Currie, B. J. (2009). Skin disorders, including pyoderma, scabies, and tinea infections. *Pediatric Clinics of North America, 56*, 1421–1440.

Burns, B. D. (2013, May 2). *Insect bites*. Retrieved from http://emedicine.medscape.com/article/769067-overview

Calianno, C. (2013). Bedbugs (*Cimex lectularius*): Identifying and managing an infestation. *Journal of the Dermatology Nurses' Association, 5*(3), 161–165.

Castellis, M. C. (2012). *Insect bites*. Retrieved from http://uptodate.com/contents/insect-bites

Centers for Disease Control and Prevention (2010). *Parasites—Scabies*. Retrieved from http://www.cdc.gov/parasites/scabies/epi.html

Cordoro, K. M. (2012, June 12). *Dermatologic manifestations of scabies*. Retrieved from http://emedicine.medscape.com/article/1109204-overview

Goldstein, A. O., & Goldstein, B. G. (2013). *Pediculosis capitis*. Retrieved from http://www.uptodate.com/contents/pediculosis-capitis

Goldstein, B. G., & Goldstein, A. O. (2011). *Scabies*. Retrieved from http://www.uptodate.com/contents/scabies

Guenther, L. (2012, February 9). *Pediculosis*. Retrieved from http://emedicine.medscape.com/article/225013-overview

Habif, T. P. (2004). *Clinical dermatology: A color guide to diagnosis and therapy* (4th ed.). Philadelphia, PA: Mosby.

James, W. D., Berger, T. G., & Elston, D. M. (2006). *Andrews' diseases of the skin: Clinical dermatology* (10th ed.). Philadelphia, PA: Saunders/Elsevier.

# Lentigo/Nevi

## LENTIGO

### OVERVIEW

A *lentigo* is a benign, small, sharply circumscribed, pigmented macule surrounded by normal-appearing skin. Lentigines result from increased activity of the epidermal melanocytes. In contrast to *ephelides* (freckles) that fade without sun exposure, lentigines are persistent. The two major types of lentigines are simple lentigo and solar lentigo (Schaffer &Bolognia, 2012).

### EPIDEMIOLOGY

In America, solar lentigines are present in almost all White people older than age 60 years. Solar lentigines are seen more in fair-skinned than dark-skinned people. However, inherited patterned lentiginosis can occur in Blacks if they have a mixed American Indian ancestry and/or relatives with red hair (Schwartz, 2012).

### PATHOLOGY/HISTOLOGY

The pathology/histology of various lentigines can include the following (Habif, 2004; James, Berger, & Elston, 2006; Schaffer & Bolognia, 2012; Schwartz, 2012):

- Lentigo simplex appears as an elongation of the rete ridges with melanocyte proliferation in the basal layer, increased melanin in both the melanocytes and the basal keratinocytes, and the presence of melanophages in the upper dermis.
- Solar lentigines have extended rete ridges and an abundance of pigmented basaloid cells, which form buds and strands. There is no presence of atypia in the melanocytes.
- Lentigines can result from PUVA (psoralen + ultraviolet-A light) therapy; these have increased melanocytes that are hypertrophic and frequently have cellular atypia. There is an elongation of the rete ridges and increased pigmentation in the basal cell region with transepidermal pigment cell excretion.
- Radiation lentigines show increased melanin deposits in basal keratinocytes, cellular atypia, increased amount of melanocytes, and decreased rete ridges.

- Oral and labial melanotic macules show epithelial hyperplasia with irregular spreading and elongation of the rete ridges. There is increased melanin in the melanocytes and keratinocytes of the basal layer and in the melanophages of the dermal papillae.
- Tanning-bed lentigines have increased density of melanocytes and some mild nuclear atypia.
- Ephelides (freckles), a type of lentigo have an increase in pigment content in the basal cell layer but do not have elongated rete ridges or an increased number of melanocytes.

## CLINICAL PRESENTATION

The appearance of lentigines varies and is dependent on race, history of exposure, genetics, and the type of lesion (James et al., 2006; Schwartz, 2012):

- Lentigo simplex is the most common type of lentigo and is not induced by sun exposure or systemic disease. The lesions are round or oval macules that are 3 to 15 mm in diameter. Their margins can be either irregular or smooth with even pigmentation that is brown to black. The lesions are usually noted in childhood but can be present at birth.
- Solar lentigines are the most common benign sun-induced lesions. They most commonly appear on the face, upper torso, and upper extremities. Initially they are smaller than 5 mm in diameter and are flat or depressed. The lesions are typically brown, but the color may range from yellow-tan to black. Solar lentigines slowly increase in number and size and can merge to form larger patches. These lesions are most common in individuals who have had increased exposure to sun tanning and artificial sources of ultraviolet light.
- Ink-spot lentigines have sharp, irregular borders that resemble a spot of ink that has bled into the skin lines. They are most often seen on sun-exposed areas of the body, and patients usually have only one ink-spot lentigo admixed with multiple solar lentigines. A differential diagnosis for an ink-spot lentigo is melanoma.
- PUVA lentigo is a chronic light-brown macule that appears about 6 months after the start of PUVA therapy for psoriasis and remains for 3 to 6 months after therapy has ceased. The presence of lesions is associated with the number of PUVA doses and may occur on all sites. The lesions are usually 3 to 8 mm in diameter, but stellate lesions can be up to 3 cm in diameter. The lentigines may persist for 3 to 6 months after therapy is discontinued.
- Radiation lentigo resembles UV-induced lentigo but includes histopathologic signs of long-term cutaneous radiation damage such as epidermal atrophy, subcutaneous fibrosis, keratosis, and telangiectasia. Radiation lentigines are relentless and typically occur 4 months after the initial exposure to radiation.
- Tanning-bed lentigines are caused by tanning bed use. These lentigines are similar to PUVA lentigines, except psoralens are not involved. They occur most often on exposed sites. The lesions are usually 2 to 5 mm in diameter, with color ranging from dark brown to black.
- Oral and labial melanotic macules are similar to each other and are smaller than 4 mm. Labial lesions occur on the vermilion of the lower lip and are brown to blue or blue-black in color. The lesions are usually solitary, symmetric, and asymptomatic. Oral lesions can appear on the gingiva, buccal mucosa, palate, and tongue.
- Vulvar and penile lentigo are benign lesions similar to labial melanotic macules. The most common sites in men are the glans penis, corona, corona sulcus, and penile shaft. The lesions have irregular borders, vary in color from tan to dark brown, and may have a diameter as large as 15 mm. In women, the lesions appear on the genital

mucosa as a mottled, pigmented patch. The diameter can be 5 to 15 mm or larger. Lentigines involving the external genitalia are also reported in LAMB (lentigines, atrial myxoma, and blue nevi) syndrome.

## DIFFERENTIAL DIAGNOSIS

- Actinic keratosis
- Ephelides (freckles)
- Melanoma (if pigmented)
- Seborrheic keratosis

## TREATMENT/MANAGEMENT

Treatment options for lentigines are as follows:

- Tretinoin and hydroquinone creams can lighten lentigines but require several months of treatment.
- Cryotherapy and trichloroacetic acid are effective for the treatment of solar lentigines, but postinflammatory hyperpigmentation is a risk of treatment.
- Bleaching solution containing 2% mequinol (4-hydroxyanisole, 4HA) and 0.01% tretinoin (Solagé) applied twice daily for 3 months on solar lentigines has shown efficacy.
- Treatment of solar lentigines with a focal medium-depth chemical peel can help to fade solar lentigines.
- Cryosurgery is used to treat isolated lentigines.
- Lasers are effective in the treatment of various lentigines. A short-pulsed, pigment-specific laser will destroy the pigment within a solar lentigo and show significant clinical improvement with a low risk of adverse effects and high patient acceptance. (Schwartz, 2012; Schaffer & Bolognia, 2012)

## SPECIAL CONSIDERATIONS

Abnormal presentations of lentigines include the following:

- Inherited patterned lentiginosis
- Nevus spilus
- Lentigines profuse
- Agminated lentiginosis
- Xeroderma pigmentosa
- Multiple lentigines syndrome (formerly LEOPARD syndrome)
- Peutz-Jeghers syndrome
- Laugier-Hunziker syndrome
- LAMB syndrome
- NAME (nevi, atrial myxoma, and neurofibromaephelides) syndrome
- Carney syndrome (James et al., 2006; Schwartz, 2012)

## WHEN TO REFER

A biopsy should be performed or the patient referred to a dermatologist for suspicious lentigo (abnormal pigmentation or irritation) or when signs of abnormal lentigo syndromes are present.

## PATIENT EDUCATION

- Apply sunscreen to prevent new solar lentigines and to prevent the darkening of existing solar lentigines.
- Avoid sun exposure or the use of tanning beds and wear sun-protective clothing and hats.

# NEVI

## OVERVIEW

Intradermal, compound, and junctional nevi are classified as common acquired melanocytic nevi (Figure III.35). They are also termed *moles* (Robbins, 2013). Common melanocytic nevi are acquired in early childhood. They usually begin as brown to black macules and can remain macular or progress to papular lesions. Common acquired nevi appear after 6 months of age and increase in number and size until the third decade, then decrease in size and lose pigment thereafter (Habif, 2004; Rao, Wang, & Murphy, 2001).

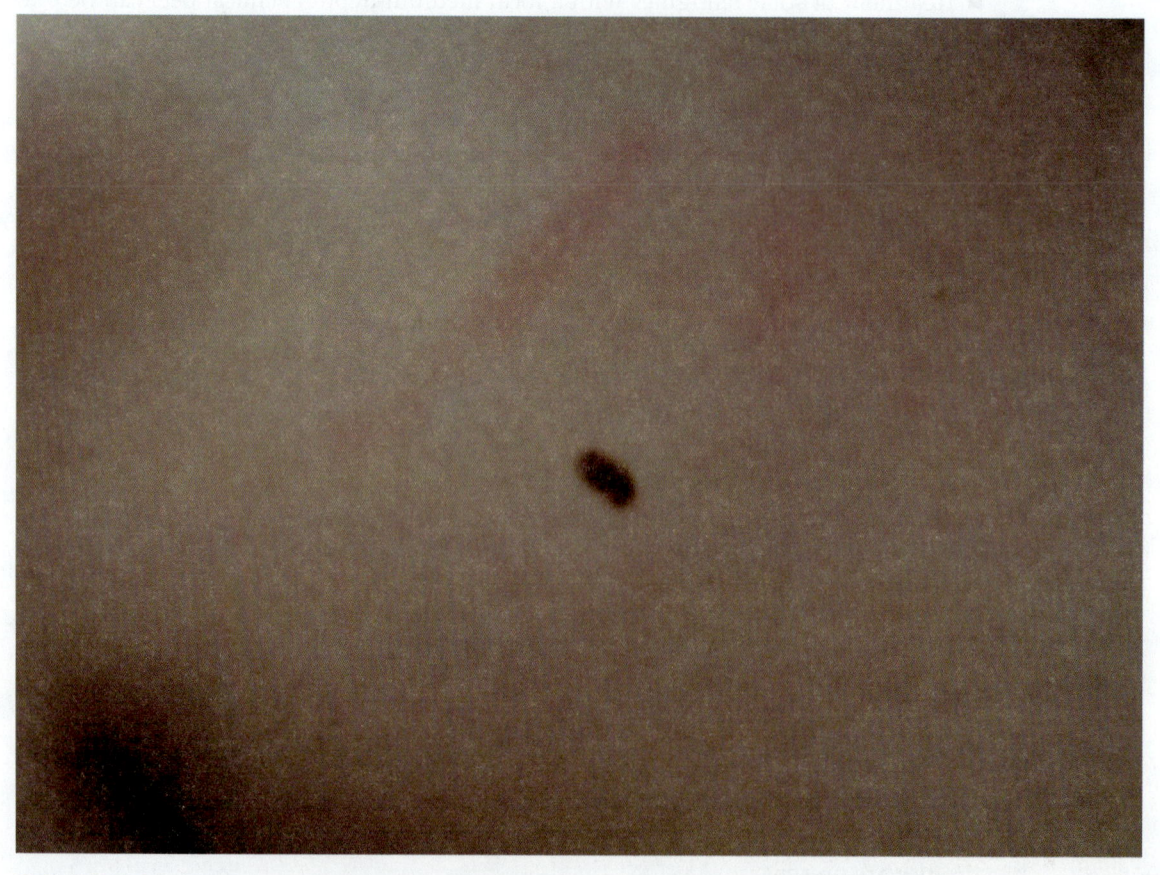

FIGURE III.35  Example of nevus, also called a mole

## EPIDEMIOLOGY

Acquired melanocytic nevi are common in the United States and worldwide and are present at equal rates in both sexes. The occurrence of nevi is related to age, race, genetic, and environmental factors (Robbins, 2013). The prevalence of nevi in ethnic groups with dark skin is lower than that seen in individuals with fair skin. Some individuals of northern European extraction (e. g., Germany, Holland, Belgium, and the United Kingdom) will present with large (≥ 1 cm in largest diameter), often numerous (> 50, up to several hundred), nevi of a red-brown color (McCalmont, 2013).

Melanocytic nevi are not gender specific; however, the melanocytes respond to hormonal activity because they change pigmentation during pregnancy (McCalmont, 2013). Congenital melanocytes are present at birth with new melanocytic nevi appearing throughout the first 3 decades of life (Habif, 2004; McCalmont, 2013).

## PATHOLOGY/HISTOLOGY

The different classification of nevi are as follows (Habif, 2004; McCalmont, 2013; Robbins, 2013):

- *Conventional (acquired) melanocytic nevi* develop as a proliferation of single melanocytes along the dermoepidermal junction. As the melanocytes grow, small groups of cells develop in the lower layer of the epidermis, which results in a lesion called junctional melanocytic nevus. As the nevus grows, nests continue along the junction, and within the superficial dermis; this is called a compound melanocytic nevus. As a nevus ages, the junctional component will disappear. The resultant nevus is termed an *intradermal melanocytic nevus*.
- *Congenital melanocytic nevi* are similar to the acquired nevi in that junctional, compound, and intradermal patterns are observed. The congenital nevi extend into the dermis, with melanocytes positioned in the interstitial dermis between collagen bundles (Figure III.36). The depth of growth into the dermis is variable.

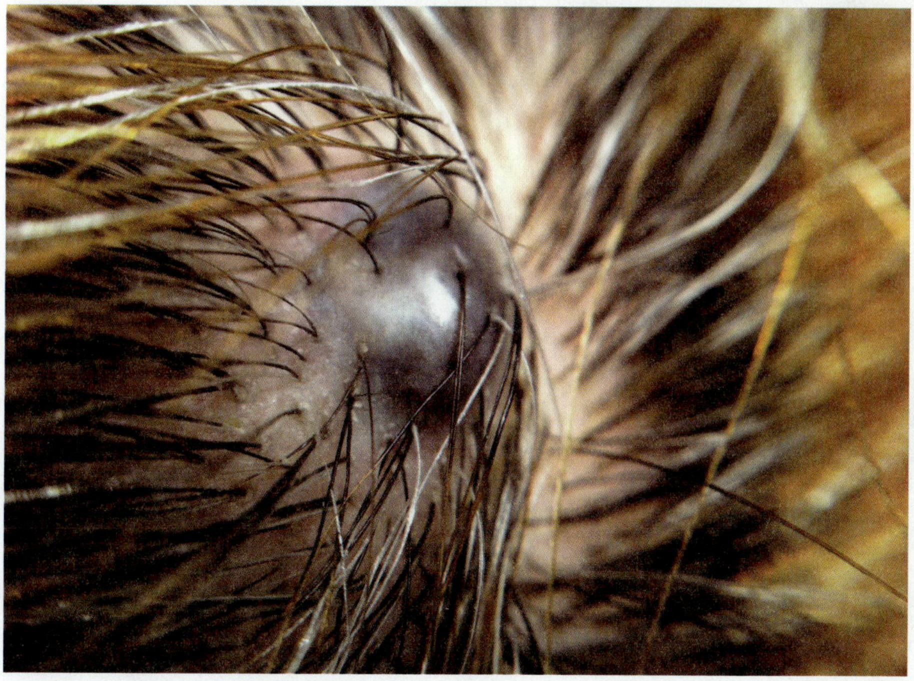

**FIGURE III.36**
A congenital nevus on the scalp
Courtesy of Ron Landreth

218 ■ III. Common Dermatologic Conditions

- *Spitz nevi* are usually acquired melanocytic nevi, and they can have a pattern that is junctional, compound, or intradermal. Spitz nevi are benign, small, symmetric, and demarcated but differ from conventional nevi in that nucleomegalic cells are common and predominate in some lesions.
- *Blue nevi* are dermal melanocytic neoplasms composed of spindled and/or dendritic melanocytes with heavy cytoplasmic pigmentation. Although named *blue nevi*, they can appear as tan, brown, gray, or skin colored.

## CLINICAL PRESENTATION

Common melanocytic nevi are well-circumscribed round or oval lesions with a diameter ranging from 2 to 6 mm (Figure III.37). These nevi are often, but not always, pigmented. There are three basic types of typical melanocytic nevi (Habif, 2004; Rao et al., 2001):

- *Junctional nevi* are macular, light to dark brown, symmetric, and smoothly textured. The center is typically darker than the periphery.

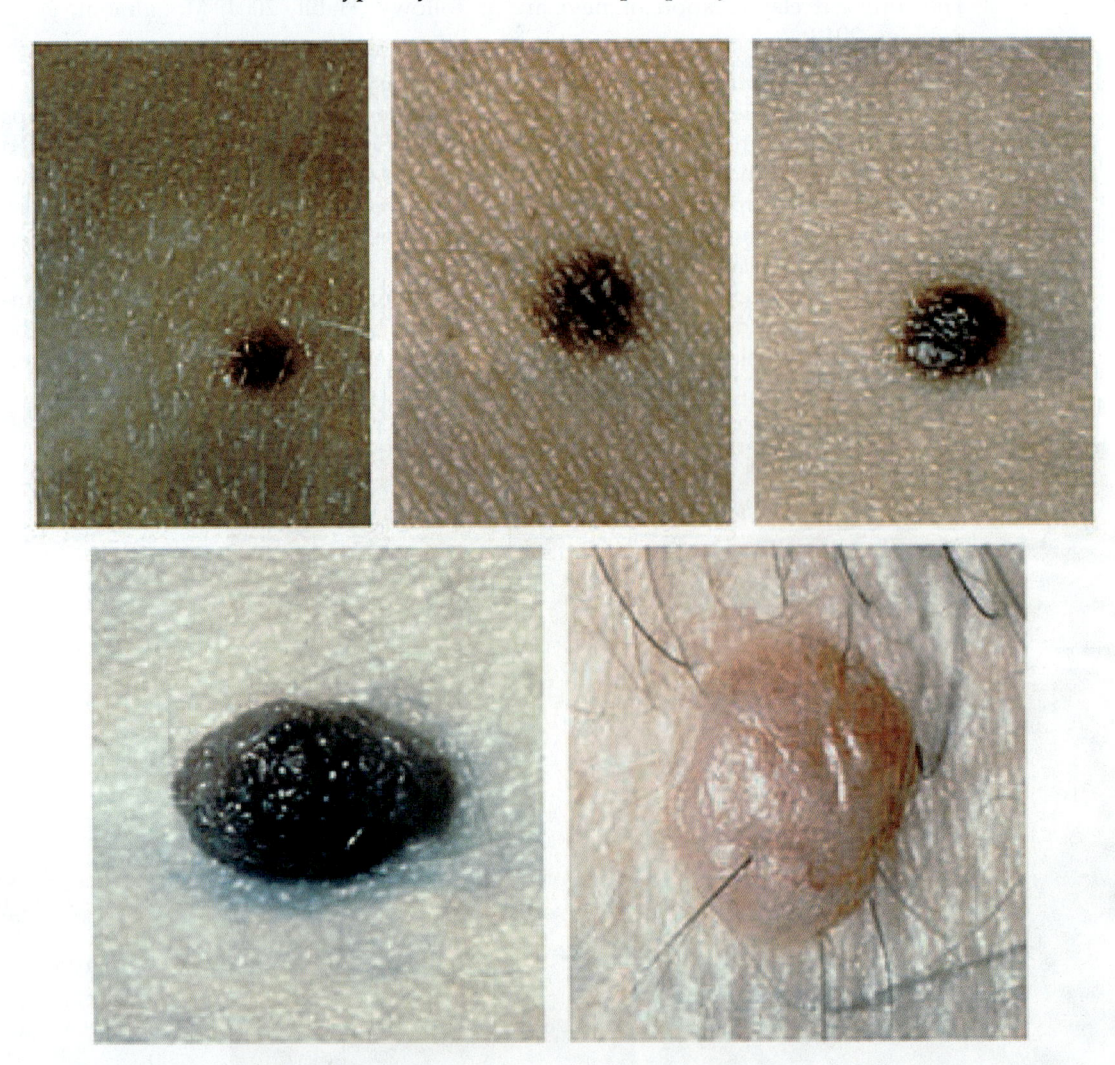

FIGURE III.37  Examples of normal nevi

- *Compound nevi* are slightly raised with colors ranging from uniform light to dark brown. During adolescence, these nevi usually become thicker, change color, and sometimes sprout terminal hair.
- *Intradermal nevi* are elevated, dome-shaped, sessile, or pedunculated papules or nodules that are light brown. Some may present with overlying telangiectatic vessels and a few terminal hairs. Two variants of intradermal nevi are the Unna and Miescher nevi. Unna nevi are polypoid or sessile lesions commonly located on the trunk, neck, shoulders, or arms. Miescher nevi are dome-shaped papules or nodules found on the face.

Clinical presentations of different classifications of nevi are:

- Melanocytic nevi are usually tan to brown, but the color can vary from nonpigmented to jet black.
- Dysplastic nevi will present as a flat pigmented macule or thin papule. The center will appear as a papular area, whereas the surrounding pigmented area will be macular.
- Spitz nevi tend to appear as pink papules on the head of a child, although many Spitz nevi exhibit a lot of vascular ectasia and will appear as hemangioma-like. Spitz nevi vary in size, but they generally are smaller than 1 cm in diameter.
- Blue nevi are typically heavily pigmented because of the presence of deep pigmentation within a refracting colloidal medium; the brownish-black pigment present contributes a bluish cast to such lesions. The optical effect that causes the clinical blueness is known as the Tyndall phenomenon. Not all blue nevi are blue; some present with various shades of gray, brown, or black. Blue nevi are usually small and symmetric, but some may be large and nodular with high cellularity when viewed under a microscope. Blue nevi typically occur on the distal extremities or scalp but can occur anywhere on the body. Blue nevi usually measure 2 cm or greater in diameter. This is particularly true of cellular lesions (cellular blue nevi) that occur at sun-protected sites, such as the buttocks.
- Congenital melanocytic nevi vary considerably in size and are commonly classified as small (<1 cm), intermediate (1–3 cm), or large/giant (> 3 cm). They are evenly pigmented and range in color from tan to brown. In some congenital nevi, the cells extend from the level of the epidermis to the subcutaneous fat, which causes an array of colors that can often be confused with melanoma. (James et al., 2006; McCalmont, 2013)

## DIFFERENTIAL DIAGNOSIS

- Atypical mole (dysplastic nevus)
- Malignant melanoma
- Nevi of Ota and Ito

## TREATMENT/MANAGEMENT

Patients with questionable lesions should have thorough visual inspection and full body skin examinations. Document the size and color of nevi evaluated and record the exact location (McCalmont, 2013). Clinical features of normal nevi are as follows (Cyr, 2008):

- Are present anywhere on the body, less commonly on sun-protected sites
- May number from 0 to 100

- Are typically greater than 6 mm in diameter
- Have orderly, symmetric distribution
- Exhibit even pigmentation; no more than two shades of brown
- Have a round or oval shape
- Have smooth, regular, well-demarcated borders

No laboratory or imaging studies are required for patients with common acquired melanocytic nevi. Children with multiple congenital melanocytic nevi involving the skin on the scalp and back should be evaluated for neurocutaneous melanosis (McCalmont, 2013).

## SPECIAL CONSIDERATIONS

- Melanocytic nevi commonly darken and/or enlarge during pregnancy.
- A single atypical mole does not increase the lifetime risk of melanoma; however, multiple atypical moles indicate increased risk. The greatest risk of melanoma is when multiple atypical moles are present (> 50) and two or more family members have a history of melanoma (Cyr, 2008; McCalmont, 2013).
- Immunocompromised patients have a higher incidence of atypical nevi (Cyr, 2008).

## WHEN TO REFER

Dermatology referral is recommended for routine evaluations if there are abnormal nevi presentations and if biopsy results confirm atypia (McCalmont, 2013).

## PATIENT EDUCATION

Cyr (2008) and McCalmont (2013) recommended educating patients on the following:

- Patients should be taught self-skin examination techniques. Teach patients about the ABCDE rule: asymmetry, border, color, diameter, and evolution. *F* can be added for "funny looking," which indicates a nevus that looks different from other surrounding nevi. Changes in size, shape, and color or itching or bleeding of the nevus should be evaluated.
- Sun avoidance and skin protection should be reviewed, especially the importance of avoiding sunburns in childhood.
- Teach patients that using a blow dryer on the hair helps to visualize nevi on the scalp.

## REFERENCES

Cyr, P. R. (2008). Atypical moles. *American Family Physician, 78*(6), 735–742.
Habif, T. P. (2004). *Clinical dermatology: A color guide to diagnosis and therapy* (4th ed.). Philadelphia, PA: Mosby.
James, W. D., Berger, T. G., & Elston, D. M. (2006). *Andrews' diseases of the skin: Clinical dermatology* (10th ed.). Philadelphia, PA: Saunders/Elsevier.
McCalmont, T. (2013, June 3). *Melanocytic nevi*. Retrieved from http://emedicine.medscape.com/article/1058445-overview#a0104

Rao, B. K., Wang, S. Q., & Murphy, F. P. (2001). Typical dermoscopic patterns of benign melanocytic nevi. *Dermatologic Clinics, 19*(2), 269–284.

Robbins, K. (2013, May). Skin-colored papules. *Clinical Advisor*, 85–88.

Schaffer, J. V., & Bolognia, J. L. (2012).*Benign pigmented skin lesions other than melanocytic nevi (moles)*. Retrieved from http://www.uptodate.com/benign-pigmented-skin-lesions-other-than-melanocytic-nevi-(moles)

Schwartz, R. A. (2012, June 19). *Lentigo*. Retrieved from http://emedicine.medscape.com/article/1068503-overview

# Lichen Planus

## OVERVIEW

*Lichen planus* (LP) is a rare, pruritic, inflammatory disease of the skin, mucous membranes, and hair follicles. The lesions are characteristically purple, shiny, flat-topped (Latin *planus*, "flat") papules on the skin (Goodheart, 2011). The disease course may be short or chronic, although most cases resolve within 1 year. Buccal mucosal or genital involvement can be severe and debilitating in some patients because of pain (Figure III.38; Goldstein & Goldstein, 2013; Habif, 2004; James, Berger, & Elston, 2006).

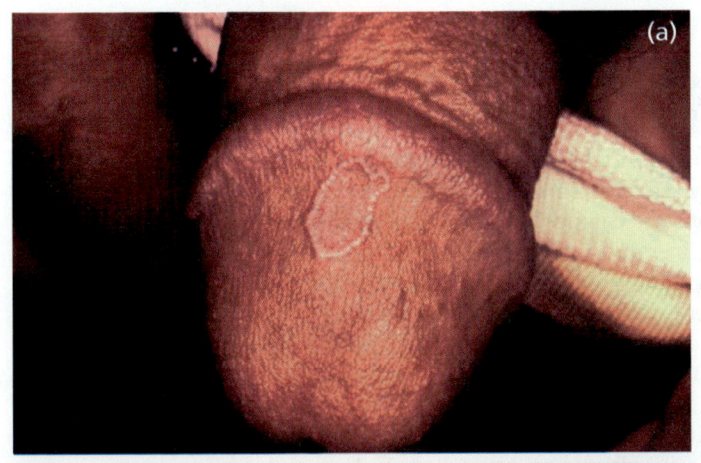

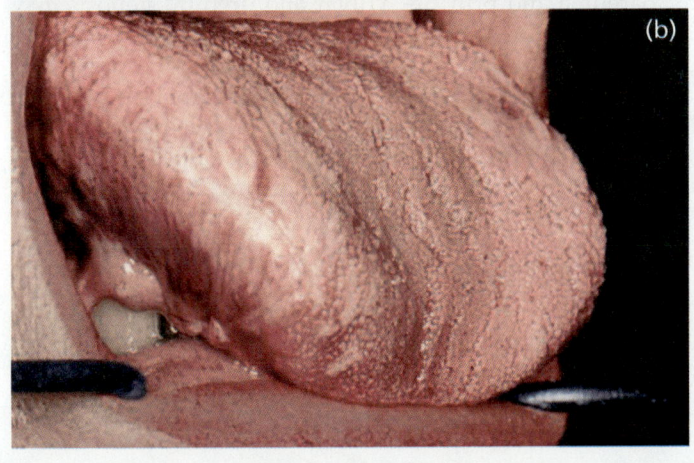

**FIGURE III.38** Examples of **(a)** genital (Courtesy of Dr. N.J. Fiumara, CDC) and **(b)** buccal (Courtesy of Robert E. Sumpter, CDC) lichen planus

## EPIDEMIOLOGY

In the United States, LP is reported to have higher incidence in the wintertime. It occurs throughout the world, in all races, and most commonly affects middle-aged adults (aged 30–60 years). No significant differences in incidence for LP are noted between male and female patients, but in women, LP may present as desquamative inflammatory vaginitis (Chuang, 2013).

## PATHOLOGY/HISTOLOGY

LP is a cell-mediated immune response of unknown source. It is often associated with other autoimmune conditions such as ulcerative colitis, alopecia areata, vitiligo, dermatomyositis, morphea, lichen sclerosis, and myasthenia gravis. There is also a link between LP and hepatitis C virus infection, chronic active hepatitis, and primary biliary cirrhosis (Chuang, 2013; James et al., 2006).

The histopathologic features distinguish LP based on the presence of irregular acanthosis and colloid (Civatte) bodies in the epidermis with destruction of the basal layer. The upper dermis has a band-like ("lichenoid") infiltrate of lymphocytes and histiocytes. The inflammatory reaction pattern is typical. The epidermis is hyperkeratotic with irregular acanthosis and focal thickening in the granular layer (Chuang, 2013).

## CLINICAL PRESENTATION

LP most commonly occurs on the flexural surfaces of the extremities, with a generalized eruption within 2 to 16 weeks. Pruritus is common in LP but can vary in severity depending on lesion type and areas involved. LP can also affect the mucous membranes, the genitalia, the nails, and the scalp as follows:

- Mucous membranes commonly have LP on the tongue and the buccal mucosa; they appear as white or gray streaks forming a linear or reticular pattern on a violaceous background. Oral lesions are categorized as reticular, plaque like, atrophic, papular, erosive, and bullous. Ulcerated oral lesions have had a higher incidence of malignant transformation in men, which is attributed to smoking and chewing tobacco. Other mucosal membrane involvement is found on the conjunctivae, the larynx, the esophagus, the tonsils, the bladder, the vulva, and the vaginal vault; throughout the gastrointestinal tract; and around the anus.
- Genital lesions in men appears as annular lesions on the glans with Wickham striae on the lesions. Vulvar involvement can range from reticulate papules to severe erosions, with associated dyspareunia and pruritus. Vulvar and urethral stenosis may be a complication.
- Nail LP appears as longitudinal grooving and ridging. LP can cause hyperpigmentation, subungual hyperkeratosis, onycholysis, and longitudinal melanonychia.
- Skin lesions can include lesions on the scalp, which may be violaceous, scaly, and pruritic papules. These lesions can progress to atrophic cicatricial alopecia, known as lichen planopilaris. Pseudopelade can be a final endpoint. (Chuang, 2013, Goldstein & Goldstein, 2013; Habif, 2004)

Variations in LP include the following:

- Hypertrophic LP is very pruritic and appears on the extensor surfaces of the legs, especially around the ankles. These lesions can be chronic with resultant pigmentation changes and scarring when the lesions finally clear.

- Atrophic LP is the result of annular or hypertrophic LP.
- Erosive/ulcerative LP is found on the mucosal surfaces and evolves from sites of previous LP involvement.
- Follicular LP (also known as Lichen planopilaris) is characterized by keratotic papules that may merge into plaques. This condition is more common in women. This can result in a scarring alopecia.
- Annular LP presents with an atrophic center and is seen on the buccal mucosa and the male genitalia.
- Linear LP may form a zosteri form lesion, or they may develop as a Köebner effect.
- Vesicular and bullous LP develops on the lower limbs or in the mouth from preexisting LP lesions.
- Actinic LP occurs in regions such as Africa, the Middle East, and India. The nails, scalp, mucosa, and covered skin are spared. Lesions appear as round patches with a hyperpigmented center surrounded by a hypopigmented area.
- LP pigmentosus is a rare variant of LP but can be more common in persons with darker-pigmented skin. It usually appears on the face and neck.
- LP pemphigoides is rare. Blisters will develop on existing LP lesions. Clinically, histopathologically, and immunopathologically, it has features of LP and bullous pemphigoid but has a much better prognosis than pemphigoid. (Chuang, 2013; Habif, 2004)

## DIFFERENTIAL DIAGNOSIS

The differential diagnosis is:

- Atopic dermatitis or discoid eczema
- Graft-versus-host disease
- Herpes zoster
- Insect bites (e.g., fleas)
- Lichen nitidus
- Lichen simplex chronicus
- Lichenoid eruptions
- Pityriasis rosea
- Psoriasis, guttate
- Psoriasis, plaque
- Syphilis
- Systemic drug reactions
- Tinea corporis (Chuang, 2013)

## TREATMENT/MANAGEMENT

LP usually resolves without treatment in 8 to 12 months. Topical steroids may be used for pruritus. Severe cases, especially those with scalp, nail, and mucous membrane involvement, require more intensive therapy. Treatments for LP are as follows:

- The first-line treatments of cutaneous LP are topical steroids (class I or II ointments). Systemic steroids may be used for symptoms and for a quicker resolution. Intramuscular triamcinolone 40 to 80 mg every 6 to 8 weeks is also used, and oral metronidazole and oral acitretin have been shown to be effective.
- For LP of the oral mucosa, topical steroids are usually tried first. Topical and systemic cyclosporin, topical calcineurin inhibitors, and oral or topical retinoids are also used.
- Psoralen with UV-A (PUVA) therapy for 8 weeks has shown efficacy. (Chuang, 2013; Goldstein & Goldstein, 2013; Habif, 2004)

## SPECIAL CONSIDERATIONS

- Men are at higher risk of developing malignancy because of increased oral tobacco use.
- Medications used for the treatment of LP may cause infection, osteoporosis, adrenal insufficiency, bone marrow suppression, renal damage, hyperlipidemia, and growth retardation in children.
- Permanent alopecia may be the result of scalp involvement.
- Hypertrophic lesions can cause residual hyperpigmentation.
- Vulvar lesions can be pruritic and painful.
- Hepatitis C virus infection may be present.
- The prognosis for LP is good because most cases regress within 18 months. Some cases recur. (Chuang, 2013; Goldstein & Goldstein, 2013; Habif, 2004)

## WHEN TO REFER

Dermatology referral is warranted for all types of LP.

## PATIENT EDUCATION

- Patients should be told about the self-limiting nature of LP.
- Patients should be told that recurrences are rare.
- Patients should be told about the potential side effects of various treatments.

### CLINICAL PEARLS

High (2011) described the primary skin lesions of LP by "P" words, and Goodheart (2011) referred to the seven Ps:

- Plentiful
- Pruritic but may be asymptomatic
- Polished; shiny
- Purple; violaceous in color
- Polygonal
- Planar; flat-topped
- Papules and plaques

Other presentations include:

- Lesions are pleomorphic in shape and configuration (even on the same patient). LP lesions have a tendency to heal with postinflammatory hyperpigmentation.
- Oral lesions differ from skin lesions, displaying Wickham striae (a white reticular netlike or lacy pattern), which lacks the papules seen on the skin (High, 2011). The presence of Wickham striae of oral mucosa is essentially diagnostic for LP (Habif, Campbell, Chapman, Dinulos, & Zug, 2011).
- According to High (2011, p. 87), "Lichenoid drug eruption may be indistinguishable from idiopathic LP."
- Diseases such as hepatitis C or drug-associated lichenoid reactions must be ruled out (Goodheart, 2011).

## REFERENCES

Chuang, T. Y. (2013, February 25). *Lichen planus*. Retrieved from http://emedicine.medscape.com/article/1123213-overview#aw2aab6b2b2.

Goldstein, B. G., & Goldstein, A. O. (2013). *Lichen planus*. Retrieved from http://www.uptodate.com/contents/lichen-planus?view.

Goodheart, H. (2011). *Goodheart's same-site differential diagnosis: A rapid method of diagnosing and treating common skin disorders*. Philadelphia, PA: Lippincott Williams & Wilkins.

Habif, T. P. (2004). *Clinical dermatology: A color guide to diagnosis and therapy* (4th ed.). Philadelphia, PA: Mosby.

Habif, T. P., Campbell, J., Chapman, M., Dinulos, J., & Zug, K. (2011). *Skin disease diagnosis and treatment* (3rd ed.). Philadelphia, PA: Elsevier/Saunders.

High, W. (2011). Lichenoid skin eruptions. In J. Fitzpatrick & J. Morelli (Eds.). *Dermatology secrets plus* (4th ed, pp. 84–89). Philadelphia, PA: Elsevier/Saunders.

James, W. D., Berger, T. G., & Elston, D. M. (2006). *Andrews' disease of the skin: Clinical dermatology* (10th ed.). Philadelphia, PA: Saunders/Elsevier.

# Molluscum Contagiosum

**OVERVIEW**

*Molluscum contagiosum virus* (MCV) is a large DNA-containing benign viral infection that affects humans (Figure III.39; Goodheart, 2011). It is caused by four closely related types of poxvirus, MCV-1 to -4, and their variants. MCV-1 infections are the most common, representing 90% of cases in the United States. MCV causes characteristic skin lesions consisting of multiple, rounded, dome-shaped, flesh-colored, waxy papules that are 2 to 5 mm in diameter (Bhatia, 2012; Gelmetti, Frasin, & Restano, 2010; Isaacs, 2012; James, Berger, & Elston, 2006).

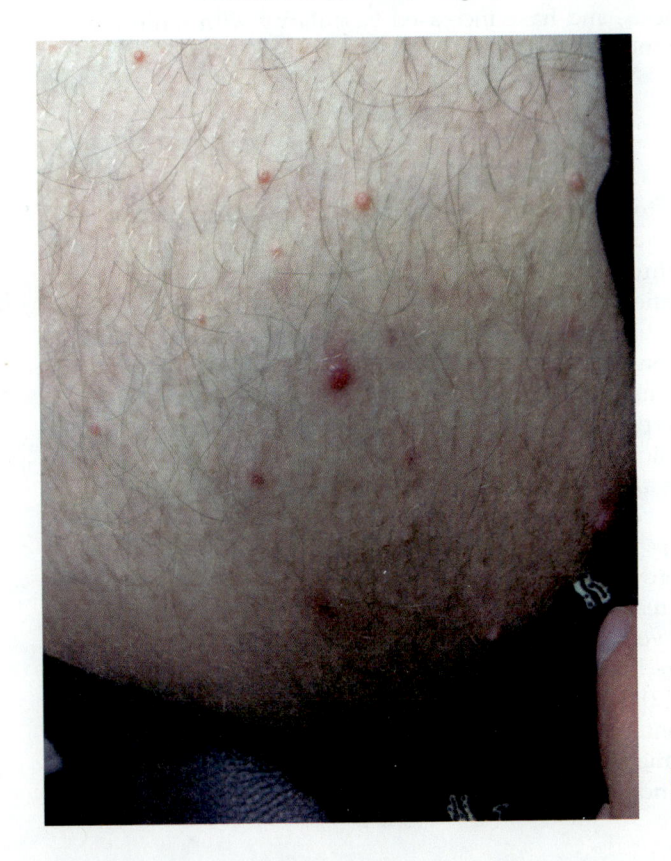

FIGURE III.39   Molluscum contagiosum virus infection

## EPIDEMIOLOGY

In the United States, MCV accounts for approximately 1% of all skin disorders (Isaacs, 2012). In patients infected with HIV/AIDS with a CD4 cell count less than 100 cells/μL, the prevalence of MCV-2 is as high as 33% (Bhatia, 2012).

Several studies have shown that males are affected by MCV more than females. MCV is rare in children younger than age 1 year. The greatest incidence is in children younger than age 5 years, in young sexually active adults, and in HIV patients. The frequency among children is attributed to casual contact, whereas the peak in young adults correlates with sexual contact (Bhatia, 2012; Isaacs, 2012).

## PATHOLOGY/HISTOLOGY

MCV reproduces in the cytoplasm of epithelial cells, producing cytoplasmic inclusions and enlargement of infected cells. This virus infects only the epidermis when there is contact with infected persons or contaminated objects. The initial infection seems to occur in the basal layer, and the incubation period is usually 2 to 6 weeks (Bhatia, 2012; Isaacs, 2012).

MCV has a characteristic histopathology. Lesions affect primarily the follicular epithelium. The lesion is acanthotic and cup shaped. In the cytoplasm of the prickle cells, numerous small eosinophilic and later basophilic inclusion bodies, called molluscum bodies or Henderson–Patterson bodies, are formed. Eventually their bulk compresses the nucleus to the side of the cell. In the fully developed lesion, each lobule empties into a central crater. Characteristic brick-shaped poxvirus particles are seen on electron microscopy in the epidermis. Sometimes the lesions expand beyond local cellular involvement and become inflamed, edematous, and have increased vascularity with infiltration by neutrophils, lymphocytes, and monocytes (Bhatia, 2012; James et al., 2006).

## CLINICAL PRESENTATION

MCV is spread by direct skin-to-skin contact and can occur anywhere on the body. The virus can be transmitted via autoinoculation by scratching or touching a lesion. Infection can also be spread through bath sponges or towels or skin contact during contact sports. If MCV is identified in the genital skin areas of an adult, it is considered a sexually transmitted disease (Habif, Campbell, Chapman, Dinulos, & Zug, 2011).

MCV is usually asymptomatic; however, individual lesions may be tender or pruritic. Patient history may include infected sexual partners, family members, or other contacts. Parents may report recent exposure to other children affected with MCV at school, camp, or public recreational facilities (e.g., gymnasiums, swimming pools; Bhatia, 2012; Gelmetti et al., 2010; Isaacs, 2012; James et al., 2006).

If the patient has skin conditions that disrupt the epidermal layer (*atopic dermatitis*), molluscum tends to spread more rapidly. Atopic dermatitis must be treated simultaneously with MCV to prevent autoinoculation related to the altered skin barrier (Habif et al., 2011). MCV may resolve spontaneously in 6 to 9 months, although some cases may persist for several years. Immunosuppressed patients or patients taking immunosuppressive drugs (prednisone, methotrexate) may have more extensive and resistant infections (Bhatia, 2012).

Lesions are solitary, nontender, flesh-colored, dome-shaped papules with a central umbilication. Lesions may be grouped or spread out. Healthy patients may have fewer than 20 lesions. Underneath the umbilicated center is a white, curd-like core that contains molluscum bodies. Lesions may be located anywhere; however, a preference for the face, trunk, and extremities is seen in children and a preference for the groin and genitalia is observed in adults. Lesions are rarely found on the palms, soles, oral mucosa, or conjunctiva (Bhatia, 2012; James et al., 2006; Isaacs, 2012).

Other characteristics of MCV to consider include the following:

- Intertriginous areas: Hundreds of lesions may develop in intertriginous areas, such as the axillae and intercrural region.
- Atopic dermatitis: Patients with atopic dermatitis usually have a large number of lesions that are typically seen in areas of lichenified skin.
- Eczema: Approximately 10% of patients develop eczema around the lesions, with this being attributed to toxic substances produced by the virus or to a hypersensitivity reaction to the virus. Eczema that is associated with molluscum lesions subsides spontaneously following initial exposure to the virus.
- Inflammatory changes: After trauma, or spontaneously after several months, inflammatory changes result in suppuration, crusting, and eventual resolution of the lesion. (Bhatia, 2012; Isaacs, 2012)

Disfiguring lesions may occur in patients with the following conditions:

- AIDS: Facial and perioral MCV most commonly observed as a manifestation of HIV infection.
- Immunocompromised: Lesions often occur more on the face and neck
- Sarcoidosis
- Lymphocytic leukemia
- Congenital immunodeficiency
- Selective immunoglobulin M deficiency
- Thymoma
- Treatment with prednisone and methotrexate
- Disseminated malignancy
- Refractory atopic dermatitis

## DIFFERENTIAL DIAGNOSIS

- Basal cell carcinoma
- Condyloma acuminatum
- Cryptococcosis
- Keratosis pilaris
- Milia
- Pearly penile papules
- Pyogenic granuloma
- Surgical treatment of basal cell carcinoma
- Varicella-zoster virus

## TREATMENT/MANAGEMENT

Goals of treatment include prevention of lesion spread to other sites, decreasing the risk of transmission to others, resolution of pruritus, and prevention of scarring that can result from lesions that become inflamed, traumatized, or secondarily infected. Adolescents and adults with sexually transmitted MCV should be treated to avoid the spread of the disease to others. Early treatment is also indicated for immunocompromised individuals, in whom infections can become severe. However, for healthy children with MCV, treatment is optional. Parents and guardians should be informed of the expected course of the disease without treatment and the potential adverse effects of each treatment option (Isaacs, 2012).

In most instances, a diagnosis is easily established because of the distinctive, central umbilication of the dome-shaped lesion. The following techniques can aid in the diagnosis of MCV:

- Biopsies may be warranted if diagnosis is uncertain. Characteristic intracytoplasmic inclusion bodies (molluscum bodies, or Henderson–Paterson bodies) are seen with MCV.
- Express the pasty core of a lesion by crushing the lesion between two microscope slides; staining with crystal violetto reveals the particulate virions, which are present in abundance. (Bhatia, 2012; James et al., 2006)

Therapeutic options for MCV can be divided into broad categories, including the following:

- Benign neglect
- Direct lesional trauma
- Antiviral therapy
- Immune response stimulation (Bhatia, 2012; Isaacs, 2012; James et al., 2006)

Therapy is dependent on the clinical situation. In healthy children, treatment is aimed at limiting discomfort either by choosing no treatment or minimal trauma. However, in adults who usually want treatment, cryotherapy or curettage of individual lesions is effective and tolerated (Bhatia, 2012).

Clinical success has been reported with the use of the following topical agents, which may act as irritants, stimulating an immunologic response (Bhatia, 2012; Isaacs, 2012; James et al., 2006).

- Imiquimod cream (can be used in conjunction with cantharidin)
- Tretinoin
- Bichloracetic acid
- Trichloroacetic acid
- Salicylic acid
- Lactic acid
- Glycolic acid
- Silver nitrate

## SPECIAL CONSIDERATIONS

Those who are immunocompromised or have AIDS with low CD4 T-lymphocyte counts usually present with widespread, persistent, atypical presentation of MCV (Bhatia, 2012; Isaacs, 2012). Treatment for extensive molluscum in advanced HIV disease is resistant because the lesions are numerous and likely to recur (Turiansky & James, 2011).

## WHEN TO REFER

The prognosis in MCV is good because the disease is benign and self-limited. However, resistant cases or patients with immunity concerns should be evaluated by an infectious disease specialist (Bhatia, 2012).

## PATIENT EDUCATION

According to Bhatia (2012), providers should include the following in patient education:

- Educate patients or parents about MCV, prognosis, transmission to others, treatment options, and risk of therapy.
- Advise patients that good hand washing and limited physical contact will reduce transmission. Instruct the patient to avoid scratching, which will prevent spread of lesions.
- Inform parents that removing children from school is not necessary. They should keep affected areas covered, avoid sharing of clothes, and discourage physical contact to help prevent transmission.
- Educate about all sexually transmitted diseases even though MCV is benign and can be treated. Emphasize abstinence until lesions resolve. Patients with multiple sexual partners should be tested for HIV.

## CLINICAL PEARLS

- Children diagnosed with MCV should not bathe with their siblings (Habif et al., 2011).
- Cantharone (cantharidin 0.7%) should not be used on a child's face (Habif et al., 2011).
- The treatments effective in treating warts are often effective for treating MCV (Reed, 2011).
- An anecdotal treatment for MCV is cimetidine and oral griseofulvin (Goodheart, 2011).

## REFERENCES

Bhatia, A. C. (2012, January 5). *Molluscum contagiosum*. Retrieved from http://emedicine.medscape.com/article/910570-overview

Gelmetti, C., Frasin, A., & Restano, L. (2010). Innovative therapeutics in pediatric dermatology. *Dermatology Clinics, 28*, 619–629.

Goodheart, H. (2011). *Goodheart's same-site differential diagnosis: A rapid method of diagnosing and treating common skin disorders*. Philadelphia, PA: Lippincott Williams & Wilkins.

Habif, T., Campbell, J., Chapman, M., Dinulos, J., & Zug, K. (2011). *Skin disease diagnosis and treatment* (3rd ed.). Philadelphia, PA: Saunders/Elsevier.

Isaacs, S. N. (2012). *Molluscum contagiosum*. Retrieved from http://uptodate.com/contents/molluscum-contagiosum

James, W. D., Berger, T. G., & Elston, D. M. (2006). *Andrews' diseases of the skin: Clinical dermatology* (10th ed.). Philadelphia, PA: Saunders/Elsevier.

Reed, B. (2011). Warts and molluscum contagiosum. In J. E. Fitzpatrick & J. G. Morelli (Eds.), *Dermatology secrets plus* (4th ed., pp. 182–187). Philadelphia, PA: Elsevier/Mosby.

Turiansky, G., & James, W. (2011). Cutaneous manifestation of AIDS. Warts and molluscum contagiosum. In J. E. Fitzpatrick & J. G. Morelli (Eds.), *Dermatology secrets plus* (4th ed., pp. 280–286). Philadelphia, PA: Elsevier/Mosby.

# Nail Conditions

## INGROWN NAILS

### OVERVIEW

*Ingrown toenail (onychocryptosis)* occurs when the lateral nail plate pierces the lateral nail fold and enters the dermis (Figure III.40). The great toenail is most commonly affected. Common signs and symptoms include pain, edema, exudate, and granulation tissue. The condition is often caused by poorly fitting shoes, excessive trimming of the lateral plate, pincer nail deformity, and trauma (Goldstein & Goldstein, 2012b; James, Berger, & Elston, 2006; Tolen, 2013).

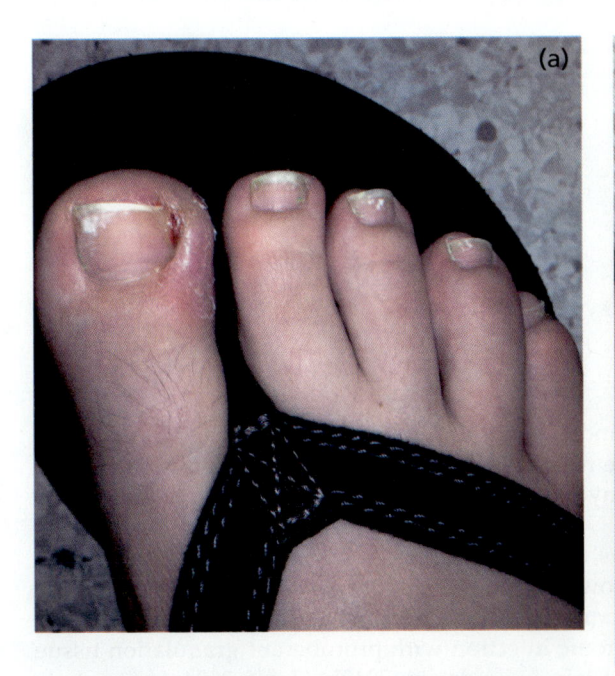

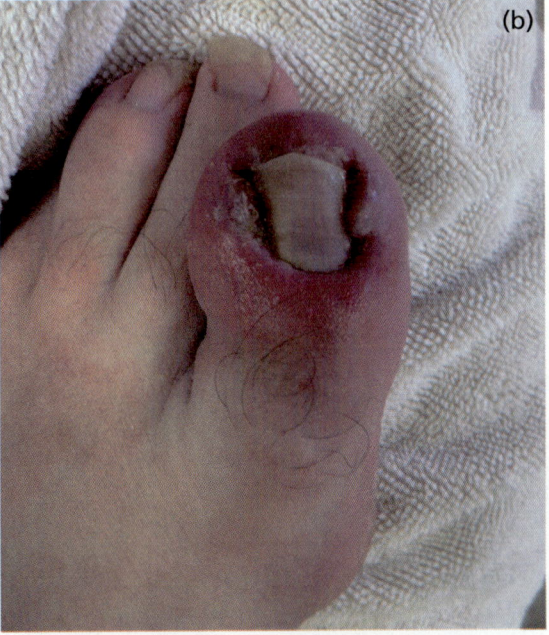

FIGURE III.40 Examples of **(a)** mild to moderate and **(b)** moderate to severe ingrown toenails

## EPIDEMIOLOGY

In the United States, ingrown toenails are the most common nail problem. The lateral margins of the great toe are most frequently affected. In general, morbidity is usually the result of infection of the tissues; if not treated, abscess formation (paronychia) may occur or spread, leading to osteomyelitis, systemic infection, sepsis, or amputation. No racial predilection is noted, and there is a reported male-to-female ratio of three to one. Ingrown toenails can occur at any age but are most common at 20 to 30 years. Children are most commonly affected when they begin to walk and wear shoes; at this stage, congenital onychocryptosis can occur (Tolen, 2013).

## PATHOLOGY/HISTOLOGY

Ingrown nails result from an abnormal fit of the nail plate in the usual nail groove. Sharp spicules of the lateral nail margin develop and are slowly driven into the dermis of the nail groove. The nail acts as a foreign body, causing an inflammatory response in the area of penetration; erythema, edema, purulence, and development of granulation tissue occurs (Tolen, 2013).

## CLINICAL PRESENTATION

Patients present with complaints of sharp, focal pain adjacent to the nail bed of the affected digit. When the toenail is involved, the discomfort worsens with weight bearing and ambulation. Signs and symptoms of an ingrown toenail are as follows (Goldstein & Goldstein, 2012b; Habif, 2004; James et al., 2006; Tolen, 2013):

- Mild to moderate lesions characterized by minimal to moderate pain, little erythema, and no discharge
- Moderate to severe lesions characterized by substantial erythema and pus

## DIFFERENTIAL DIAGNOSIS

- Impetigo
- Lymphangitis
- Obesity
- Osteomyelitis
- *Staphylococcus aureus* infection
- Streptococcal infection, Group A

## TREATMENT/MANAGEMENT

Usually, no laboratory studies are indicated in patients with ingrown nails. Potassium chloride (KOH) and fungal culture may be needed if a fungal infection is suspected. If fracture, foreign body, or osteomyelitis is suspected, radiography is recommended (Tolen, 2013).

Treatment options in patients with ingrown nails depend on the stage of onychocryptosis. Development of ingrown nails is divided into three stages: (1) erythema, edema, and focal tenderness; (2) crusting and expressible purulence at the nail fold and nail plate junction; and (3) chronic infection with protuberant granulation tissue extending over the nail plate (Goldstein & Goldstein, 2012b; Habif, 2004; James et al., 2006; Tolen, 2013).

- Stage 1 can be treated by recommending shoes with a comfortable wide toe or open-toed shoes. Patients should be instructed to cut the nail straight across and avoid cutting back the lateral margins. The nail edge should extend past the tissue.
- Stage 2 can be treated by pulling the soft skin away from the side of the nail, elevating the affected edge of nail from the soft skin, and placing a small pledget of cotton under the nail edge to lift it back into the nail grove. Children should be kept from participating in excessive activity, the foot should be elevated, and warm foot soaks should be given.
- Stage 3 should be treated by removing the nail margin in a minor surgical outpatient procedure: Perform a digital block with lidocaine 1% without epinephrine; 2.5% lidocaine mixed with 2.5% prilocaine applied topically can help with discomfort from digital block. Using nail-splitting scissors or a hemostat, insert the instrument under the nail plate and remove the involved nail wedge with nail clippers or scissors. Remove granulation tissue with a curette and/or silver nitrate sticks. Dilute hydrogen peroxide one to one with tap water and cleanse the surgical site with cotton swabs two to three times per day, followed by application of either bacitracin or mupirocin ointment. Often secondary infections are treated with oral antibiotics, especially in patients with diabetes or those who are immunocompromised. Follow-up in 2 to 3 days is recommended.

For recurrent ingrown toenails, consider permanent nail ablation of the lateral nail horn. This is best achieved with a combination of surgical excision plus phenol ablation (chemical matrixectomy).

## SPECIAL CONSIDERATIONS

The nail plate can be forced out of the nail groove by inappropriate fitting shoes, trauma, or cutting the nail back in a curvilinear fashion. Other causes include the following:

- Heredity (Some people are genetically predisposed to inwardly curved nails with distortion of one or both nail margins.)
- Underlying bony pathology causing deformation of the nail
- Obesity causing deepening of the nail groove
- Antiviral therapy for HIV (Indinavir has also been reported to have an association with increased incidence of ingrown nails.)
- Previous trauma resulting in an irregularly shaped nail
- Drugs such as isotretinoin and lamivudine, which may induce periungual granulation tissue, mimicking an ingrown toenail (James et al., 2006; Tolen, 2013)

## WHEN TO REFER

The following situations warrant a referral:

- Consult a podiatrist, dermatologist, or orthopedic surgeon for removal of the ingrown nail or for patients who have had previous unsuccessful removal.
- Referral to an orthopedist is required if inflammatory osteophytic changes are observed or if evidence of osteomyelitis is present. Immediate antibiotic treatment should begin, and inpatient treatment may be needed for osteomyelitis.
- Follow-up care is recommended for immunocompromised patients or patients with diabetes. Antibiotics may be started in those who are immunosuppressed. (Tolen, 2013)

## PATIENT EDUCATION

- All patients should be educated about proper nail trimming. They should allow the lateral plate to grow well beyond the lateral nail fold before trimming horizontally.
- Inform patients that good hygiene and wearing appropriately sized footwear are important. They should not wear shoes with narrow, pointed toe boxes that compress the toes.

# MELANONYCHIA

## OVERVIEW

Melanonychia is a brown or black pigmentation of the nail caused by the presence of melanin in the nail plate. Melanonychia commonly presents lengthwise along the nail, which is referred to as longitudinal melanonychia (LM) or melanonychiastriata (Adigun, 2012; Rich & Jefferson, 2012).

## EPIDEMIOLOGY

Physiologic melanonychia is more common in darker-skinned individuals. Black individuals older than 20 years have a 77% incidence of melanonychia, whereas those older than 50 years have a greater than 90% chance of developing the condition. Japanese individuals have 10% to 20% incidence of LM, whereas Whites have only a 1.4% chance of developing LM. The morbidity and mortality of melanonychia depends on the underlying cause. If subungual melanoma is the source, morbidity and mortality is higher compared with other bodily areas affected by melanoma sites. Melanonychia is not gender specific; males and females are affected equally. As noted earlier, older individuals are affected more often than younger. In children, melanonychia is often caused by melanocytic nevi, and subungual melanoma and melanoma in situ are rare (Adigun, 2012).

## PATHOLOGY/HISTOLOGY

Melanonychia occurs because of increased manufacture of melanin by melanocytes in the nail matrix. Adults commonly have approximately 200 melanocytes per square millimeter in the nail matrix. When these melanocytes are activated, melanosomes filled with melanin are moved to differentiating matrix cells, which travel distally as they become nail plate oncocytes. The result is a visible band of pigmentation in the nail plate (Adigun, 2012).

LM can be caused by melanocytic activation or melanocytic hyperplasia. Melanocytic activation is an increased synthesis of melanin with a normal number of melanocytes. Melanocytic hyperplasia (including melanocytic nevi and melanoma) is an increased synthesis of melanin with an increased number of melanocytes. Nevi account for 12% of LM cases in adults and 50% of LM cases in children.

The histopathologic findings vary based on the etiology of melanonychia. Nail matrix nevi can have an unusual appearance histologically, and they are considered "special site nevi," a subset of acral-pigmented lesions. The majority of nail matrix nevi are junctional. Histologically, nail matrix nevi can be highly cellular; can have hyperchromatic, large cells that do not form discrete nests; and can possess prominent, abundant, and uneven cytoplasmic dendrites. A Fontana–Masson stain highlights melanin and thus may be useful in the determination of location of pigment within the nail matrix epithelium. Of note, 20% to 30% of subungual melanomas may be amelanotic, and immunostains for melanocytes, such as S-100, Melan-A, HMB-45, and microphthalmia transcription factor (MITF), may provide important diagnostic information (Adigun, 2012).

## CLINICAL PRESENTATION

Patients with melanonychia usually present with an asymptomatic pigmentation of the nail plate. Obtain a careful history about medications, previous treatments, hobbies, medical history, family history, previous trauma to the area, history of biopsy of the nail and the results, whether any cultures for fungal or bacterial infections been done, the number of nails affected, changes to the nail over time, and the ethnicity of the patient (Adigun, 2012).

Melanonychia appears as a tan, brown, or black discoloration of the nail unit that is observed in the nail plate. The nail plate can be totally involved, or only a single longitudinal band may be present. Transverse melanonychia is possible, and more than one nail can be affected (Adigun, 2012).

## DIFFERENTIAL DIAGNOSIS

- Melanotic macule of the nail unit
- Nail matrix nevus
- Onychomycosis
- Subungual hematoma
- Subungual melanoma (Adigun, 2012)

## TREATMENT/MANAGEMENT

If an infectious cause is suspected, a nail plate clipping should be evaluated for histologic analysis and appropriate cultures. Laboratory tests are recommended if systemic and/or dermatologic cause is suspected (Adigun, 2012).

In cases of subungual melanoma, the patient may describe a long-standing history of LM but has noticed a change in appearance. Changes in color, size, pattern, ulceration; new onset of pain; or the presence of blood under the nail plate should be evaluated. Subungual nevi have parallel lines, whereas subungual melanoma has irregular lines that are not parallel (Adigun, 2012).

If melanonychia is secondary to systemic and/or dermatologic disease, treatment of the underlying condition is helpful. If melanonychia is secondary to a drug, discontinuation of the offending agent may result in clearance (Adigun, 2012). Close monitoring of the affective nail is recommended, especially if patients refuse to have a nail biopsy.

## SPECIAL CONSIDERATIONS

Characteristics of melanonychia that should warrant concern for subungual melanoma (e.g., Hutchinson sign) are described with the acronym ABCDEF:

- Age (peak incidence of subungual melanoma, age 50–70 years)
- Brown-black band with range greater than 3 mm with multicolored borders
- Change in nail band morphology despite treatment
- Digit involved (thumb often affected more than the great toe, and the great toe is frequently affected more than the index finger by subungual melanoma)
- Extension of the dark hyperpigmentation of the nailbed, nail matrix, and/or nail plate onto the adjacent cuticle and proximal and/or lateral nail folds (Hutchinson sign)
- Family or personal history of dysplastic nevus or melanoma (Adigun, 2012)

Peutz–Jeghers syndrome or Laugier–Hunziker syndrome can be identified by examining the oral and genital mucosa.

## WHEN TO REFER

LM is associated with multiple systemic conditions that may require referral to a specific specialist to manage the primary disease. Subungual melanoma has a poor prognosis; consultation with a hematologist/oncologist regarding management options is recommended (Adigun, 2012).

## PATIENT EDUCATION

Patients should be instructed to closely monitor LM lesions for any change in color, pattern, size of the band, or new-onset pain and/or ulceration because these can be signs of subungual melanoma (Adigun, 2012).

# ONYCHOMYCOSIS

## OVERVIEW

*Onychomycosis* (OM) is a fungal infection that can affect any part of the nails (Figure III.41). OM can cause pain, discomfort, and deformity of the nail, which may produce serious physical and occupational limitations (Tosti, 2013).

## EPIDEMIOLOGY

The proliferation of fungal infections in the United States can be attributed to the large immigration of dermatophytes, especially *Trichophyton rubrum*, from West Africa and Southeast Asia. The incidence of OM has been reported to be 2% to 13% in North America. OM accounts for half of all nail disorders and frequently affects adults.

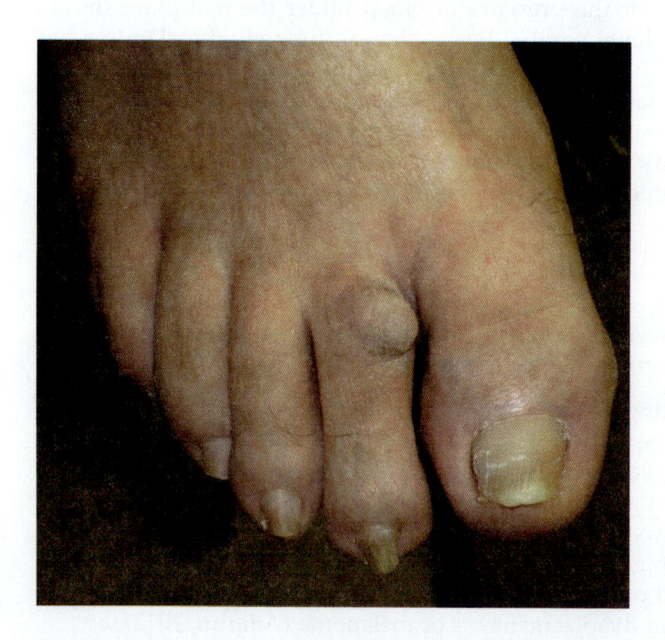

FIGURE III.41  Onychomycosis infection

OM affects toenails more than fingernails. One third of patients with skin fungal infections also have OM. The incidence of OM has been increasing, owing to such factors as diabetes, heredity, immunosuppression, and increasing age (Tosti, 2013).

OM affects persons of all races and affects males more commonly than females, whereas candidal infections are more common in women than in men. Aging adults are affected more often than children younger than 18 (2.6% incidence; Tosti, 2013).

## PATHOLOGY/HISTOLOGY

The main subtypes of OM are distal lateral subungualonychomycosis (DLSO), white superficial onychomycosis (WSO), proximal subungualonychomycosis (PSO), endonyxonychomycosis (EO), and candidalonychomycosis. Patients may have a blend of these subtypes. Total dystrophic onychomycosis refers to the most advanced form of any subtype (Goldstein & Goldstein, 2012a; Habif, 2004; James et al., 2006; Tosti, 2013).

The pathogenesis of OM depends on the clinical subtype. In DLSO, the most common form of OM, the fungus spreads from the plantar foot and invades the hyponychium of the nailbed; as a result, inflammation occurs. WSO is rare and caused by direct invasion of the surface of the nail plate. In PSO, the least common subtype, the fungus invades the nail matrix through the proximal nail and grows deep into the proximal nail plate. EO is a variation of DLSO in which the fungus is present on the skin and invades the nail plate. Total dystrophic onychomycosis involves the entire nail (Goldstein & Goldstein, 2012a; Habif, 2004; James et al., 2006; Tosti, 2013).

*Candida* infection of the nail is rare because the yeast needs an individual with altered immunity to be able to penetrate the nails. The yeast infects the nail plate and eventually the proximal and lateral nail folds (Goldstein & Goldstein, 2012a; Habif, 2004; James et al., 2006; Tosti, 2013).

Histologic examination of the nail is preferred over a culture or KOH testing. Nail clippings (sent in formalin-filled container) or an incisional nail biopsy should be sent. Specimens should be checked with periodic acid–Schiff stain (PAS) or methenamine silver to evaluate for fungal elements (James et al., 2006; Tosti, 2013).

## CLINICAL PRESENTATION

OM is caused by three main classes of fungi: dermatophytes, yeasts (e.g., *Candida*), and nondermatophytic molds (Goldstein & Goldstein, 2012a; Habif, 2004; James et al., 2006; Tosti, 2013).

- Dermatophytes: *T. rubrum* accounts for 70% of all cases, and *Trichophyton mentagrophytes* accounts for 20%. *T. rubrum* is the most common pathogen in DLSO. PSO as a result of *T. rubrum* infection is typical of immunosuppressed patients, and PSO with periungual inflammation is usually caused by molds. WSO is usually caused by *T. mentagrophytes*.
- Yeasts: OM from *Candida* is rare, seen in premature children, immunocompromised patients, and persons with chronic mucocutaneous candidiasis.
- Nondermatophytic molds (e.g., *Fusarium* species, *Scopulariopsis brevicaulis*, *Aspergillus* species): These are becoming more common worldwide, accounting for up to 10% of cases. Nondermatophytic molds cause deep WSO.

Risk factors for OM include family history, advancing age, presence of comorbidities, previous trauma, hot climate, participation in fitness activities, immunosuppression (e.g., HIV, drug induced), diabetes, psoriasis, tinea pedis, genetic predisposition, communal bathing, and occlusive footwear (Goldstein & Goldstein, 2012a; Tosti, 2013).

OM is usually asymptomatic and patients will seek care because of cosmetic concerns, which can affect self-esteem and social interaction because of paresthesia, pain, discomfort, and loss of dexterity (Goldstein & Goldstein, 2012a; Tosti, 2013).

The subtypes of OM may be distinguished on the basis of their usual presenting clinical features (Goldstein & Goldstein, 2012a; James et al., 2006; Tosti, 2013).

- DLSO appears as a subungual hyperkeratosis and onycholysis on the nail, which is usually yellow-white in color. Yellow streaks and/or yellow onycholytic areas in the central portion of the nail plate are common.
- EO presents as a milky white discoloration of the nail plate, without subungual hyperkeratosis or onycholysis.
- WSO is confined to the toenails and manifests as small, white, speckled or powdery patches on the surface of the nail plate. The nail is rough and crumbles easily. Molds produce a deep variety of WSO characterized by a larger and deeper nail plate invasion.
- PSO presents as an area of leukonychia in the proximal nail plate that moves distally with nail growth. Periungual inflammation is present when PSO is caused by mold.
- Total dystrophic onychomycosis presents as a thickened, opaque, and yellow-brown nail.
- In *Candida*, OM associated with chronic mucocutaneous candidiasis, or immunodepression, several or all digits are affected by total dystrophic onychomycosis associated with periungual inflammation. The fingers or toes may often take on a bulbous or drumstick appearance.

## DIFFERENTIAL DIAGNOSIS

Goldstein and Goldstein (2012a), Habif (2004), James et al. (2006), and Tosti, (2013) cited the following as the differential diagnosis for OM:

- Contact dermatitis, irritant
- Lichen planus
- Malignant melanoma
- Psoriasis, nails
- Traumatic onycholysis

## TREATMENT/MANAGEMENT

Treatment of OM depends on the clinical type of the OM and the number and severity of affected nails. Systemic treatment is required in PSO and in DLSO. Topical therapy can be used for WSO. Topical therapies used alone should be limited to cases involving less than half the nail plate or if patients cannot tolerate systemic therapies. The agent commonly used in the United States is cyclopiroxolamine 8% nail lacquer solution (Goldstein & Goldstein, 2012a; Habif, 2004; James et al., 2006; Tosti, 2013).

The oral antifungal agents (itraconazole and terbinafine) are used for the treatment of OM because of shorter treatment duration and higher efficacy as compared to topical medications, with minimal adverse effects. Itraconazole is given at a dosage of 200 mg daily for 12 weeks for toenails and 6 weeks for fingernails, and terbinafine is given at a dosage of 250 mg daily for 12 weeks for toenails and 6 weeks for fingernails. Evidence shows better efficacy with terbinafine than with other oral agents. To decrease the adverse effects and duration of oral therapy, topical treatments and nail avulsion may also be part of the treatment plan (Goldstein & Goldstein, 2012a; Habif, 2004; James et al., 2006; Tosti, 2013).

Several laser devices are used to treat OM, including Nd:YAG lasers, diode lasers, and photodynamic therapy. Evidence-based data on efficacy of the different lasers are still poor. Surgical approaches to OM treatment can also include mechanical, chemical, or surgical nail avulsion. Chemical removal by using a 40% to 50% urea compound is painless and useful in patients with thick nails. Removal of the nail plate should be done as an adjunct in patients who are also on oral therapy (Tosti, 2013).

Although hepatotoxic reactions are unlikely, patients undergoing oral antifungal therapy should have a complete blood cell count and measurements of liver enzyme levels approximately every 4 to 6 weeks. Treatment may be discontinued after standard dosing with terbinafine or itraconazole when no evidence of fungal infection (by microscopy or culture) is present. After antifungal therapy, nails usually grow at a rate of 2 mm a month and can take a year to appear normal. If the outgrowth distance slows or stops after discontinuing antifungal therapy, another course of oral medication may be needed (James et al., 2006; Tosti, 2013).

## SPECIAL CONSIDERATIONS

In the elderly, persons with diabetes, and immunocompromised patients, skin injury adjacent to the nail may allow organisms to colonize, thereby increasing the risk of infectious complications such as cellulitis, osteomyelitis sepsis, and tissue necrosis (Tosti, 2013).

## WHEN TO REFER

Dermatology or podiatry referral for complicated presentation or resistant-to-treatment OM is recommended.

## PATIENT EDUCATION

Tosti (2013) recommended informing patients of the following:

- Patients should use footwear, especially in high-exposure areas such as communal bathing facilities and health clubs.
- Following treatment, nails may take up to a year to appear normal, and prophylactic antifungal therapy may be required to prevent reinfection of the skin and the nails. Patients can use topical terbinafine cream twice daily for 1 or 2 weeks for maintenance and prevention of tinea pedis.

# PARONYCHIA

## OVERVIEW

*Paronychia* is a superficial painful infection of the epithelium lateral and proximal to the nail plate (Figure III.42). The purulent infection is most frequently caused by trauma to the nail fold and staphylococci infection but usually has mixed aerobic and anaerobic flora. Patients' symptoms are substantially improved by simply draining the area. Chronic paronychial infections usually are fungal rather than bacterial in nature (Hickin, 2008; James et al., 2006; Murphy-Lavoie, 2012; Rich & Jefferson, 2012).

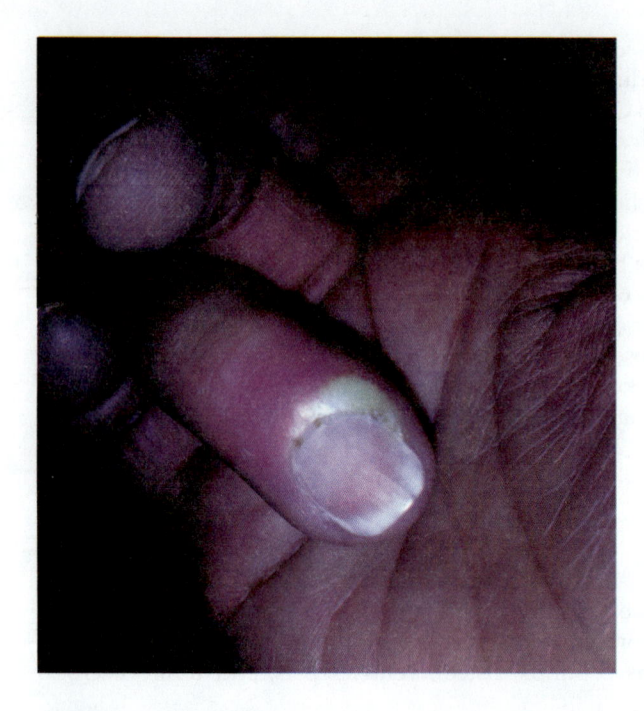

**FIGURE III.42** Paronychia infection
Courtesy of Dr. Joann Lubrano, DO

## EPIDEMIOLOGY

In the United States, paronychia is the most common of all hand infections, accounting for 35% of cases. If not properly treated, paronychia can result in hand infections, and occasionally, systemic infection from hematogenous extension. Paronychia is more common in females than in males (3:1) (Murphy-Lavoie, 2012).

## PATHOLOGY/HISTOLOGY

The lateral nail fold is usually affected first with paronychia infection because of cracks, fissures, or trauma (extreme manicuring, nail biting, thumb sucking), which allows bacterial entry through the skin barrier. The causative bacteria are usually *S. aureus, Streptococcus pyogenes, Pseudomonas* species, *Proteus* species, or anaerobes. The pathogenic yeast is most frequently *Candida albicans*. Patients at risk include those with diabetes mellitus, dyshidrotic eczema, or contact dermatitis and those with occupations that cause chronic dry, irritated hands. Sometimes, the infection involves the complete margin of skin around the nail plate, which causes mechanical separation of the nail plate from the perionychium (Goldstein & Goldstein, 2012b; James et al., 2006; Murphy-Lavoie, 2012).

## CLINICAL PRESENTATION

Patients present with complaints of a sudden onset of pain and swelling around the nail. Subjective history will often include nail biting, finger sucking, or trauma; exposure to chemical irritants, acrylic nails, or nail glue; or frequent water exposure to hands. Inquire as to the duration of symptoms, history of nail infections and previous treatment, and exposure to chemicals or water. Painless or severe swelling that radiates requires an expanded differential diagnosis. Chronic and recurrent paronychial infections should be evaluated thoroughly to rule out malignancy or fungal infection (Goldstein & Goldstein, 2012b; Murphy-Lavoie, 2012).

Possible physical findings of paronychia include the following:

- Erythema
- Edema
- Tenderness along the lateral nail fold
- Abscesses
- Infection
- Tissue irregularity (indicative of a malignancy)
- Vesicles on an erythematous base (indicative of herpetic whitlow)
- Green coloration of the nail (suggestive of *Pseudomonas* species infection)
- Hypertrophy of the nail plate (indicative of a fungal infection) (Goldstein & Goldstein, 2012b; Murphy-Lavoie, 2012)

The digital pressure test is used to evaluate for abscesses. Apply pressure to the palmar surface of the affected finger, and, if there is an abscess, the area will blanch. Infection is usually present only in the lateral nail fold; however, the entire finger and hand should be evaluated for extension of the infection.

## DIFFERENTIAL DIAGNOSIS

Goldstein and Goldstein (2012b) and Murphy-Lavoie (2012) cited the following for differential diagnosis.

- Cutaneous candidiasis
- Dermatitis, contact
- Dyshidrotic eczema
- Felon (pulp space infection)
- Fingertip injuries
- Hand infections
- Herpetic whitlow
- Nail cosmetics
- Onychomycosis
- Pseudomonal nail infection
- Psoriasis

## TREATMENT/MANAGEMENT

The only laboratory studies for paronychia are a Gram stain and culture or fungal culture. These can be done if bacterial infection or candidal infection is suspected. Laboratory studies are not routinely necessary for this paronychia process. If herpetic whitlow is suspected, a Tzanck smear or viral culture is recommended; a skin biopsy may be indicated in chronic cases in which malignancy is in question. Obtain a plain film radiograph of the fingertip to rule out foreign body, fracture, or sign of osteomyelitis (recurrent infection, elevated erythrocyte sedimentation rate, or presence of risk factors for osteomyelitis) (James et al., 2006; Murphy-Lavoie, 2012).

Treatment is as follows (Goldstein & Goldstein, 2012; James et al., 2006; Murphy-Lavoie, 2012):

- For acute paronychia:
  - Provide warm compresses or soaks with half-strength hydrogen peroxide. The digit should be anesthetized with an appropriate digital nerve block.

- Clean the nail plate and finger with antiseptic. The tip of a sharp instrument or point of a surgical blade is used to raise the lateral nail fold. The lateral fold of skin should be elevated slightly and irrigated with isotonic sodium chloride solution using a catheter tip syringe. Purulent drainage may be present.
- Severe paronychia extends along the medial and lateral nail edges. Treatment consists of splinting the cavity with a small wick to prevent adhesion and reformation.
- If purulence has progressed under the nail, excision of the ipsilateral nail may be warranted.
- The presence of a subungual abscess formation requires nail plate removal. Debridement of the nailbed may be necessary.
- The presence of a finger pulp abscess may require an additional incision of the pad of the fingertip to adequately drain. Referral to a hand surgeon is recommended because of the multiple neurovascular bundles that are present in the edges of the finger.
- Most paronychia infections can be managed without antibiotics unless cellulitis is present. Culture is recommended to rule out methicillin-resistant *Staphylococcus aureus* (MRSA) infection. Over-the-counter analgesics are usually sufficient.
- Chronic paronychial infections are usually managed with oral antifungals such as ketoconazole, itraconazole, or fluconazole.

## SPECIAL CONSIDERATIONS

Patients with diabetes mellitus, a history of steroid use, or a history of retroviral agent use related to HIV infection and those who are immunocompromised are at a greater risk for paronychia. Indinavir and lamivudine have been associated with an increased incidence of paronychia formation (Goldstein & Goldstein, 2012b; Murphy-Lavoie, 2012).

## WHEN TO REFER

Consult a hand surgeon if cellulitis, deep infection, glomus tumor, mucous cyst, or osteomyelitis are a possibility (Murphy-Lavoie, 2012).

## PATIENT EDUCATION

Providers should instruct patients to do the following:

- Cut hangnails to a semilunar smooth edge with a clean sharp nail trimmer.
- If frequently washing hands, use antibacterial soap and thoroughly dry hands.
- Do not push cuticles back or pick at cuticles.
- Wear rubber or latex-free gloves.
- Keep diabetes mellitus under control.

## CLINICAL PEARL

Three percent Thymol in alcohol applied topically three times daily to the affected nail fold is effective treatment for paronychia.

# REFERENCES

Adigun, C. (2012, May 31). *Melanonychia*. Retrieved from http://emedicine.medscape.com/article/785158-overview

Goldstein, A. O., & Goldstein, B. G. (2012a). *Onychomycosis*. Retrieved from http://uptodate.com/contents/onychomycosis

Goldstein, B. G., & Goldstein, A. O. (2012b). *Paronychia and ingrown toenails*. Retrieved from http://uptodate.com/contents/paronychia-and-ingrown-toenails

Habif, T. P. (2004). *Clinical dermatology: A color guide to diagnosis and therapy* (4th ed.). Philadelphia, PA: Mosby.

Hickin, L. (2008). Infections of the skin and nails. *Practice Nurse, 35*(9), 14–19.

James, W. D., Berger, T. G., & Elston, D. M. (2006). *Andrews' diseases of the skin: Clinical dermatology* (10th ed.). Philadelphia, PA: Saunders/Elsevier.

Murphy-Lavoie, H. (2012, May 31). *Paronychia*. Retrieved from http://emedicine.medscape.com/article/785158-overview

Rich, P., & Jefferson, J. A. (2012). *Overview of nail disorders*. Retrieved from http://uptodate.com/contents/overview-of-nail-disorders

Tolen, R. W. (2013, April 5). *Ingrown nails*. Retrieved from http://emedicine.medscape.com/article/909807-overview

Tosti, A. (2013, February 15). *Onychomycosis*. Retrieved from http://emedicine.medscape.com/article/1105828-overview#aw2aab6b2b2

# Pemphigus

## OVERVIEW

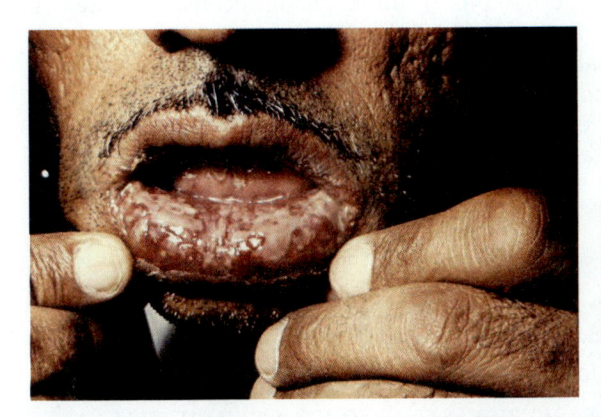

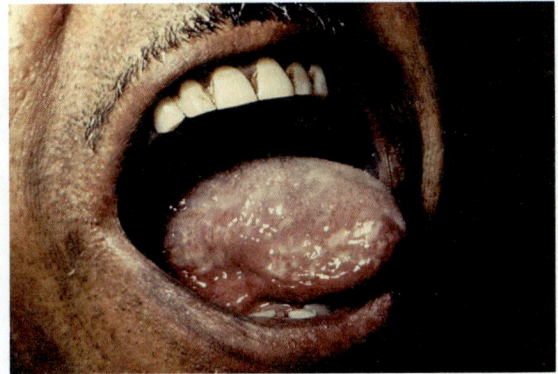

**FIGURE III.43** Examples of pemphigus vulgaris, the most common type of pemphigus
Courtesy of Dr. J. Lieberman, CDC, and Dr. Freideen Farzin, University of Tehran

*Pemphigus* commonly refers to a group of autoimmune blistering diseases on the skin and mucous membranes (Figure III.43). There are three types of pemphigus: pemphigus vulgaris, pemphigus foliaceus, and paraneoplastic pemphigus. Each of these types has specific presentations and immunopathologic qualities. Pemphigus vulgaris is the most common, accounting for 70% of all pemphigus cases (Herti & Sitaru, 2013; Zeina, 2013). Pemphigus vulgaris typically begins in the oral mucosa, and it can be months before cutaneous lesions develop (Wolff, Johnson, & Saavedra, 2013). Pemphigus foliaceous, the second most common type of pemphigus, has no mucosal lesions and begins with scaly, crusted lesions on an erythematous base (Wolff et al., 2013).

## EPIDEMIOLOGY

Pemphigus vulgaris can be a life-threatening autoimmune mucocutaneous disease with a mortality rate of approximately 5% to 15%. Mortality in individuals with pemphigus vulgaris is three times higher than in the general population. Morbidity and mortality in pemphigus vulgaris is related to the severity of the disease, the amount of steroids used to induce remission, and the presence of other comorbidities. The prognosis is poor in patients with severe disease and the elderly (Zeina, 2013).

All races can be affected with pemphigus vulgaris; however, the Jewish population shows predominance. Pemphigus vulgaris is not gender-specific, although in adolescence, girls are affected more than boys. The average onset of pemphigus vulgaris is in the fifth and sixth decades of life (Herti & Sitaru, 2013; Zeina, 2013).

## PATHOLOGY/HISTOLOGY

Pemphigus vulgaris (immunoglobulin G [IgG] directed against desmoglein-3 [DSG3] and DSG1) is an autoimmune, intraepithelial, blistering disease that affects the skin and mucous membranes (Kobayashi & David-Bajar, 2011). It is caused by circulating autoantibodies targeted against keratinocyte cell surfaces. When IgG autoantibodies bind to the keratinocyte cell surfaces, blisters are formed. These intercellular antibodies adhere to keratinocyte desmosomes and desmosome-free areas of the keratinocyte cell membrane. The binding of autoantibodies causes loss of cell-to-cell adhesion, a process called acantholysis. The antibody alone is capable of causing blistering without complement or inflammatory cells (Habif, 2004; Herti & Sitaru, 2013; Zeina, 2013).

Histopathology shows an intradermal blister. Initial changes consist of intercellular edema in the basal layer with loss of intercellular attachments. Suprabasal epidermal cells separate from the basal cells to form clefts and blisters. The basal cells are separated from one another and appear as a row of tombstones attached to the basement membrane. Blister cells contain some acantholytic cells. Histopathology helps differentiate pemphigus vulgaris from other forms of pemphigus (Habif, 2004; Zeina, 2013).

## CLINICAL PRESENTATION

Although the exact cause of pemphigus vulgaris is unknown, multiple possible causes have been identified, including the following:

- Genetics: Certain major histocompatibility complex (MHC) Class II molecules—in particular, alleles of human leukocyte antigen DR4 (DRB1*0402) and human leukocyte antigen DRw6 (DQB1*0503)—are common in patients with pemphigus vulgaris.
- Age: The most common age for pemphigus vulgaris is in the fifth and sixth decade of life.
- Autoimmune diseases: Pemphigus commonly occurs in patients with other autoimmune diseases, particularly myasthenia gravis and thymoma.
- Drugs: Those reported most significantly in association with pemphigus vulgaris include penicillamine, captopril, cephalosporin, pyrazolones, nonsteroidal anti-inflammatory drugs, and other thiol-containing compounds. Rifampin, emotional stress, thermal burns, ultraviolet rays, and infections (e.g., coxsackievirus, *Herpesviridae* family) have also been reported as triggers for pemphigus vulgaris. (Herti & Sitaru, 2013; Ruocco et al., 2013; Zeina, 2013)

Mucous membranes are usually the first sign of pemphigus vulgaris. Patients with mucosal lesions often consult dentists, oral surgeons, or gynecologists. Oral lesions occur in 50% to 70% of all mucosal lesions, and the majority of all pemphigus vulgaris patients will have mucosal involvement. The diagnosis of pemphigus vulgaris should be considered in any patient with persistent oral erosive lesions. Characteristics of mucous membrane involvement are as follows:

- Intact bullae in the mouth are rare; usually patients will have widespread oral erosions that are painful and slow to heal. The painful erosions may spread to involve the esophagus and larynx, which will cause hoarseness and inability to eat or drink. In adolescents with pemphigus vulgaris, stomatitis is the presenting complaint in approximately half of cases.
- The nasal mucosa, conjunctiva, labia, vagina, cervix, vulva, penis, urethra, or anus may be affected.
- One or multiple fingers or toes may be affected with paronychia, subungual hematomas, and nail dystrophies. (Herti & Sitaru, 2013; Zeina, 2013)

Most patients with pemphigus vulgaris develop skin lesions that appear as a fragile blister with a positive Nikolsky sign. This sign is confirmed by applying a finger on the blister; this separates the normal-appearing epidermis and produces erosion. Nikolsky sign can be positive for pemphigus vulgaris as well as other blistering diseases. Also, the Asboe–Hansen sign is positive when lateral pressure is applied at the edge of the blister and the blister spreads to normal unaffected skin (Herti & Sitaru, 2013; Zeina, 2013).

Vegetations may develop on pemphigus vulgaris erosions. Lesions in skin folds easily form vegetating granulations. For some, erosions will form excessive granulation tissue and crusting in intertriginous areas and on the scalp or face. These lesions are resistant to treatment and are often present for long periods (Herti & Sitaru, 2013; Zeina, 2013).

It is rare to have pemphigus during pregnancy. If present, maternal autoantibodies cross the placenta, resulting in neonatal pemphigus. Neonatal pemphigus is temporary and resolves with clearance of maternal autoantibodies. The treatment during pregnancy is with oral corticosteroids; however, because this drug crosses the placenta, there is a risk of low birth weight, prematurity, infection, and adrenal insufficiency (Herti & Sitaru, 2013; Zeina, 2013).

## DIFFERENTIAL DIAGNOSIS

- Bullous pemphigoid
- Dermatitis herpetiformis
- Erythema multiforme
- Familial benign pemphigus (Hailey–Hailey disease)
- Linear immunoglobulin A (IgA) dermatosis
- Pemphigus erythematosus
- Pemphigus foliaceus
- Pemphigus herpetiformis
- Pemphigus, drug-induced
- Pemphigus, IgA
- Pemphigus, paraneoplastic

## TREATMENT/MANAGEMENT

To establish a diagnosis of pemphigus vulgaris, a histopathology sample is taken from the edge of a blister. Skin biopsy specimens placed in transport media may yield false-negative results; therefore, a direct immunofluorescence (DIF) specimen from normal-appearing skin is recommended. If DIF is positive, than serum indirect immunofluorescence (IDIF) should be done (Habif, 2004; Herti & Sitaru, 2013; Zeina, 2013):

The goal of treatment in pemphigus vulgaris is to decrease blister formation, support healing, and medicate with the least amount of medication necessary to control the disease. Therapy is individualized, taking into account preexisting and coexisting conditions (Habif, 2004; Herti & Sitaru, 2013; Ruocco et al., 2013; Zeina, 2013):

- High-dose steroids are used; however, adverse effects of therapy must be monitored.
- Immunosuppressive drugs should be considered initially in the course of the disease. Epidermal growth factor may excel healing of localized lesions. Rituximab is considered first-line therapy. The antitumor-necrosis-factor drugs sulfasalazine and pentoxifylline are effective adjunctive treatments for clinical improvement by reducing serum level of tumor. Dapsone has been used in the maintenance phase of pemphigus vulgaris treatment.
- Intravenous immunoglobulin therapy has been used effectively.
- For resistant ulcerations, photodynamic therapy has been suggested as an adjunctive treatment.

## SPECIAL CONSIDERATIONS

Pemphigus in the elderly, young children, pregnant women, and immunocompromised patients can be detrimental. Treatment options are limited for these populations. For the elderly caution and consideration must be applied with use of immunosuppressive drugs due to possible impaired liver and renal function. Children's medication use is limited because of potential toxicity and impact on kidney function. Pregnant women are extremely limited to what drugs should be used, and immunocompromised patients (HIV) should not be prescribed medications that would further compromise their immune systems.

## WHEN TO REFER

Refer all suspected cases to a specialist (Habif, Campbell, Chapman, Dinulos, & Zug, 2011). Management of patients with pemphigus vulgaris requires a multidisciplinary approach, involving the following:

- An ophthalmologist should evaluate patients with suspected ocular involvement and those requiring continued high-dose steroids.
- A dentist and/or an otolaryngologist should be consulted for evaluation and management of oral disease.
- A dietitian and/or nutritionist are needed for patients on systemic steroids. These patients will require diets and supplements that maintain adequate vitamin D and calcium intake. Patients with a history of kidney stones should not receive calcium carbonate.
- A rheumatologist is needed to evaluate for osteoporosis in patients who have received long-term systemic steroids. (Zeina, 2013)

## PATIENT EDUCATION

Ruocco et al. (2013) and Zeina (2013) recommended the following advice.

- Patients should avoid taking unnecessary medications, prolonged exposure to ultraviolet light, and emotional stress.
- Patients with oral disease should avoid foods that can irritate the oral mucosa (e.g., spicy foods, tomatoes, orange juice, nuts, chips, hard vegetables, and acidic fruit).

- Patients should avoid activity that could further traumatize the skin and cause blistering.
- Patients should be aware of dental plates, dental bridges, or contact lenses, which may cause or worsen mucosal disease.
- Patients' understanding of the disease and education about pemphigus vulgaris should be emphasized because of the chronic nature of this disorder.
- Patients should be knowledgeable regarding their medications. They should know about dose, adverse effects, and symptoms of toxicity so they can report adverse effects to the physician.
- Patients should understand appropriate wound care.

## CLINICAL PEARLS

- Pemphigus: ICD-9, 694.4; ICD-10, L10
- Pemphigus vulgaris may present with oral lesions only (Habif et al., 2011).
- Early lesions of pemphigus vulgaris may reveal suprabasal acantholysis (Wolff et al., 2013).
- Mortality from pemphigus vulgaris is substantial (Habif et al., 2011).
- Pemphigus foliaceus may demonstrate subcorneal acantholysis (Wolff et al., 2013).
- Pemphigus foliaceus that presents early can resemble seborrheic dermatitis (Habif et al., 2011).
- Gradual tapering of prednisone and other agents is required to sustain remission of bullous pemphigoid (Habif et al., 2011).

## REFERENCES

Habif, T. P. (2004). *Clinical dermatology: A color guide to diagnosis and therapy* (4th ed.). Philadelphia, PA: Mosby.

Habif, T., Campbell, J., Chapman, M., Dinulos, J., & Zug, K. (2011). *Skin disease diagnosis and treatment* (3rd ed.). Philadelphia, PA: Elsevier, Saunders.

Herti, M., & Sitaru, C. (2013). *Pathogenesis, clinical manifestations, and diagnosis of pemphigus*. Retrieved from http://www.uptodate.com/contents/pathogenesis-clinical-manifestations-and-diagnosis-of-pemphigus

Kobayashi, T., & David-Bajar, K. (2011). Vesiculobullous disorders. In J. E. Fitzpatrick & J. G. Morelli (Eds.), *Dermatology secrets plus* (4th ed., pp. 70–77). Philadelphia, PA: Elsevier/Saunders.

Ruocco, E., Wolf, R., Ruocco, V., Brunetti, G., Romano, F., & Schiavo, A. L. (2013). Pemphigus: Associations and management guidelines: Facts and controversies. *Clinics in Dermatology, 31*(4), 382–390.

Wolff, K., Johnson, R., & Saavedra, A. (2013). *Fitzpatrick's color atlas and synopsis of clinical dermatology* (7th ed.). Philadelphia, PA: McGraw-Hill Medical.

Zeina, B. (2013, May 10). *Pemphigus vulgaris*. Retrieved from http://emedicine.medscape.com/article/1064187-overview

# Perioral Dermatitis

## OVERVIEW

*Perioral dermatitis* (POD) is a common inflammatory disorder of facial skin that is more frequent in patients with rosacea (Figure III.44; Lipozencic, 2011). Women and children are most often affected. Histologically, POD lesions are similar to those of rosacea. Patients often require topical treatment, oral medications, evaluation of history to detect underlying causes, and support (Kammier, 2012).

## EPIDEMIOLOGY

POD occurs on the face, which can cause emotional complications as a result of the nature and chronic course of the disease. In 90% of cases, POD affects young females, aged 20 to 45 years. POD is becoming more common in male patients, which is attributed to cosmetic habits. POD is also common in children (James, Berger, & Elston, 2006; Kammier, 2012; Reichenberg, 2012).

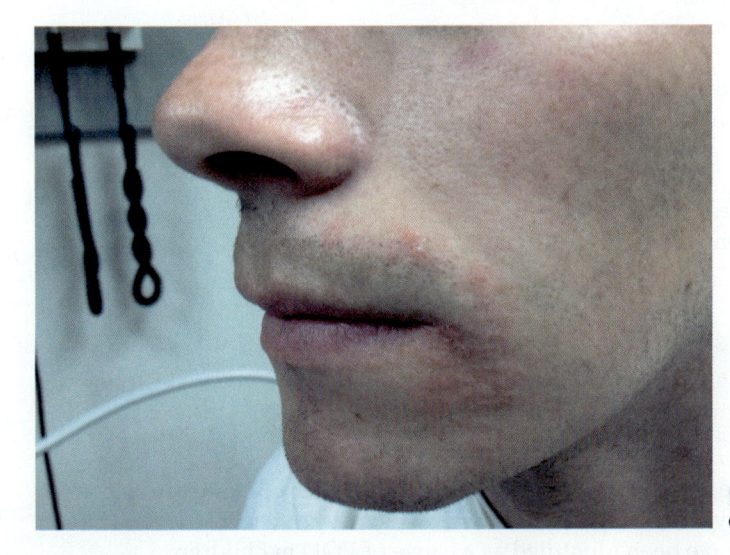

FIGURE III.44 Perioral dermatitis
Courtesy of Jeri Brehm, FNP, APRN-BC

## PATHOLOGY/HISTOLOGY

The etiology of POD is unknown; however, the use of topical steroids on the face is often the cause of POD. Neurogenic inflammation has also been proposed as a pathogenic cause of POD (Kammier, 2012; Reichenberg, 2012).

Histologic findings show a lymphohistiocytic infiltrate with perifollicular localization in all stages and a marked granulomatous inflammation. Papules and pustules often cause perifollicular abscesses (Kammier, 2012).

## CLINICAL PRESENTATION

Subjective symptoms of POD consist of a sensation of burning and tension with minimal itching. POD can be chronic, which can cause lifestyle restrictions because of the disfiguring facial lesions (Kammier, 2012).

POD lesions present as a cluster of erythematous follicular papules, papulovesicles, and papulopustules on an erythematous base. The lesions have a distinct perioral distribution with dermatitis confined symmetrically around the mouth and a clear zone of about 5 mm between the vermillion border and the affected skin. Other locations that can be affected are the nasolabial folds and the parts of the lower eyelids. Other associated presentations include vulvar involvement in young girls with POD and dorsal hand lesions (James et al., 2006; Kammier, 2012; Reichenberg, 2012). The duration of the lesions is weeks to months (Wolff et al., 2013).

## DIFFERENTIAL DIAGNOSIS

According to Kammier (2012), Lipozencic (2011), and Reichenberg (2012), differential diagnosis should take the following into account.

- Acne vulgaris
- Allergic contact dermatitis
- Basal cell carcinoma
- Contact dermatitis, allergic
- Contact dermatitis, irritant
- Dermatophyte infections
- Impetigo
- Irritant contact dermatitis
- Lupus miliaris disseminates faciei
- Rosacea
- Seborrheic dermatitis
- Steroid-induced rosacea
- Systemic lupus erythematosus

## TREATMENT/MANAGEMENT

An underlying cause of POD cannot be detected in all patients. However, the following are known causes (Kammier, 2012).

- When used in excess, topical steroids can cause POD.
- Fluorinated toothpaste, skin care ointments and creams that contain petrolatum or paraffin base, and the vehicle isopropyl myristate are causative factors.
- Recently, sunscreens have been identified as a cause of POD in children.

- Ultraviolet light, hot climates, and wind worsen POD.
- Fusiform spirilla bacteria, *Candida* species, and other fungi have been cultured from POD lesions.
- Hormonal factors may cause POD because of changes noted premenstrually.
- Tooth whiteners have been implicated as a cause (Goodheart, 2011).

Anti-inflammatory medication such as that used for rosacea is required. Small studies have shown efficacy of photodynamic therapy (PDT) for POD. Treatment should be modified to the severity and extent of the disease (James et al., 2006; Kammier, 2012; Lipozencic, 2011; Reichenberg, 2012).

- Topical therapy is recommended for mild cases of POD, children, and pregnant women. Topical anti-inflammatory agents (e.g., metronidazoleand erythromycin) are given in a nongreasy base (e.g., gel, lotion, cream). Pimecrolimus cream is the most effective treatment for steroid-induced POD. Topical antiacne medications such as adapalene and azelaic acid also have been used. Ointments should be avoided.
- Perioral dermatitis responds readily to oral tetracycline (250–500 mg daily) or its derivatives, doxycycline and minocycline (100 mg twice daily; Goodheart, 2011). Isotretinoin is used for granulomatous forms. Pediatric patients with severe or resistant forms of POD may be treated with erythromycin.
- Withdrawing all topical medications and cosmetics to eliminate potential causes for POD is an option for compliant patients who do not want antibiotics.

Inevitably, POD symptoms will worsen when initializing treatment if topical steroids are withdrawn. The patient should be made aware of this complication. In cases with preceding long-term use of topical steroids, steroid weaning with low-dose 0.1% to 0.5% hydrocortisone cream can be used (Kammier, 2012).

## SPECIAL CONSIDERATIONS

POD can cause emotional problems because of the disfiguring character of the facial lesions and the potential for prolonged course of disease. In cases of lupus-like POD, there is potential for scarring in the affected areas (Kammier, 2012).

## WHEN TO REFER

Consult a dermatologist for evaluation and treatment options.

## PATIENT EDUCATION

According to Kammier (2012), patients should be made aware that:

- The affected skin area should be gently cleaned twice daily.
- Symptoms may worsen initially, especially if the cause of POD was the use of topical steroids.
- Except for prescribed medications, the use of all topical preparations, including cosmetics, should be avoided.
- Improvement may not occur for weeks, despite correct treatment.

Providing and educating patients about POD will help them with compliance, help them cope with their altered appearance, and decrease recurrences.

## CLINICAL PEARLS

- Perioral dermatitis: ICD-9, 695.3; ICD-10, L71.0
- If the etiology of POD is topical corticosteroids, the dermatitis may flare before it begins to improve—"one step forward, two steps back" (Goodheart, 2011, p. 68).
- It is uncommon for POD to recur after effective treatment (Goodheart, 2011).
- POD is rare in men except after topical steroid use (Goodheart, 2011).

## REFERENCES

Goodheart, H. (2011). *Goodheart's same-site differential diagnosis: A rapid method of diagnosing and treating common skin disorders.* Philadelphia, PA: Lippincott Williams & Wilkins.

James, T. P., Berger, T. G., & Elston, D. M. (2006). *Andrews' diseases of the skin: Clinical dermatology* (10th ed.). Philadelphia, PA: Saunders/Elsevier.

Kammier, H. J. (2012, July 11). *Perioral dermatitis.* Retrieved from http://emedicine.medscape.com/article/1071128-overview

Lipozencic, J. (2011). Perioral dermatitis. *Clinical Dermatology, 29*(2), 157–161.

Reichenberg, J. (2012). *Perioral (periorificial) dermatitis.* Retrieved from http://www.uptodate.com/perioral-periorificial-dermatitis

Wolff, K., Johnson, R., & Saavedra, A. (2013). *Fitzpatrick's color atlas and synopsis of clinical dermatology* (7th ed.). New York, NY: McGraw-Hill Medical.

# Pityriasis Rosea

## OVERVIEW

*Pityriasis rosea* (PR) is a benign rash that is often seen in healthy children and adults. It is an acute papular eruption that usually lasts 1 to 2 months (Figure III.45). PR has a sudden onset with a primary lesion called a *herald patch*. The rash usually requires only symptomatic treatment (Goldstein & Goldstein, 2013; Schwartz, 2013).

## EPIDEMIOLOGY

In the United States, PR usually occurs in spring and winter. Worldwide, PR has been estimated to account for 2% of dermatologic outpatient visits. PR affects people of all age groups but occurs most often in persons aged 10 to 35 years and is infrequent in infants and the elderly (Goodheart, 2011). In the United States, PR occurs about twice as often in females as males, and there is no racial predominance. The appearance of lesions in African Americans is darker and does not have a rose color (Schwartz, 2013).

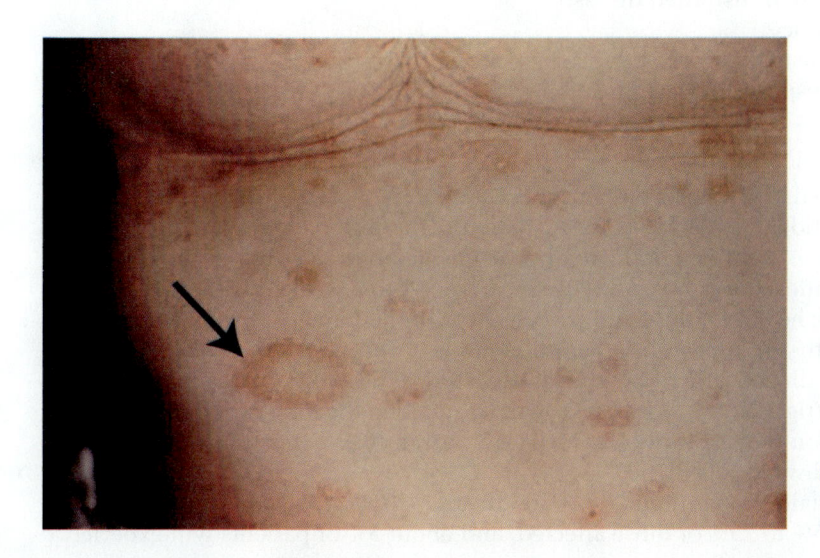

**FIGURE III.45** *Pityriasis rosea*
Courtesy of Centers for Disease Control and Prevention

## PATHOLOGY/HISTOLOGY

PR is said to be caused by a viral etiology; this is supported by the seasonal occurrence, its acute course, the potential for epidemics, the onset of prodromal symptoms, and the low recurrence rate (Goodheart, 2011). The decreased response of natural killer cells and B-cells has been recognized in PR, suggesting that T-cell-mediated immunity is primarily responsible in the development of PR. Increased amounts of CD4 T cells and Langerhans cells appear in the dermis, which suggest viral antigen processing and presentation. Anti-immunoglobulin M (IgM) to keratinocytes is also found in patients with PR (Schwartz, 2013).

The herald patch is noted in 50% to 90% of PR cases at least 7 to 10 days before the secondary eruption. This secondary eruption will appear in groups following the skin folds on the skin, which accounts for the Christmas tree pattern seen on the back (Schwartz, 2013).

PR-like eruptions can also occur in association with many drugs (e.g., acetylsalicylic acid, barbiturates, bismuth, captopril, clonidine, gold, imatinib, isotretinoin, ketotifen, levamisole, metronidazole, omeprazole, D-penicillamine, terbinafine, rituximab, nortriptyline, and clozapine), as well as certain vaccines (e.g., bacille Calmette-Guérin and diphtheria). Antitumor-necrosis-factor alpha agents such as adalimumab and etanercept have also been implicated. PR-like drug eruptions may be difficult to distinguish from non-drug-induced cases. However, drug-induced PR often lasts longer than non-drug-induced cases. Lesions are also thought to be increased in individuals with high levels of stress (Schwartz, 2013).

Histologic specimens of the epidermis show superficial perivascular dermatitis. Focal parakeratosis in mounds, hyperplasia, and focal spongiosis are also observed in the epidermis, which may show exocytosis of lymphocytes, variable spongiosis, mild acanthosis, and a thinned granular layer as well. In the dermis, extravasated red blood cells are a useful finding, with associated perivascular infiltrate of lymphocytes, histiocytes, eosinophils, and monocytes (Schwartz, 2013).

## CLINICAL PRESENTATION

Taking the patient's history should include asking questions about:

- Medication intake
- Previous sexually transmitted disease
- Possible pregnancy
- Dermatologic history
- Recent upper respiratory tract infection
- Travel history
- Occupational exposure (Schwartz, 2013)

The disease usually starts with a solitary, salmon-colored, fine-scaled lesion that heralds the eruption. On darker-skinned patients, the lesions are often dark brown. The herald patch is localized and can appear on the abdomen, the groin, the axilla, the distal extremities, the palms, and the soles. After 1 to 2 weeks, a generalized exanthem will appear; however, the eruption can occur immediately after the herald patch or can take months to appear. The herald patch is a dermatologic mystery in that it does not occur with any other known skin diseases. The secondary lesions appear as bilateral, symmetric macules, with scale positioned along the long axes of the cleavage lines. This eruption will typically last for 1 or 2 months (Goldstein & Goldstein, 2013; Monroe, 2013; Schwartz, 2013).

PR is usually asymptomatic (Goodheart, 2011). Pruritus is present in approximately 25% to 75% of those affected, and about 5% of patients will experience mild malaise and lymphadenopathy before the herald patch. Approximately 20% of patients present with atypical or variant forms of PR, such as the following:

- In drug-induced PR, the herald patch may be absent or may present with multiple lesions in unusual areas. Sometimes the patch will not be followed by an eruption.
- Inverse PR occurs on the face, hands, and feet. The face is commonly affected in young children, pregnant women, and Black people. In these cases, secondary syphilis should be ruled out, especially if the palms and soles of feet are involved.
- A morphologic variant produces individual patches that are 3 to 6 cm in diameter, with central clearing and collarette of scale with surrounding erythema. This variant is often referred to as *pityriasis circinata et marginata* of Vidal or limb-girdle PR. Common sites of occurrence are the axillae and the groin. (Schwartz, 2013)

## DIFFERENTIAL DIAGNOSIS

Goldstein and Goldstein (2013), James et al. (2006), and Schwartz (2013) suggest the following considerations for differential diagnosis.

- Drug eruptions
- Erythema annulare centrifugum
- Erythema dyschromicum perstans
- Erythema multiforme
- Guttate psoriasis
- Kaposi sarcoma
- Lichen planus
- Nummular dermatitis
- Parapsoriasis
- Pityriasis lichenoides
- Pityriasis lichenoides chronica
- Pityriasis rubra pilaris
- Psoriasis, guttate
- Seborrheic dermatitis
- Syphilis
- Tinea corporis
- Tinea versicolor

## TREATMENT/MANAGEMENT

PR is usually diagnosed on clinical presentation; therefore, laboratory tests are generally not warranted. However, there are a few exceptions that should be considered.

- If only a herald patch is present, a potassium hydroxide test should be done to rule out tinea corporis
- A rapid plasma reagin or venereal disease research laboratory test should be done to rule out secondary syphilis
- HIV test
- Lyme disease (Goldstein & Goldstein, 2013; Schwartz, 2013)

   Treatments include:

- Pruritus can be treated with bland emollients, oral antihistamines, or topical preparations containing calamine, menthol-phenol, pramoxine, colloidal starch, or oat-

meal. For a severe rash, topical steroids can be used to relieve the pruritus only; steroids do not typically aid in resolving the rash.
- Systemic steroids may exacerbate PR. However, the use of prednisone (0.5–1 mg/kg/d for 7 days) in patients with severe pruritus, vesicular lesions, or the potential for significant postinflammatory hyperpigmentation should be considered.
- Ultraviolet (UV)-B phototherapy, beginning at 80% of the minimum erythrogenic dose, may provide quick relief of pruritus in resistant cases. The dose can be increased by 20% increments until itching is controlled. There is a potential for postinflammatory pigmentation, so an alternative therapy is to use low-dose UV-A1 phototherapy two to three times a week until resolved.
- Dapsone (20 mg twice daily) has been used in atypical PR.
- To shorten the duration of PR in adults, acyclovir (1 g) orally five times a day for 7 days has shown efficacy except for HHV-6 and HHV-7.
- PR patients with Group A streptococcal infection require treatment to prevent scarlet fever and poststreptococcal sequelae. (Goldstein & Goldstein, 2013; James et al., 2006; Monroe, 2013; Schwartz, 2013)

Multiple antibiotics (erythromycin, azithromycin) have been attempted without improvement of PR.

## SPECIAL CONSIDERATIONS

Schwartz (2013) noted that:

- An increased risk of PR occurs among patients who are immunocompromised and who are treated with ampicillin.
- PR during the first trimester of pregnancy may cause premature delivery and fetal demise.
- Black people experience widespread forms of the disease and associated lymphadenopathy, with postinflammatory hyperpigmentation. Black children are prone to having papular lesions and scalp or facial involvement with a shorter duration of the disease, often with resolution within 2 weeks.

## WHEN TO REFER

According to Schwartz (2013), referral should be sought in the following cases.

- Patients with severe pruritus or disease that requires systemic steroid therapy or UV-B therapy or with atypical appearances of PR should have a dermatologic consult (Habif, Campbell, Chapman, Dinulos, & Zug, 2011).
- Patients who are immunocompromised or those who have had transplants should have consults with infectious disease specialists.
- Pregnant women with PR need to be referred to an obstetrician for high-risk management.

## PATIENT EDUCATION

Schwartz (2013) suggested the following:

- Instruct patients to avoid contact with irritants (e.g., harsh soaps, fragrances, hot water, wool, synthetic fabrics, and tight clothing).
- Educate about the benign and noncontagious nature of PR and the length and course of the disease.

## CLINICAL PEARLS

- Ultraviolet radiation exposure from the sun speeds the disappearance of PR lesions (Klenk & Travers, 2011).
- In Black skin, PR may present uncharacteristically in either a papular or vesiculobullous form (High & Grammer-West, 2011).
- PR appearance may mimic secondary syphilis (Habif et al., 2011).

## REFERENCES

Goldstein, A. O., & Goldstein, B. G. (2013). *Pityriasis rosea*. Retrieved from http://www.uptodate.com/contents/pityriasis-rosea

Goodheart, H. (2011). *Goodheart's same-site differential diagnosis: A rapid method of diagnosing and treating common skin disorders*. Philadelphia, PA: Lippincott Williams & Wilkins.

Habif, T., Campbell, J., Chapman, M., Dinulos, J., & Zug, K. (2011). *Skin disease diagnosis and treatment* (3rd ed.). Philadelphia, PA: Elsevier/Saunders.

High, W., & Grammer-West, N. (2011). Special considerations in skin of color. In J. E. Fitzpatrick & J. G. Morelli (Eds.), *Dermatology secrets plus* (4th ed., pp. 427–434). Philadelphia, PA: Elsevier/Mosby.

James, W. D., Berger, T. G., & Elston, D. M. (2006). *Andrews' disease of the skin: Clinical dermatology* (10th ed.). Philadelphia, PA: Saunders/Elsevier.

Klenk, A., & Travers, J. (2011). Papulo squamous skin eruptions. In J. E. Fitzpatrick & J. G. Morelli (Eds.), *Dermatology secrets plus* (4th ed., pp. 50–56). Philadelphia, PA: Elsevier/Mosby.

Monroe, J. R. (2013). Dermadiagnosis. *Clinician Reviews, 23*(2), 17.

Schwartz, R. A. (2013, March 25). *Pityriasis rosea*. Retrieved from http://emedicine.medscape.com/article/1107532-overview

# Psoriasis

## OVERVIEW

*Psoriasis* is a persistent, noncommunicable, systemic, inflammatory disease. Patients with psoriasis have a genetic susceptibility for the disorder. Lesions typically appear on the scalp, torso, elbows, and knees (Figure III.46). The joints may be affected with psoriatic arthritis, which occurs in approximately 30% of patients with psoriasis. Psoriasis has the tendency to be intermittent with exacerbations that occur with systemic or environmental stressors. Patients with psoriasis are susceptible to depression because of the effect of psoriasis on quality of life (James, Berger, & Elston, 2006; Meffert, 2013).

## EPIDEMIOLOGY

Psoriasis is the most common autoimmune disease in the United States; as many as 7.5 million Americans have it (National Psoriasis Foundation, 2013). According to the National Institutes of Health (NIH), approximately 2.2% of the United States population has psoriasis. Overall, approximately 2% to 3% of people are affected by psoriasis worldwide. Psoriasis is not gender specific and can begin at any age, with the prevalence of onset in the second and third decade of life and again in the fifth and sixth decade of life. New-onset psoriasis affects approximately 10% to 15% of children aged 10 years and younger. The occurrence of psoriasis in a person is related to the temperature of their climate, family history, and genetic makeup. Those who are dark-skinned and live in warmer climates have less incidence of psoriasis. The frequency of psoriasis in African Americans versus Caucasians is 1.3% to 2.5% (Feldman, 2012; Meffert, 2013).

## PATHOLOGY/HISTOLOGY

Psoriasis is a complicated disorder that is determined by personal genetic makeup and immune-mediated factors. This is verified by the effective treatment of psoriasis with immune-mediating, biological medications (Meffert, 2013). Psoriasis has long been known to occur in families. The possible role of genetic factors can be illustrated by the following (Feldman, 2012).

- Approximately 40% of patients with psoriasis or psoriatic arthritis have a family history of these conditions in first-degree relatives.

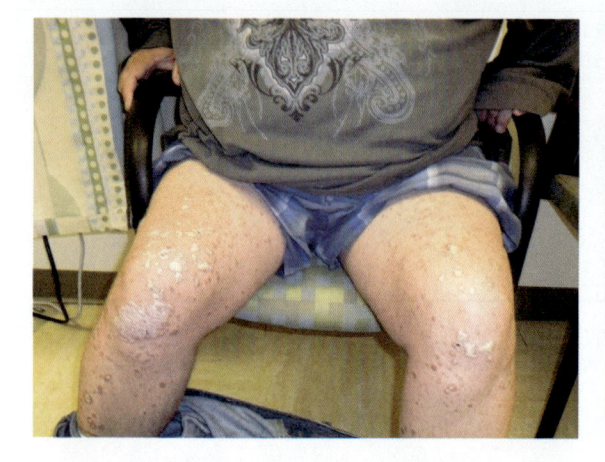

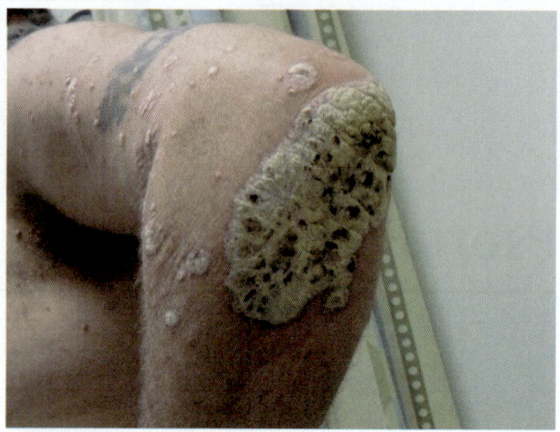

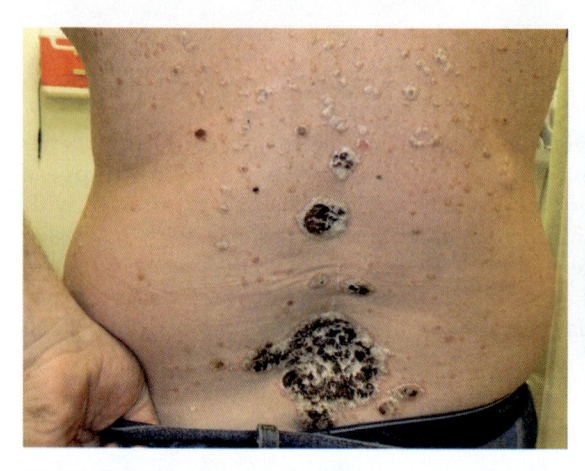

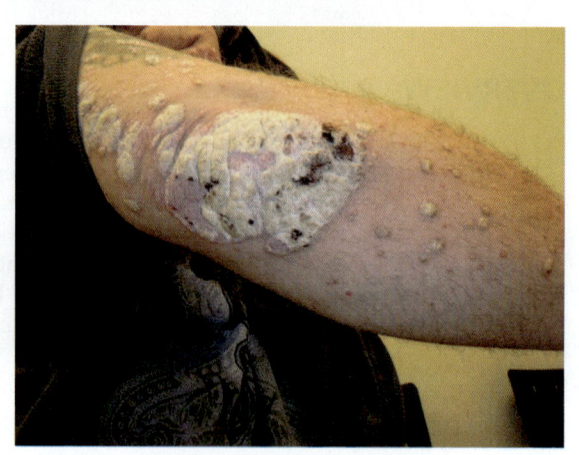

**FIGURE III.46**   Psoriasis lesions
Courtesy of Sue Reed, FNP

- Family studies in psoriatic arthritis have demonstrated that the disease is 100 times more likely to occur among family members than among unrelated controls.
- Psoriasis tends to be concordant among monozygotic twins more commonly than among dizygotic twins.

The pathogenesis of psoriasis is not well known. Possible causes of psoriasis are infection, trauma, and stressors. However, once activated, there is an influx of leukocytes to the dermal and epidermal layers of the skin that result in psoriatic plaques (Feldman, 2012; Meffert, 2013).

Many of the clinical elements of psoriasis are clarified by the substantial amount of cytokines (tumor necrosis factor-alpha [TNF-α], interferon-gamma, and interleukin-2) produced. Elevated levels of TNF-α specifically are found to correlate with flares of psoriasis. Specific findings in the psoriatic lesions include vascular distention as a result of superficial blood vessel dilation and distorted epidermal cell cycle. Epidermal hyperplasia results in an accelerated cell turnover rate, which causes improper cell maturation. Cells that normally shed their nuclei in the stratum granulosum will keep their nuclei, a condition known as *parakeratosis*. In addition, affected epidermal cells do not release enough lipids, which normally bond adhesions of corneocytes. This cause's poorly adherent stratum corneum to be formed, which leads to the flaky, scaled appearance of psoriasis lesions. The surface of the lesion will appear as silver scales.

Conjunctival impression cytology demonstrated a higher incidence of squamous metaplasia, neutrophil clumping, and nuclear chromatin changes in patients with psoriasis (Meffert, 2013).

## CLINICAL PRESENTATION

Environmental, genetic, and immunologic factors appear to play a role in hyperproliferation of keratinocytes in psoriasis. These include:

- Environmental factors: Cold, trauma, infections (e.g., streptococcal, staphylococcal, HIV), alcohol, and drugs (e.g., iodides, steroid withdrawal, aspirin, lithium, beta-blockers, botulinum A, antimalarials) have been observed to trigger exacerbations. Perceived stress may exacerbate psoriasis as well. Hot weather, sunlight, and pregnancy may be advantageous.
- Genetic factors: Patients with psoriasis have a genetic predisposition for the disease.
- Immunologic factors: Research suggests that psoriasis is an autoimmune disease. Psoriatic lesions have increased T-cell activity in the affected skin layers. Some of the most recent drugs used to treat moderate to severe psoriasis directly change the function of lymphocytes. Also of importance, 2.5% of people with HIV infection have worsening of psoriasis as their CD4 counts decrease. Certain immunologically active events, such as streptococcal pharyngitis, cessation of steroid therapy, and use of antimalarial drugs can cause a type of psoriasis known as guttate psoriasis. (Feldman, 2012; Meffert, 2013)

The most frequent skin characteristics of psoriasis are scaled erythematous macules, papules, and plaques. Typically, the macules are seen first, and these progress to maculopapules and ultimately to well-demarcated, noncoherent, silvery plaques overlying a glossy homogeneous erythema. The area of skin involvement varies with the form of psoriasis (Meffert, 2013). Psoriasis can usually be recognized without difficulty, but atypical or nonclassic forms are more difficult to identify and treat. There are several clinical types of psoriasis (Feldman, 2012; Meffert, 2013):

- *Fixed immobile psoriasis* (psoriasis vulgaris) is the most frequent type. This type involves the scalp, extensor surfaces, genitals, umbilicus, and lumbosacral and retroauricular regions.
- *Plaque psoriasis* is manifested by raised, inflamed lesions surfaced with a silvery white scale. If the scale is scraped off, the skin underneath is inflamed. This type occurs on the extensor surfaces of the knees, elbows, scalp, and trunk.
- *Guttate psoriasis* appears as petite, mildly scaled, salmon-pink papules, 1 to 10 mm in diameter, predominately on the trunk. Two to 3 weeks after an acute episode of an infection with Group A beta-hemolytic streptococci, guttate psoriasis may occur.
- *Inverse psoriasis* appears as a smooth, inflamed lesion, without scale because of moisture in the areas affected. This type is prominent on the flexural surfaces, armpit, groin, under the breast, and in the skin folds.
- *Pustular psoriasis* has sterile pustules on the palms and soles or widespread on the body. Pustular psoriasis may rotate through erythema, pustules, and then scaling. Multiple variants of pustular psoriasis include von Zumbusch variant and acrodermatitis continua of Hallopeau.
- *Erythrodermic psoriasis* has symptoms of erythema, pain, pruritus, and thin scaling that involves nearly the entire body. Associated symptoms include fever, chills, hypothermia, and dehydration because of the great amount of skin affected. Hospitalization may be needed for management of pain, dehydration, hypotension, and potential cardiac instability.

- *Scalp psoriasis* presents with erythematous, thick plaques with silvery scales. This disorder affects about half of patients who have psoriasis.
- *Nail psoriasis* causes thickening and pitting of the nails with associated yellow color. Nails may lift from the nailbed. Affected nails are often misdiagnosed as onychomycosis. Still, patients with nail psoriasis can have concomitant fungal infection.
- *Psoriatic arthritis* can affect up to 30% of those who have cutaneous disease. Usually the joints affected are in the hands and feet, with associated stiffness, pain, and joint damage.
- *Oral psoriasis* appears as whitish lesions on the oral mucosa. It also may appear on the lip as a severe cheilosis.
- *Eruptive psoriasis* is seen on the upper torso and extremities. This type is seen more at younger ages.
- In addition to skin manifestations, psoriasis may also affect the eyelid, conjunctiva, or cornea and give rise to ocular manifestations, including ectropion and trichiasis, conjunctivitis and conjunctival hyperemia, and corneal dryness with punctate keratitis and corneal melt. Blepharitis is the most common ocular finding in psoriasis. Erythema, edema, and psoriatic plaques may develop, and they can result in madarosis, cicatricialectropion, trichiasis, and even loss of the eyelid tissue. A chronic nonspecific conjunctivitis is fairly common. It usually occurs in association with eyelid margin involvement. Psoriatic plaques can extend from the eyelid onto the conjunctiva.

## DIFFERENTIAL DIAGNOSIS

- Adult blepharitis
- Atopic dermatitis
- Atopic keratoconjunctivitis
- Contact dermatitis
- Diaper dermatitis
- Dry eye syndrome
- Gout and pseudogout
- Lichen planus
- Lichen simplex chronicus
- Mycosis fungoides
- Nummular eczema
- Onychomycosis
- Pityriasis alba
- Pityriasis rosea
- Pustular eruptions
- Reactive arthritis
- Seborrheic dermatitis
- Siccakeratoconjunctivitis
- Squamous cell carcinoma
- Subcornealpustulosis
- Syphilis
- Tinea

## TREATMENT/MANAGEMENT

Although most cases of psoriasis are diagnosed clinically, a dermatologic skin biopsy is recommended for difficult presentations. Uric acid levels and rheumatoid serology may be needed to differentiate gout or rheumatoid arthritis from psoriatic arthritis in inflamed joints. Fungal studies are useful for hand and foot psoriasis that are resistant to topical steroids (Meffert, 2013).

Treatment options for psoriasis are:

- Emollients
  - Feldman (2011) stated that hydration and emollients are an important and inexpensive option for psoriasis treatment. Keeping psoriatic skin soft and moist decreases symptoms of itching and tenderness. Also, keeping the skin hydrated prevents irritation and reduces the potential for consequent *Koebnerization* (development of new psoriatic lesions at sites of trauma).
  - Naldi and Chalmers (2008) stated that emollients help soften psoriatic scale and decrease pruritus. There are few benefits to using emollients alone for the treatment of psoriasis.
- Topical steroids
  - Feldman (2011) stated that topical corticosteroids remain the foundation for topical psoriasis treatment despite the development of newer therapies. Although ointments are thought to be more effective because of their occlusive properties, this may not be appropriate for certain types of psoriasis lesions. In practice, the efficacy and potency of a topical steroid is dependent on many factors, including skin type, plaque thickness, and, most important, compliance.
  - Naldi and Chalmers (2008) found that potent and very potent topical steroids significantly improved psoriasis severity scores in comparison to placebo. Topical steroids in combination with occlusion therapy, vitamin D derivatives, and oral retinoids were more effective than steroids alone for the treatment of psoriasis.
- Topical vitamin D analogs
  - Feldman (2011) stated that analogs may be effective as monotherapy for some patients. Systematic reviews, however, have found that combination therapy with a topical steroid is more effective than either treatment alone.
- Tar
  - Feldman (2011) and Naldi and Chalmers (2008) noted that tar can be a useful adjunct to topical steroids.
- Topical retinoids
  - According to Feldman (2011), tazarotene, a topical retinoid, was found to be safe and effective in two randomized, vehicle-controlled trials that included 1,303 patients with psoriasis.
- Calcineurin inhibitors
  - Feldman (2011) stated that topical tacrolimus and pimecrolimus are generally well tolerated when used to treat facial and intertriginous psoriasis, which can prevent long-term topical steroid use.
- Methotrexate or cyclosporin
  - Methotrexate has been used for the past 30 years for the effective treatment of psoriasis, and it continues to play an important role in the management of severe psoriasis, despite the advent of newer agents. It is particularly valuable for patients with concomitant arthritis (Naldi & Chalmers, 2008).
  - Cyclosporin is effective in patients with severe psoriasis. The efficacy of methotrexate and cyclosporine for the treatment of psoriasis is similar (Feldman, 2011).
- Systemic retinoids
  - Systemic retinoids are indicated in patients with severe psoriasis, including pustular and erythrodermic forms, and in patients with HIV-associated psoriasis. The retinoid of choice is acitretin (Soriatane). Acitretin has become a valuable modality when used in conjunction with ultraviolet (UV) - B or psoralen + UVA (PUVA) therapy (Feldman, 2011).

- Biologic immune modifying agents
  - Feldman (2011) stated that immunomodulatory agents (*biologics*) are becoming treatment alternatives for moderate to severe plaque-type psoriasis.
- UV light
  - UV irradiation has been recognized as beneficial for the control of psoriasis. UV radiation has antiproliferative effects (slowing keratinization) and anti-inflammatory effects (inducing cell death of pathogenic T cells in psoriasis plaques). There are different types of phototherapy and photochemotherapy that can be used (UVB, narrowband UVB, and PUVA; Feldman, 2011).
  - Naldi and Chalmers (2008) noted that phototherapy (UVB) is suitable for inducing remission of psoriasis, but not for long-term maintenance of remission. PUVA is effective for the clearance of psoriasis, but the risk of skin cancer limits the number of lifetime exposures that may be offered safely to people with psoriasis.

## SPECIAL CONSIDERATIONS

The diagnosis of psoriasis can directly affect a person's life. The emotional and physical impairments experienced with this disease can be greater than that found in other chronic illnesses such as cancer, arthritis, hypertension, heart disease, diabetes, and depression (Meffert, 2013).

## WHEN TO REFER

Psoriasis is a chronic problem, and evaluation with a dermatologist or a rheumatologist is recommended. Determining the severity of psoriasis requires combining objective measures (body surface area involvement) and disease location.

## PATIENT EDUCATION

Psoriasis can be a frustrating disease for patients, families, and providers. Compliance is often an issue if treatment is centered on topical therapies. For treatment planning, patients need to be grouped into mild to moderate and moderate to severe disease categories (Feldman, 2011).

Those with psoriasis are at higher risk for developing other chronic diseases such as heart disease, inflammatory bowel disease, and diabetes. Severe cases of psoriasis increase an individual's risk of psoriatic arthritis, cardiovascular disease, obesity, and other immune-related conditions (National Psoriasis Foundation, 2013).

Patients with psoriasis should be advised to seek medical care in the following situations (Harvey, 2011):

- They develop significant joint pain, stiffness, or deformity
- They develop signs of infection, such as red streaks or pus from the red areas, fever with no other cause, or increased pain

    A number of lifestyle factors are related to psoriasis (Feldman, 2012).

- Smoking is associated with an increased risk of psoriasis and also with increased severity of psoriasis.
- Psoriasis has been associated with obesity and higher body mass index in adults and children. Increased levels of proinflammatory cytokines, including TNF-α, in tissue or serum in obese patients may contribute to the relationship between obesity and psoriasis.

Vitamin D deficiency may be associated with increased risk of autoimmune disorders, including type 1 diabetes, multiple sclerosis, inflammatory bowel disease, and psoriasis.

## CLINICAL PEARLS

- Psoriasis: ICD-9, 696; ICD-10, L40
- Scaley plaques psoriasis on the elbows, knees, and scalp is the most common presentation (Habif, 2011).
- Psoriasis frequently begins during childhood, this dermatosis can be provoked after a streptococcal pharyngitis (Habif, 2010).
- Psoriasis can be more of an emotional disability than a physical one hence, "the heartbreak of psoriasis."
- Nail pitting is a common change associated with psoriasis (Fitzpatrick & Morelli, 2011).
- Three drugs that can exacerbate psoriasis include beta blockers, antimalarials, and lithium. Caution should be used if prescribing them to a patient with psoriasis.

## REFERENCES

Feldman, S. R. (2011). *Treatment of psoriasis*. Retrieved from http://www.uptodate.com/treatment-of-psoriasis

Feldman, S. R. (2012). *Epidemiology, clinical manifestations, and diagnosis of psoriasis*. Retrieved from http://www.uptodate.com/contents/epidemiology-clinical-manifestations-and-diagnosis-of-psoriasis

Fitzpatrick, J. & Morelli, J. (2011). *Dermatology secrets plus* (4th ed.). Philadelphia, PA: Elsevier Mosby.

Habif, T. (2010). *Clinical dermatology: A color guide to diagnosis and therapy* (5th ed.). China: Elsevier.

Habif, T. (2011). *Skin disease diagnosis & treatment* (3rd ed.). Edinburgh, Scotland: Elsevier.

Harvey, L. (2011, August 22). *Psoriasis. When to seek medical care*. Retrieved from http://www.emedicinehealth.com/psoriasis/page4_em.htm#when_to_seek_medical_care

James, W. D., Berger, T. G., & Elston, D. M. (2006). *Andrew's diseases of the skin: Clinical dermatology* (10th ed.). Philadelphia, PA: Saunders/Elsevier.

Meffert, J. (2013, April 22). *Psoriasis*. Retrieved from http://emedicine.medscape.com/article/1943419-overview#aw2aab6b2b2

Naldi, L., & Chambers, R. J. (2008). Psoriasis. In H. Williams, M. Bigby, T. Diepgen, A. Herxheimer, L. Naldi, & B. Rzany (Eds.), *Evidence-based dermatology* (2nd ed., pp. 171–185). Malden, MA: Blackwell.

National Psoriasis Foundation. (2013). *Health conditions associated with psoriasis*. Retrieved from http://www.psoriasis.org/about-psoriasis-related-conditions

# Rosacea

## OVERVIEW

*Rosacea* is a common chronic and relapsing inflammatory skin condition characterized by symptoms of facial flushing and clinical signs, including erythema, telangiectasia, roughness of skin, and inflammatory acne-like eruptions (Figure III.47). Persistent erythema on the central face for longer than 3 months is the definition of rosacea (Banasikowska, 2012; Dahl, 2012; Maier, 2012).

## EPIDEMIOLOGY

In the United States, the incidence of rosacea is estimated to be about 1.5%; however, this is not accurate because of the variable clinical appearances and the multiple skin disorders that exhibit similar clinical features. Rosacea is a common skin condition that disproportionately affects persons of fair-skinned European and Celtic origin (Banasikowska, 2012; Brodsky, 2009; Dahl, 2012).

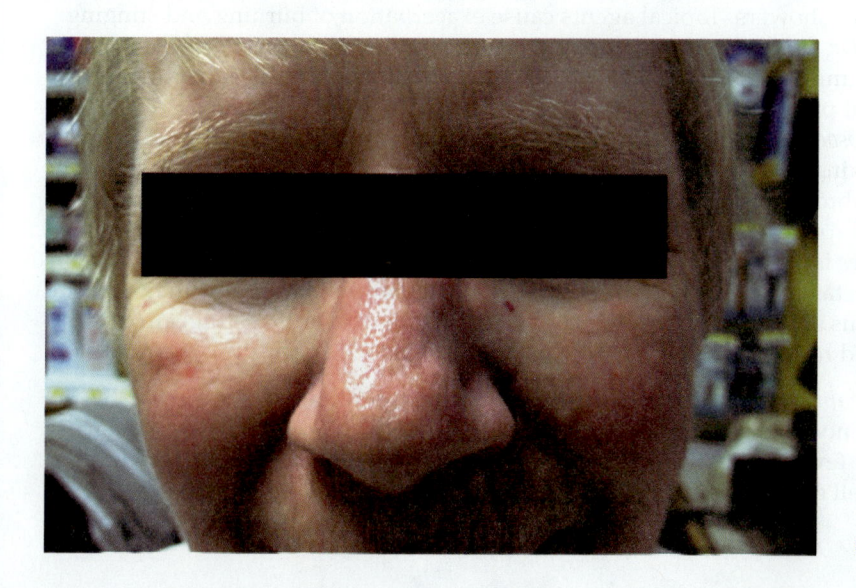

**FIGURE III.47** Rosacea

## PATHOLOGY/HISTOLOGY

The histologic aspects of rosacea rest on the stage of disease. Nonpustular lesions show a nonspecific perivascular and perifollicular lymphohistiocytic infiltrate, accompanied by occasional multinucleated cells, plasma cells, neutrophils, and eosinophils. Papulopustular lesions are more pronounced granulomatous inflammation and sometimes perifollicular abscesses. *Demodex folliculorum* may be present in nearby follicles. The histologic features of granulomatous rosacea show caseating and noncaseating granulomata with negative stains for mycobacteria and fungi (Banasikowska, 2012).

## CLINICAL PRESENTATION

Individuals with rosacea usually have a history of facial flushing as a child or as an adolescent. As an adult, the flushing is triggered by hot drinks, heat, emotion, alcohol, and stress (Banasikowska, 2012).

The disease involves a variety of signs and symptoms, including (Banasikowska, 2012):

- Erythema and telangiectasia on the cheeks and the forehead are present.
- Inflammatory papules and pustules are usually prominent on the nose, forehead, and cheeks.
- The neck and the upper chest may also have erythema and flushing.
- Enlarged sebaceous glands are often present, with the development of thick skin and deformity of the nose (rhinophyma) in severe cases.
- Patients may experience drying and peeling of the skin. The absence of comedones helps differentiate rosacea from acne.
- Ocular lymphedema may be prominent but is uncommon.

There are four types of rosacea.

- *Erythematotelangiectatic rosacea* includes facial flushing, which may be accompanied by burning. The erythema usually does not affect periocular skin. Over time, the areas on the face will become rough with scale. Increased flushing can be triggered by emotional stress, hot drinks, alcohol, spicy foods, exercise, cold or hot weather, and hot baths and showers. Topical agents cause exacerbation of burning and stinging.
- *Papulopustular rosacea* is the most common presentation of rosacea. Patients usually affected are middle-aged women who have complaints of facial redness, papules, and pinpoint pustules. Telangiectasias are admixed with the erythema.
- *Phymatous rosacea* occurs when the nose, chin, ears, eyelids, and the forehead develop thickened skin and nodular skin surfaces. Four specific histologic variants can occur: glandular, fibrous, fibroangiomatous, and actinic. The usual treatments are isotretinoin topical application and surgical correction.
- *Ocular rosacea* is associated with conjunctival irritation, blepharitis, keratitis, lid margin telangiectasia, abnormal tearing, and styes. Ocular manifestations may precede the cutaneous signs by years. Patients often complain of eyes that sting, are dry and irritated, and have a gritty feeling. (Dahl, 2012; Maier, 2012)

*Rosacea fulminans* (pyoderma faciale) is a rare complication manifested by the occurrence of nodules and abscesses with sinus tract development. Patients usually have malaise, fever, elevated erythrocyte sedimentation rate, and possibly elevated white blood cell count (Banasikowska, 2012; Dahl, 2012).

A rare granulomatous variant of rosacea (acne agminate/lupus miliaris disseminatus faciei) can present with inflammatory erythematous or flesh-colored papules spread symmetrically across the upper face. The lesions tend to be discrete, and surrounding erythema is not a marked feature but may be present. These patients often do not have a history of flushing. This pattern of rosacea is sometimes associated with scarring and may be resistant to conventional treatment (Banasikowska, 2012).

## DIFFERENTIAL DIAGNOSIS

- Lupus erythematosus, acute
- Perioral dermatitis
- Sarcoidosis
- Seborrheic dermatitis

## TREATMENT/MANAGEMENT

Before the initiation of therapy, patients should identify and avoid triggers that cause rosacea flares. Common triggers include hot or cold temperatures, wind, hot drinks, caffeine, exercise, spicy food, alcohol, emotions, topical therapies, or medications (Banasikowska, 2012; Maier, 2012).

Treatments for rosacea include:

- Topical therapies
  - Rebora (2008) stated that azelaic acid and sulfa preparations have been found to be effective in the treatment of papulopustular rosacea.
  - Maier (2012) stated that topical metronidazole and azelaic acid are considered first-line therapies in mild to moderate disease because of evidence from randomized trials in support of their efficacy and the relative safety of these medications. Other agents, such as sulfacetamide sulfur may also be beneficial. Although an informal relationship between Demodex mites and rosacea is uncertain, topical permethrin cream may have some benefit in the treatment of rosacea.
  - Serdar (2011) stated that 1% terbinafine cream is an effective treatment for papulopustular rosacea and is an option for patients who cannot tolerate other therapies.
  - Kim (2011) concluded that pimecrolimus 1% cream is an effective and well-tolerated treatment for patients with mild to moderate inflammatory rosacea.
  - Banasikowska (2012) stated that topical metronidazole is used as a first-line agent. Other therapies suggested aretopical azelaic acid, sulfacetamide products, and topical acne medications.
- Pharmacologic agents
  - Maier (2012) reported that clonidine, beta-blockers, antidepressants, gabapentin (Neurontin), and topical oxymetazoline have been used in attempts to control flushing. However, data are limited on their efficacy in rosacea. Brimonidine tartrate, a vasoconstrictive alpha-adrenergic receptor agonist used in the treatment of open angle glaucoma, has appeared as a potential treatment for rosacea-associated facial erythema.
  - Campbell (2008) stated that cinnamon supplements commonly used to help lower blood sugar and cholesterol can cause vasodilation and worsen rosacea symptoms.
  - Banasikowska (2012) described strong evidence showing that beta-blockers, clonidine, naloxone, ondansetron, and selective serotonin reuptake inhibitors reduce

facial flushing. Oral contraceptive therapy can be useful if patients have flares of rosacea in conjunction with their hormonal cycles. For severe and persistent cases of rosacea, isotretinoin can be used, or dapsone can be used for patients who cannot tolerate isotretinoin. Retinoids are used to decrease adhesion of atypical hyperproliferative keratinocytes and can reduce the potential for malignant degeneration.
- Oral antibiotics
    - According to Rebora (2008), doxycycline is the most popular medication for papulopustular rosacea; also used are clarithromycin, ampicillin, and azithromycin. Oral metronidazole was also found to be effective in the treatment of papulopustular rosacea.
    - Maier (2012) stated that tetracycline, doxycycline, and minocycline have been used for many years for the treatment of papulopustular rosacea. Because there is no bacterial component associated with rosacea, the efficacy of these oral antibiotics in rosacea treatment is often credited to their anti-inflammatory properties. Other antibiotics considered but not often used are clarithromycin, azithromycin, erythromycin, and metronidazole. For recalcitrant disease that is unresponsive to topical or oral therapies, oral isotretinoin is used. Although improvement in inflammatory lesions and facial erythema has been reported, high-quality data of the efficacy of isotretinoin for rosacea are lacking, and the ideal regimen for treatment has not been established.
    - According to Banasikowska (2012), antibiotics, especially the tetracyclines, are used for their anti-inflammatory properties. In patients with ocular involvement, oral therapy is recommended. For those patients, oral antibiotics can help with symptoms. Doxycycline 20 to 50 mg twice daily is effective treatment.
- Laser and intense pulsed light therapies
    - Maier (2012) stated that improvement in both facial erythema and telangiectasia can occur after treatment with pulsed dye lasers, potassium titanyl phosphate (KTP) crystal lasers, or intense pulsed light. All of these modalities were found to be effective in the treatment of facial erythema and telangiectasia associated with rosacea. Light-based modalities do not cure rosacea, and periodic treatments to maintain improvement are often required.
    - Banasikowska (2012) noted that vascular laser therapy is effective treatment for rosacea. However, laser therapy is expensive and requires multiple treatments with 1 to 2 months between treatments for optimal benefit.

## SPECIAL CONSIDERATIONS

Childhood rosacea is managed similarly to rosacea in adults. However, the use of oral tetracyclines should be avoided in children under age 9 years (Maier, 2012).

## WHEN TO REFER

Ocular rosacea can result in damage to the ocular tissues. Patients with signs or symptoms of ocular involvement should be referred to an ophthalmologist for evaluation (Maier, 2012).

Patients with refractory papulopustular rosacea may benefit from treatment with oral isotretinoin, which requires referral to a dermatologist who manages this drug according to iPledge guidelines (Maier, 2012).

## PATIENT EDUCATION

Patients should be advised to avoid known exacerbating factors, such as hot or cold temperatures, wind, hot drinks, caffeine, exercise, spicy food, alcohol, strong emotions, topical products that irritate the skin and decrease the barrier, and medications that cause flushing. Patients should be encouraged to use a noncomedogenic, high-factor sunscreen when exposed to sunlight and wind. A sunscreen that contains both ultraviolet-A and ultraviolet-B block with titanium dioxide and zinc oxide is recommended. Green-tinted sunscreens provide coverage for erythema (Banasikowska, 2012).

## CLINICAL PEARLS

- Rosacea: ICD-9, 695.3
- Other rosacea: ICD-10, L71.8, Rosacea unspecified: ICD-10, L71.9
- Avoid sun exposure and known triggers (Gupta, 2013)

## REFERENCES

Banasikowska, A. K. (2012, July 11). *Rosacea*. Retrieved from http://emedicine.medscape.com/article/1071429-overview

Brodsky, J. (2009). Management of benign skin lesions commonly affecting the face: Actinic keratosis, seborrheic keratosis, and rosacea. *Current Opinion in Otolaryngology & Head and Neck Surgery, 17,* 315–320.

Campbell, T. M. (2008). Severe exacerbation of rosacea induced by cinnamon supplements. *Journal of Drugs in Dermatology, 7*(6), 586–587.

Dahl, M. V. (2012). *Rosacea: Pathogenesis, clinical features, and diagnosis*. Retrieved from http://www.uptodate.com/contents/rosacea-pathogenesis-clinical-features-and-diagnosis

Gupta, A. K. (2013). *Acne rosacea*. Retrieved from http://www.unboundmedicine.com/5minute/view/5-minute-clinical-consultation

Kim, M. B. (2011). Pimecrolimus 1% cream for the treatment of rosacea. *Journal of Dermatology, 38*(12), 1135–1139.

Maier, L. E. (2012). *Management of rosacea*. Retrieved from http://www.uptodate.com/contents/management-of-rosacea

Rebora, A. (2008). Papulopustular rosacea. In H. Williams, M. Bigby, T. Diepgen, A. Herxeimer, L. Naldi, & B. Rzany (Eds.), *Evidence-based dermatology* (2nd ed., pp. 105–109). Malden, MA: Blackwell.

Serdar, Z. A. (2011). Efficacy of 1% terbinafine cream in comparison with 0.75% metronidazole gel for the treatment of papulopustular rosacea. *Cutaneous Ocular Toxicology, 30*(2), 124–128.

# Skin Cancer

## OVERVIEW

The skin is the largest organ in the body. It provides protection from the external environment, temperature regulation, sensation, fluid management, immunologic inspection, and ultraviolet (UV) protection (Arora & Attwood, 2009). Skin cancer is the most common form of cancer in the United States, and more than 3.5 million skin cancers are diagnosed annually. In fact, each year, there are more new cases of skin cancer than cancers of the breast, prostate, lung, and colon combined (Skin Cancer Foundation, 2011).

The most common types of skin cancer are basal cell carcinoma (BCC), squamous cell carcinoma (SCC), and melanoma (Skin Cancer Foundation, 2011). Nearly 800,000 Americans are living with a history of melanoma, and 13 million are living with a history of nonmelanoma skin cancer, typically diagnosed as BCC and SCC. It is predicted that one in five Americans will develop BCC or SCC in their lifetime (Urist & Soong, 2007). Between 40% and 50% of Americans who live to age 65 will encounter BCC or SCC at least once (Skin Cancer Foundation, 2011).

## ACTINIC KERATOSIS

### OVERVIEW

An *actinic keratosis* (AK), also known as a solar keratosis, is a cutaneous lesion that is the result of chronic UV exposure from the sun, tanning beds or booths, or UV therapy, which cause abnormal production of atypical epidermal keratinocytes (Englert & Hughes, 2012; Padilla, 2012). AKs present as erythematous, scaled macules, and papules. They are found on fair-skinned adults, primarily on the sun-exposed areas of the face, ears, balding scalp, dorsal hands, and forearms (Figure III.48; James, Berger, & Elston, 2006).

### EPIDEMIOLOGY

In the United States, AKs are among the most common reasons for dermatologist visits. It is estimated that since approximately 2000, 14% of dermatology visits in the United States were related to AKs (Padilla, 2012). Englert and Hughes (2012) stated

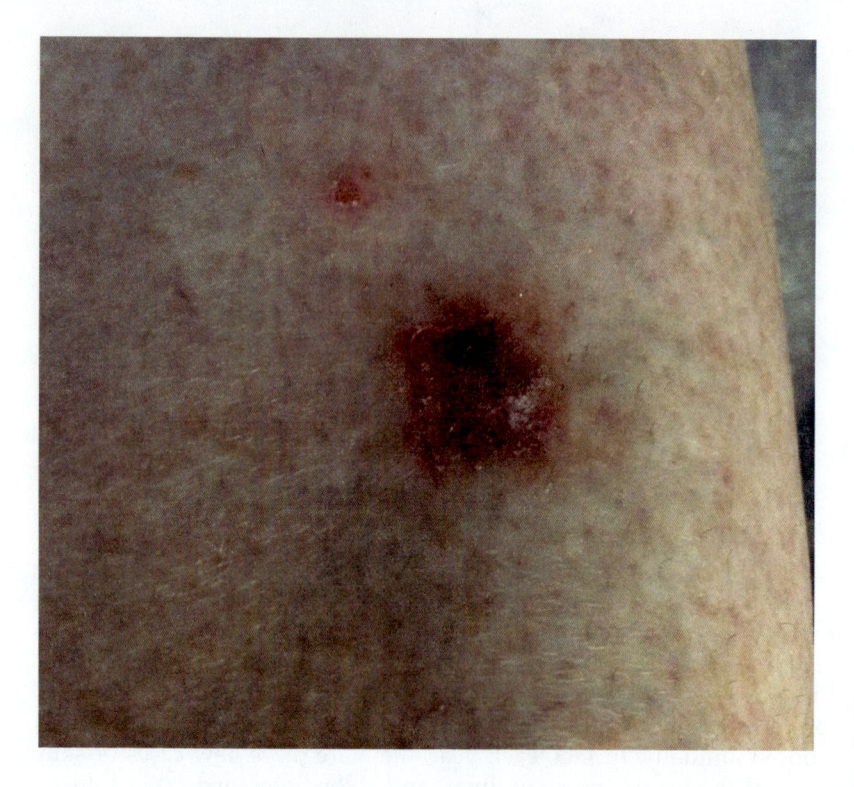

**FIGURE III.48** Example of actinic keratosis

that U.S. prevalence of AK is estimated to be 39.5 million, and in 2003, approximately 5.2 million U.S. physician visits were for AK lesions; the treatment cost was an estimated $1.1 billion in 2004. Brodsky (2009) cited that the incidence of AKs in the United States and Europe is approximately 10% to 15%; these lesions are important to recognize because of a nearly 15% progression to SCC. Also, reappearance of AKs after treatment can be 40% or higher depending on the initial treatment (Chiarello, 2000).

Typically seen in persons older than 50 years of age, AKs may occur in patients in their 20s or 30s who live in areas of high solar irradiation and who are fair skinned (James et al., 2006). Countries that have an abundance of data on the epidemiology and risk factors for AKs are Australia, northern European countries, and the United States. The amount of UV and certain phenotypic features have been associated with the development of AK. Risk factors for AKs include the following:

- UV radiation is believed to contribute to the development of AKs through the introduction of mutations in epidermal keratinocytes that lead to increased survival and production of atypical cells.
- A history of sunburns is said to increase risk.
- Not using sun protection can increase the risk of developing AKs.
- A patient's phenotype can have an effect as well. Skin color contributes to the risk for the development of an AK lesion. Freckling, light hair color, a tendency to sunburn easily, and an inability to tan are additional features that have been associated with increased risk for AKs.
- Individuals with genetic disorders that effect DNA repair after exposure to UV radiation are at increased risk for AKs. Examples include xeroderma pigmentosum, Bloom syndrome, and Rothmund–Thompson syndrome.

- Human papillomavirus (HPV) may be associated with the development of AKs. Betapapillovirus types of HPV have been detected in AKs, SCC, and BCC; however, HPV is also detected on normal skin, and the etiologic relationship between HPV and AKs is uncertain.
- Immunosuppression has been associated with increased risk for SCC and may also increase the risk of AKs. (Engel, Johnson, & Haynes, 1988; Padilla, 2012)

## PATHOLOGY/HISTOLOGY

AKs are the most common epithelial precancerous lesion. The epidermis in AKs shows parakeratosis, abnormal architecture, nuclear pleomorphism, loss of polarity, and anaplasia, but the dermis in AKs characteristically shows evidence of solar elastosis, inflammatory infiltrates, and hypervascularity without dysplasia (Brodsky, 2009). UV exposure has many effects on skin cells, from altering signal transduction pathways, to creating pyrimidine dimers and other genomic lesions that may result in genetic mutations. Over time, these molecular changes and other environmental insults may promote the development of AKs, which can increase the risk of oncogenesis through the mutation of tumor suppressors such as the p53 oncogene (Englert & Hughes, 2012; Marrot & Meunier, 2008).

## CLINICAL PRESENTATION

AKs typically present as erythematous, hyperkeratotic plaques or papules. Actinic cheilitis is a similar condition affecting the lips and has a similar rate of malignant progression (Brodsky, 2009). Accurate diagnosis of AKs may decrease the rate of progression into SCC (Englert & Hughes, 2012).

The types of AKs that can be recognized histologically are:

- Classic AKs are erythematous, scaly macules, papules, or plaques. These lesions are a few millimeters to 2 cm in diameter.
- Actinic cheilitis, also known as solar cheilitis, is an AK found on the lip. This is usually found on the lower lip and is a persistent rough or scaly area. Patients may complain of a consistent dry lip.
- Acantholytic
- An AK with cutaneous horn appears as a keratotic projection the height of which is at least one half the diameter. This often resembles a cone or spicule formation.
- Atrophic lesions have no scale; these lesions are erythematous and smooth.
- Bowenoid
- A hypertrophic lesion presents as a thick erythematous scaled patch with an erythematous base.
- Lichenoid
- A pigmented lesion often appears as a scaled lentigo; pigmented AKs are usually scaled, hyperpigmented macules or patches. (James et al., 2006; Padilla, 2012)

## DIFFERENTIAL DIAGNOSIS

Differential diagnosis comprises a number of possible conditions such as:

- Discoid lupus erythematosus
- Deep fungal infections
- Lichenoid keratosis and other benign inflammatory disorders

- Malignant melanoma/lentigo maligna
- Porokeratosis
- Seborrheic keratosis
- SCC
- Superficial BCC
- Verruca vulgaris (Berman, Bienstock, Kuritzky, Mayeaux, & Tyring, 2006; Padilla, 2012; Schwartz, Bridges, Butani, Ehrlich, 2008)

## TREATMENT/MANAGEMENT

Treatment considerations include duration, size, location, and number of lesions present, and the patient's age, immune status, occupation, lifestyle, and likelihood of treatment faithfulness (Schwartz et al., 2008). There are multiple lesion-directed methods for treating AKs (Berman et al., 2006).

- Cryotherapy destroys AKs in epithelium with liquid nitrogen. This is the most common procedure used for management of AKs, although it is limited because of patient discomfort, operator technique, and frequent localized skin damage, including blistering, scarring, and pigmentation changes.
- Laser therapy uses $CO_2$ or Er:YAG lasers.
- Dermabrasion is a superficial peel that involves the removal of skin layers down to the lower papillary or upper reticular dermis. This is effective for multiple disseminated AKs, although treatment may be painful and requires inpatient care for postoperative pain.
- Chemical peels use a variety of chemicals (e.g., trichloroacetic acid) to induce the destruction of the epidermal layer.
- Curettage and/or electrosurgery is the surgical removal of abnormal tissue and is effective for small AKs and superficial lesions, although this may cause scarring and often retreatment.
- Photodynamic therapy (PDT) uses a photosensitizing agent (e.g., 5-aminolevulinic acid) followed by irradiation. This is highly effective, but requires multiple sessions and is painful. Patients must avoid sunlight initially after treatments.

Topical therapies that are available for the treatment of AKs include:

- 5-fluorouracil inhibits DNA synthesis, causing tumor cell death. This treatment is highly effective and is usually first line for the treatment of multiple AKs in one area. However, patient tolerance is poor because of irritation and pigment changes.
- Diclofenac sodium is an anti-inflammatory agent that works via cyclooxygenase-2 inhibition. It is typically used for 2 to 3 months. Side effects include erythema, itching, and skin irritation.
- Imiquimod gel is a topical immune-response modifier. Treatment is 1 to 4 months depending on location and amount of AK damage. This treatment is also poorly tolerated because of association with local skin reactions that range from erythema to weeping, crusting, and erosion. (Berman et al., 2006; Brodsky, 2009)

Biopsy is usually indicated in the presence of suspicious or unusual lesions that may bleed, itch, or have pronounced hyperkeratosis, erythema, or induration (Cockerell & Wharton, 2005).

## SPECIAL CONSIDERATIONS

Gender and age influence the risk for developing an AK. Men are more likely than women to develop AKs, and the prevalence of AKs increases with age (Padilla, 2012).

Immunosuppression is another risk factor. AKs and SCC are up to 65 times more likely to appear in transplant patients. Lesions appear 2 to 4 years after transplantation and increase in frequency (Habif, 2004).

## WHEN TO REFER

If treatment fails, referral to a dermatologist may be necessary for biopsy, management of recurrent or unresponsive lesions, and management of skin cancers (Englert & Hughes, 2012).

## PATIENT EDUCATION

AKs are commonly seen on body sites exposed to sunlight, such as dorsal hands, forearms, face, scalp, neck, and upper chest. However, if tanning beds are used, AKs can be in all areas exposed. AKs are often asymptomatic and appear as skin-colored to reddish-brown papules and patches ranging from 1 mm to several centimeters in diameter. There may be broken blood vessels surrounding the lesion. Lesions are often rough or scaly when palpated (Englert & Hughes, 2012). Patients should be made aware of these characteristics of AKs.

The best treatment for AKs is prevention. Wearing protective clothing, using high sun protection factor (SPF) sunscreens, and avoiding peak sun exposure times (10 a.m.– 4 p.m.) are important for preventing sun damage. Regular use of sunscreens prevents the development of solar keratosis. Sunscreens that contain a combination of ingredients to block both the UVA and UVB spectrum of UV light are the most effective. Sunscreen should be applied to all sun-exposed areas in the morning and reapplied every few hours thereafter. Hats should be worn on bald scalps (Habif, 2004). Providers should instruct patients in these precautions.

## CLINICAL PEARLS

- Actinic keratosis: ICD-9, 702.0; Basil cell carcinoma: ICD-9, 173.0; SCC: ICD-9, 232.0; Melanoma: ICD-9, 172.0
- Nurse practitioners should increase their knowledge base with regard to skin cancer and the accurate recognition of precancerous lesions and treatment.
- Practitioners should educate patients about risk factors, the importance of self skin examinations and yearly clinical skin examinations, and the prevention of chronic sun exposure through sun avoidance and the prevention of sunburns (e.g., avoiding peak sun exposure times, applying sunscreens, wearing sun-protective clothing).
- Monitoring the use of treatments and following up after treatment to determine outcomes is essential to treatment management.

# BASAL CELL CARCINOMA

## OVERVIEW

BCC is the most common skin cancer in the United States, Australia, New Zealand, and multiple other countries that have a large White, fair-skinned population (James et al., 2006). BCC is more common on sun-exposed skin; these lesions are slow growing and do not normally metastasize (Figure III.49; Baded, 2013).

**284** ■ III. Common Dermatologic Conditions

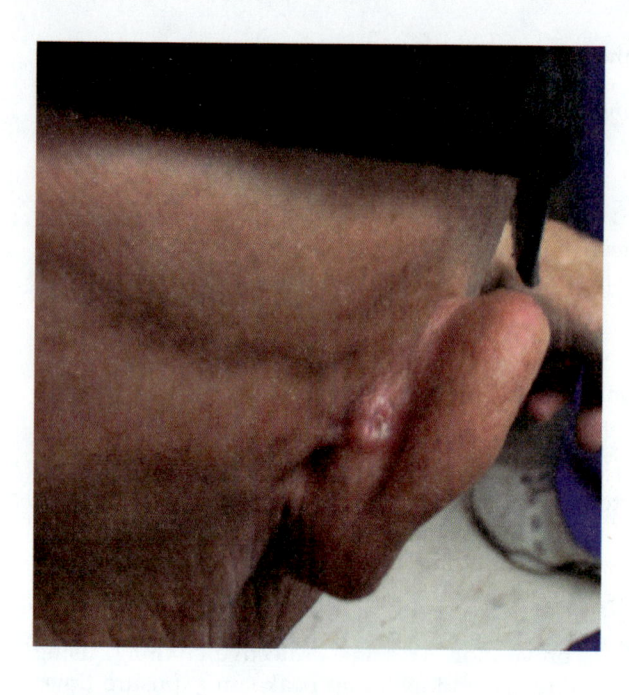

FIGURE III.49   Example of basal cell carcinoma

## EPIDEMIOLOGY

The American Cancer Society reports BCC as being the most common skin cancer in the United States, with an estimated 2.8 million cases diagnosed annually (Arora & Attwood, 2009). The projected risk for BCC in the Caucasian population is 33% to 39% for men and 23% to 28% for women in their lifetimes. BCC occurrence increase twofold every 25 years (Baded, 2013).

Although BCC is observed in people of all races and skin types, fair-skinned people (type 1 or type 2 skin) are at higher risk. Generally, the men-to-women ratio is two to one. This is attributed to the fact that men are exposed to the sun more through recreation and occupation (Baded, 2013; James et al., 2006; Nolen, Beebe, King, Bryn, & Limaye, 2011).

## PATHOLOGY/HISTOLOGY

BCC is a nonmelanocytic skin cancer that evolves from basal cells, which are small circular cells found in the lower layer of the epidermis. Basal cells attack the dermis but seldom expand to other areas of the body. Inheritance is thought to play a role in the development of BCC because the DNA of certain genes is often damaged in patients with BCC (Baded, 2013; Nolen et al., 2011).

BCC can occur on unexposed skin in some patients as a result of exposure to or contact with arsenic, tar, coal, paraffin, certain types of industrial oil, and radiation. BCC can also be associated with scars (e.g., burn complications), xeroderma pigmentosum, previous trauma, vaccinations, or even tattoos (Baded, 2013; Nolen et al., 2011). Several histologic types of BCC exist, including:

- *Nodular* BCC is the most common type and consists of large, round or oval tumor islands within the dermis, often with an epidermal connection. Artificial withdrawal of the tumor islands from the surrounding stroma is frequently seen. Ulcerations may be noted in large tumors.

- *Micronodular* BCC is another aggressive variant, which appears as small, nodular aggregates of basaloid cells.
- *Pigmented* BCC has benign melanocytes in and around the tumor that produce large amounts of melanin.
- *Morpheaform* (sclerosing) BCC has a growth pattern resulting from thin strands of tumor cells rather than round nests within a fibrous stroma. Morpheaform BCC displays islands of tumor extending into the tissue and may exhibit perineural invasion in 3% of patients.
- *Infiltrative* BCC accounts for 10% of BCCs. Tumor cells have growth patterns resulting from the strands of cells infiltrating between collagen bundles rather than round nests. The strands of infiltrating BCC tend to be thicker than those seen in morpheaform BCC, and they have a spiky, irregular appearance. Infiltrating BCC usually does not exhibit the scarlike stroma seen in morpheaform BCC.
- *Cystic* BCC consists of large, round or oval tumor islands within the dermis with mucin present in the center of the island.
- *Superficial* BCC is characterized by multiple small nests of tumor cells usually attached to the undersurface of the epidermis by a wide base. Approximately 10% to 15% of BCCs are of this type.
- The *keratotic* type resembles the solid type, with its nests of basaloid cells with peripheral palisading. The island centers display keratinization and squamous differentiation.
- The *infundibulocystic* type is rare and usually found on the face. It resembles the keratotic type. Nests are arranged in an anastomosing pattern and lack stroma. Many small, infundibular cystlike structures with keratinous material are present. Melanin is sometimes present.
- *Metatypical* BCC is rare. In this type, nests and strands of cells mature into larger and paler cells, and peripheral palisading, if any, is less developed than in other types. Prominent stroma, prominent mitotic activity, and many apoptotic cells may be present. This form may be best diagnosed when one evaluates a BCC with features between those of a nodular BCC and SCC. These tumors are often aggressive, with an increased tendency for lymphatic and perineural spread.
- The *basosquamous* type is controversial. It has been defined as a BCC with differentiation toward SCC. It is made up of basaloid cells that are larger, paler, and rounder than those of a solid BCC. It also consists of squamoid cells and intermediate cells. This type is considered to have metastatic potential and is considered an aggressive skin cancer.
- *Fibroepithelioma* of Pinkus is a fibroepithelioma type that consists of thin, anastomosing strands of basaloid cells in a prominent stroma. (Baded, 2013; Nolen et al., 2011)

## CLINICAL PRESENTATION

Patients with BCC often have a history of chronic sun exposure, including recreational sun exposure (e.g., sunbathing, outdoor sports, fishing, boating) and occupational sun exposure (e.g., farming, construction). Consider BCC if a patient has a history of a nonhealing sore that is friable and umbilicated. Characteristic features of BCC tumors include the following:

- Waxy papules with central depression
- Pearly appearance
- Erosion or ulceration, often central
- Bleeding, especially when traumatized
- Crusting
- Rolled (raised) border

- Translucency
- Telangiectases over the surface
- Slow growing (0.5 cm in 1–2 years) (Baded, 2013; James et al., 2006; Nolen et al., 2011)

Several clinicopathologic types of BCC exist, each with distinct biologic behavior (Arora & Attwood, 2009; Baded, 2013; Nolen et al., 2011).

- *Nodular* BCC usually presents as a round, pearly, flesh-colored papule with telangiectases. As it enlarges, it frequently ulcerates centrally, leaving a raised, pearly border with telangiectases. The tumor may present as a cyst, which can be mistaken for inclusion cysts of the eyelid.
- *Cystic* BCC is an uncommon variant of nodular BCC, and it is often difficult to differentiate from nodular BCC. Typically, a bluish-gray cyst-like lesion is noted. The cystic center of the tumor is filled with clear, gelatinous mucin.
- *Pigmented* BCC is an uncommon variant of nodular BCC that usually has brown-black macules within some of the tumor or covering the entire tumor. Differential diagnosis includes malignant melanoma. Some areas of these tumors do not retain pigment, and pearly, raised borders with telangiectases can be observed. This aids clinically in differentiating this tumor from a malignant melanoma.
- *Keratotic* BCC is a variant of nodular BCC.
- *Infiltrative* BCC infiltrates the dermis in thin strands between collagen fibers, making tumor margins less clinically apparent. Mohs micrographic surgery is the treatment of choice for infiltrative BCC.
- *Micronodular* BCC does not ulcerate, appears yellow-white when stretched, has a well-defined border, and is firm to palpation.
- *Morpheaform* BCC appears as flat or slightly depressed, fibrotic, and firm, with white or yellow, waxy, sclerotic plaque and margins that are difficult to differentiate. Mohs micrographic surgery is the treatment of choice for morpheaform BCC.
- *Superficial* BCC is seen mostly on the upper trunk or shoulders. This type of BCC grows slowly, is rarely invasive, and appears clinically as an erythematous, well-circumscribed patch or plaque, often with a whitish scale, and has a thin border. Erosion is not common, but pinpoint areas of hemorrhage or eschar may be present. Numerous superficial BCCs may indicate arsenic exposure.

BCC is also a feature of basal cell nevus syndrome (i.e., Gorlin syndrome), an autosomal dominant inherited condition. The lesions in these patients cannot be distinguished histologically from ordinary BCCs. Patients with this syndrome may have as many as 100 BCCs. Multiple BCCs begin to appear after puberty on the face, trunk, and extremities. In many cases, the tumors are highly invasive and may involve areas around the eyes and nose (Baded, 2013; James et al., 2006; Nolen et al., 2011).

## DIFFERENTIAL DIAGNOSIS

- AK
- Angiofibroma
- Bowen disease
- Fibrous papule of the face
- Malignant melanoma
- Molluscum contagiosum
- Nevi, melanocytic
- Psoriasis

- Sebaceous hyperplasia
- SCC

## TREATMENT/MANAGEMENT

BCC rarely metastasizes, so laboratory and imaging studies are not clinically indicated in patients presenting with localized lesions. Computed tomography (CT) scans or radiography is indicated if involvement of deeper structures, such as bone, is clinically suspected (Baded, 2013).

A skin biopsy is often required to confirm the diagnosis and determine the histologic subtype of BCC. Most often, a shave biopsy is all that is required. However, pigmented BCCs are often difficult to distinguish from melanoma, and an excisional or punch biopsy may be indicated to determine the depth of the lesion if it proves to be a malignant melanoma (Baded, 2013).

Treatment decisions should be individualized according to the patient's particular risk factors and preferences. Treatments vary according to cancer size, depth, and location. Several topical creams are used in the management of a BCC that is nonrecurring and superficial. The National Comprehensive Cancer Network (NCCN) 2011 guidelines state that low-risk patients with superficial BCC who cannot undergo surgery or radiation can be treated with topical therapies, including (Baded, 2013):

- Topical 5-fluorouracil 5% cream may be used to treat small, superficial BCCs in low-risk areas. 5-fluorouracil is not used for other types of BCC because it does not penetrate deeply enough into the dermis to eradicate all tumor cells. Irritation and crusting occurs with use, and patients experience discomfort. The recurrence rate is high. Fluorouracil is typically administered twice daily for 3 to 6 weeks, depending on areas treated (facial areas for 3 weeks and trunk areas up to 6 weeks).
- Interferon alfa-2b is a protein product manufactured using recombinant DNA technology. It has shown success in treating small (<1 cm), nodular, and superficial BCCs. Interferon is not frequently used because it is expensive, requires frequent office visits for follow-up, causes discomfort with treatment, and produces side effects similar to flulike symptoms.
- Imiquimod 5% cream (Aldara) is approved by the U.S. Food and Drug Administration for the treatment of nonfacial superficial BCC. Treatment is usually initiated at three times per week and is increased as tolerated to once, and even twice, daily to maintain mild to moderate skin irritation. A 12-week course of treatment is often used, but patients may take breaks in between applications.
- The receptor-selective acetylenic retinoid tazarotene (Tazorac) can also be used to treat small low-risk BCCs. The use of tazarotene to treat BCC is considered off label; if used, treatment is required for 5 to 8 months.

BCCs are usually radiosensitive, and radiation therapy can be used for advanced and large lesions or in those patients for whom surgery is not an option (e.g., because of allergy to anesthetics, current anticoagulant therapy, a tendency to form keloids, or facial tumors). Postoperative radiation is also used as an adjunct to therapy when patients have aggressive tumors that were treated with surgery or if surgical excision failed to clear tumor margins (Baded, 2013).

PDT is a recent treatment option for BCC in European countries. PDT uses light and prophyrins (5-aminolevulinic acid) to cause tumor destruction. The acid is applied to the tumor site and uses light therapy to activate the acid and penetrate the cancer and cause cell death (Chartier & Aasi, 2011).

## SPECIAL CONSIDERATIONS

Some studies have shown that men and people diagnosed with BCC before age 60 are at a higher risk for a second cancer, including melanoma, cancer of the lip, salivary glands, larynx, lungs, breast, kidney, and non-Hodgkin lymphoma (MD Consult, 2010).

## WHEN TO REFER

Treatment options for a patient with BCC should be evaluated jointly with a surgeon, dermatologist, and radiotherapist if warranted. For example, joint consultation is warranted if the area involved (usually the face) needs to be treated with radiation rather than surgery. If the area involved is large and deep, radiation is often used (Baded, 2013).

## PATIENT EDUCATION

Baded (2013) suggested informing patients of the following:

- Patients should avoid possible risk factors (e.g., sun exposure, ionizing radiation, arsenic ingestion, tanning beds). Recommend wearing sun-protective clothing and glasses when outdoors.
- If surgery is warranted, explain the procedure and the extent of surgery that will be required.
- Teach self-skin examinations and what to look for as signs of skin cancer.
- The American Cancer Society recommends a dermatologic examination every 3 years for people in the second through fourth decades of life and every year for people after the fourth decade of life.

# MALIGNANT MELANOMA

## OVERVIEW

Primary skin cancers are classified by the cell of origin within the skin (Fitzpartrick & Morelli, 2011). Malignant melanoma is a malignancy of the mealnocytes and although its source is most often in the skin, melanoma can occur in the eyes, ears, leptomeniges, gastrointestinal tract, and genital or oral mucous membranes (Habif, 2010; Habif et al., 2011). Melanoma is deadly but is potentially curable if diagnosed and treated early. If undetected or ignored it can metastasize to any organ. Late diagnosis creates a very poor prognosis (Habif et al., 2011).

The U.S. Surveillance, Epidemiology, and End Results (SEER) program, which is supported through the National Cancer Institute, provides cancer data in the United States through registries representative of the U.S. population. For the past several decades the SEER program has tracked the incidence of melanoma and found that there has been a steadily increasing incidence by roughly 2.8% annually from 1981 to 2008 (Little & Eide, 2012).

## EPIDEMIOLOGY

In 2009, the American Cancer Society approximated that 68,720 cases (39,080 in men and 29,640 in women) of melanoma were diagnosed in the United States (Figure III.50). Melanoma is responsible for only about 5% of skin cancers; however, it accounts for three times as many deaths each year compared with nonmelanoma skin cancers. The prevalence of melanoma rises by 5% to 7% annually. In 1935, the lifetime risk of developing melanoma was only 1 per 1,500; in 2000, the lifetime risk was estimated at 1 per 75 (Tan, 2013). Melanoma is the major cause of skin-cancer related mortality worldwide (Springer & McClary, 2013).

Queensland, Australia, has the highest incidence of melanoma in the world, with approximately 57 cases per 100,000 people per year, and Israel has approximately 40 cases per 100,000 people annually. In Hawaii and the southwestern United States, Caucasians have the highest incidence, with approximately 20 to 30 cases per 100,000 people per year (Tan, 2013).

Melanoma is more common in Whites than in Blacks and Asians. The typical patient who is at risk for melanoma has fair skin, sunburns easily, has blond or red hair, and skin that freckles easily (James et al., 2006). Melanoma is slightly more common in men than in women. In men, melanoma is the fifth most common cancer, and in women it is the sixth most common cancer (Russak & Rigel, 2012). Melanoma is not age specific but is rare in children younger than age 10. The average age for a melanoma diagnosis is 57 years (Tan, 2013).

## PATHOLOGY/HISTOLOGY

Melanocytes originate in the neural crest, travel to the epidermis, and produce melanin. Melanoma arises from the melanocytes in the skin, which may be abnormal or healthy. Melanoma can occur anywhere on the body. Certain lesions can be precursor lesions of melanoma, such as common acquired, atypical, congenital, and blue nevi (Tan, 2013).

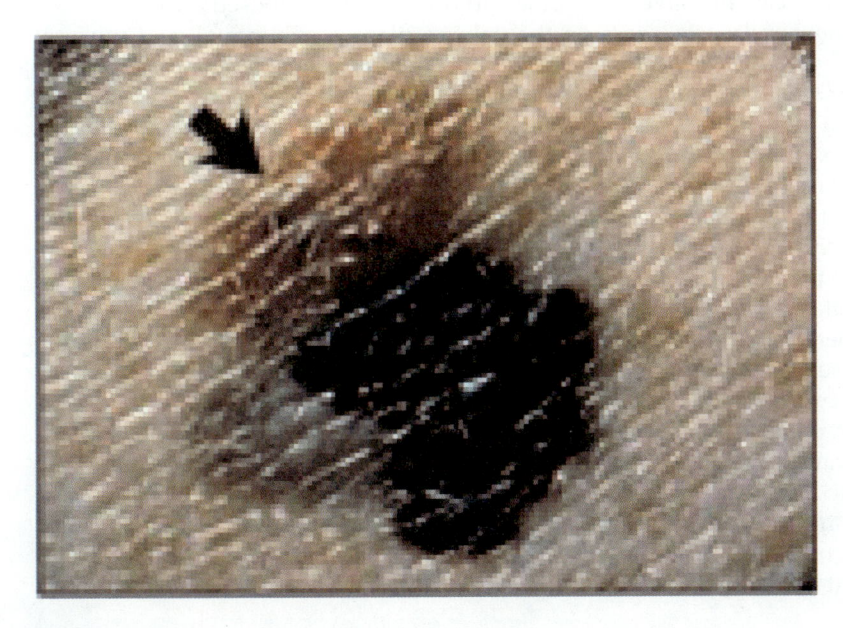

FIGURE III.50 Example of malignant melanoma
Courtesy of National Cancer Institute

Of the lesions that develop in the head and neck region, most melanomas arise in the face (47%). The remainder are found on the neck, which accounts for 29%, the scalp (14%), and the ear (10%). In addition, approximately 55% of mucosal melanomas are found in the head and neck (Herr, 2011).

Histologic examination for melanoma reveals cytologic atypia with large cells containing large, pleomorphic, hyperchronic nuclei. Multiple mitotic elements are present, as is a pagetoid growth pattern with upward growth of melanocytes outside the basal layer (Tan, 2013).

## CLINICAL PRESENTATION

Melanomas exhibit two growth stages, the radial and the vertical phase. In the radial growth phase, reproduction of malignant melanocytes is confined to the epidermis and the upper dermis. In the vertical growth phase, malignant melanocytes form nests or nodules in the dermis. Five principle histologic types of melanoma are observed including the following (Arora & Attwood, 2009; Armstrong, Liu, & Mihm, 2013; Doben & MacGillivray, 2009; Herr, 2011; Swetter & Geller, 2013):

1. *Superficial spreading melanoma* appears as a plaque that is a few millimeters to several centimeters in diameter, with irregular borders and varied colors. Malignant melanocytes spread throughout the layers of the epidermis as single cells or nests. Dermal invasion is seen in the vertical growth phase. This type of melanoma is responsible for about one half of all melanomas on the head and neck. When contained in the epidermis, the growth pattern is biphasic with an initial radial growth phase. Then the melanoma has a vertical phase, when the melanocytes invade deep into the dermal layer.
2. *Lentigo maligna melanoma* begins as a nonpalpable tan or brown macule, enlarging gradually over many years. Dermal invasion is noted by palpable areas. A dermal nodule indicates a vertical growth phase. About one fourth of head and neck melanomas are of this type. These melanomas are flat with a slow growth phase. Lentigo maligna are the least invasive melanoma and occur on sun-exposed areas.
3. *Acral lentiginous melanoma* arises on the palmar, plantar, subungual, and mucosal surfaces of the body. Mucosal melanoma is a rare form of melanoma that accounts for approximately 1% to 4% of cases of head and neck melanoma. Most of these tumors (55%) arise in the nasal cavity, followed by the oral cavity (40%). Although the growth patterns of mucosal melanoma tend to mirror the nodular pattern of their cutaneous counterparts, they differ in that tumoral thickness is not well correlated with the prognosis. Most patients present with clinically localized disease and more than 50% experience local recurrence after treatment. Prognosis is dismal, regardless of the thickness of the primary lesion.
4. *Nodular melanoma* presents as dark, sometimes ulcerated pigmented nodules. On histology, there is a nodule of neoplastic cells in the dermis, with no adjacent radial growth phase. These fast-growing lesions have only a vertical growth phase and comprise as much as one third of the head and neck melanomas.
5. *Desmoplastic melanoma* is a rare, aggressive subtype of melanoma that has a tendency to invade perineural areas and reoccur. Desmoplastic melanoma frequently occur on the head and neck of elderly men in their sixth and seventh decades of life and are often deep at the time of diagnosis because of the difficulty of clinical diagnosis with these atypical and often unpigmented lesions. Although they account for only 1% of all cutaneous lesions, more than 75% of them are

found within the head and neck region. The clinical presentation of desmoplastic melanomas is unique, and these tumors do not generally adhere to the ABCDE criteria (discussed later in this section) that typify more traditional cutaneous lesions. They are often found in conjunction with LM lesions. Desmoplastic melanoma tumors tend to be locally aggressive, highly infiltrative, and frequently associated with involvement of the cranial nerves and skull base. Approximately half of these lesions recur.

In 2002, the American Joint Committee on Cancer Melanoma Task Force reviewed the staging system for skin-involved melanomas based on research from more than 15,000 patients. Staging continues to follow the traditional tumor-node-metastasis (TNM) classification system. This system classifies melanomas on the basis of their local, regional, and distant characteristics, as follows:

- Stage I and II: localized primary melanoma
- Stage III: metastasis to single regional lymph node basin (with or without in-transit metastases)
- Stage IV: distant metastatic disease (Herr, 2011)

Two of the most frequently used staging systems for thickness of melanoma are the Clark levels and the Breslow thickness classifications.

- Clark levels: The Clark method is used to stage the melanoma according to its depth of penetration into the deep levels of skin as follows (Herr, 2011):
  - Level I: confined to the epidermis; radial growth phase
  - Level II: spread into the papillary dermis; radial growth phase
  - Level III: spread into the papillary dermis–reticular dermis junction; vertical growth phase
  - Level IV: spread into the reticular dermis; vertical growth phase
  - Level V: spread into the subcutaneous fat
- Breslow thickness: The Breslow thickness classification system is used to stage melanomas according to the thickness of the lesion, as measured from the granular layer of the epidermis to the deepest point of tumor infiltration in the vertical dimension. The system is as follows (Herr, 2011):
  - Thin lesion (T1): less than 0.76 mm
  - Intermediate thickness (T2): 0.76–1.50 mm
  - Intermediate thickness (T3): 1.51–4.00 mm
  - Thick lesion (T4): More than 4 mm

Overall, the two most important prognostic factors for cutaneous melanoma are the thickness of the tumor and the status of the regional lymph-node basin. Prognostic indicators can be further subdivided based on TNM staging.

- When considering localized disease (T classification), tumor thickness is the most significant prognostic indicator; however, the presence of ulceration has also been found to be an important predictor of outcome.
- Three statistically significant prognostic factors have been identified in regional disease (N classification). The most important indicator for patients with nodal metastasis is the number of positive lymph nodes.
- Finally, in patients with distant metastases (M classification), the anatomic site of spread is the most important indicator of prognosis. Patients with involvement of the skin, subcutaneous tissues, or distant lymph nodes have a better prognosis than those with metastases to the lungs or visceral organs. (Herr, 2011)

## DIFFERENTIAL DIAGNOSIS

- Atypical fibroxanthoma
- BCC
- Benign melanocytic lesions
- Blue nevus
- Dysplastic nevus
- Epithelioid (Spitz) tumor
- Halo nevus
- Histiocytoid hemangioma
- Lentigo maligna melanoma
- Metastatic tumors to the skin
- Mycosis fungoides
- Pigmented AK
- Pigmented spindle cell tumor
- SCC
- Sebaceous carcinoma

## TREATMENT/MANAGEMENT

Tan (2013) recommends:

- Carefully obtain any family history of melanoma, skin cancer, or abnormal appearing nevi. Patients with a family history of melanoma will have a 10% chance of having melanoma. These patients tend to have melanoma at a younger age and will have several atypical nevi.
- Inquire about any previous history of melanoma, which increases the risk for a second melanoma.
- Obtain history of sun exposure, including severe sunburns in childhood.
- Inquire about any changes (size, color, symmetry, bleeding, or ulceration) of any lesions.

Patients with newly diagnosed melanoma may require imaging to rule out metastasis. A chest x-ray may be done on patients with stage I or II melanoma. Patients with stage III melanoma, having a recurrence of melanoma, or melanoma in remission should have a chest x-ray or CT scan of the chest because the lungs are the most common site for metastatic disease (Buzaid & Gershenwald, 2013; Tan, 2013).

Blood work may be an indicator of potential metastatic disease. Elevated alkaline phosphatase level or elevated liver function test may indicate metastatic disease to bone or liver. The lactate dehydrogenase (LDH) level is not a specific indicator for melanoma but can be elevated with malignancies. LDH level is often done in follow-up monitoring for patients with melanoma. Magnetic resonance imaging of the brain should be done on patients with metastasis to check for brain involvement. A positron emission tomography scan can help stage patients who have nodal involvement or satellite lesions (Tan, 2013).

The prognosis and treatment of cutaneous melanoma depends greatly on the thickness of the lesion. Obtaining a full-thickness excisional biopsy is recommended for small lesions or in large lesions that are not in visible locations. Excisional biopsies extend down to the subcutaneous fat with 2- to 3-mm margins. Punch biopsies can also be done in the thickest part of the lesion. Techniques that do not permit a full-thickness sample, such as shave or curette biopsy, are discouraged. Do not treat pigmented lesions with laser therapy, electrocautery, or cryotherapy unless biopsy analysis proves them to be noncancerous (Herr, 2011). Once the biopsy has been confirmed as melanoma, a reexcision with appropriate margins must be done. Current recommendations for margins of excision are:

- Lesions less than 1 mm in thickness: 1-cm margin
- Lesions 1 to 4 mm in thickness: 2-cm margin
- Lesions greater than 4 mm in thickness: at least 2-cm margin (Tan, 2013)

The status of the regional lymph nodes is a powerful predictor of survival rates for melanoma. For a patient with clinical evidence of regional nodal metastases at presentation, lymph node dissection with treatment of the primary lesion is appropriate (Herr, 2011).

Malignant melanoma is known to be a relatively chemoresistant tumor. The treatment for metastatic melanoma includes several Food and Drug Administration–approved drugs. One is a chemotherapy drug, dacarbazine, a drug given intravenously, with varied response rates of 10% and 25%. Also used as a treatment option is interleukin-2, an agent that boosts the immune system by activating T cells. Response rates are 15% initially, but only 5% have a prolonged response. Another new agent, vemurafenib (Zelboraf) was the second drug approved for metastatic melanoma. These two drugs work differently to treat melanoma, and currently there are clinical trials to combine treatment with both of these drugs (Chapman, 2011). Vemurafenib was successful in shrinking the tumors of 81% of patients who had the gene defect that is present in 40% to 60% of melanomas (Skin Cancer Foundation, 2013).

The plan of care for a patient with melanoma should be based on the initial melanoma diagnosis and the realization that the patient is at increased risk for recurrence and metastasis. Follow-up guidelines from the NCCN are:

- Stage 0 in situ requires a skin examination at least annually for life.
- Stage IA calls for complete examination to include lymph node and skin examination every 3 to 12 months for 5 years, then annually as clinically indicated and skin examination at least annually for life.
- Stages IB–IV (patients with no evidence of disease) warrant complete examination to include lymph node and skin every 3 to 6 months for 2 years, then every 3 to 12 months for 2 years, then annually as clinically indicated; chest x-ray, LDH, and complete blood count every 6 to 12 months are recommended. Advise a CT scan to screen stage IIB and higher for recurrent/metastatic disease. Patients should undergo a skin examination at least annually for life. (Tan, 2013)

## SPECIAL CONSIDERATIONS

The following factors increase the risk for a person to develop skin cancer.

- Age and gender: In the United States, melanoma is more common in men than in women. However, incidence is greater in women until age 40, but by age 75, the incidence of melanoma is three times as high in men compared with women (Russak & Rigel, 2012).
- Chronic or severe skin problems: These can increase the risk of melanoma.
- Certain diseases: A number of conditions have been shown to possibly increase the risk of developing melanoma. For example, melanoma has developed in patients who received solid organ transplants from donors who had the disease. Women who have a history of endometriosis have an increased risk of developing melanoma (Gemmill, 2010). A strong association between Parkinson disease and melanoma has been suspected, perhaps based on the fact that both diseases involve cells

that metabolize tyrosine via dopaquinone intermediates (Hawryluk & Fisher, 2011). Levodopa serves as a substitute for tyrosine hydroxylase and might therefore accelerate melanoma tumor growth, but data are inconclusive for this (Gao, Simon, Han, Schwarzchild, & Ascherio, 2009). A family history of melanoma does not increase one's risk of developing Parkinson disease, but a diagnosis of Parkinson disease does increase one's risk of developing melanoma (Hawryluk & Fisher, 2011; Liu, Gao, Lu, & Chen, 2011).

- Exposure to chemicals or radiation: Radiation and some chemicals (vinyl chloride, polychlorinated biphenyls, and petrochemicals) in health care or industrial settings may increase the risk of melanoma (Leber et al., 1999; Urist & Soong, 2007).
- Being and airline pilot: Airline pilots have been found to have an increased risk for melanoma possibly because of excessive exposure to ionizing radiation at high altitudes or because they have more opportunity to spend time in sunny regions (Hawryluk & Fisher, 2011).
- Geography: Warmer climates with more sun exposure increase the risk of malignant melanoma.
- High mole count: Individuals with a large number of nevi (moles) have a strong risk factor for the development of melanoma. Studies have shown that those with a higher mole count, which are often counted on the back (greater than 40 on the back can be considered high), are at a greater risk for melanoma (Berwick, Erdei, & Hay, 2009; Russak & Rigel, 2012; Springer & McClary, 2013).
- High dysplastic nevi count: Clinically, the number of dysplastic nevi is associated with increased melanoma risk. One dysplastic nevus creates a twofold risk, whereas 10 or more dysplastic nevi induce a 12-fold increased risk of melanoma. Having many small nevi imparts an approximately twofold increased risk, and the presence of both small and large nondysplastic nevi results in a fourfold risk. Congenital nevi are not generally associated with melanoma risk; however, giant pigmented congenital nevi confer substantial melanoma risk (Hawryluk & Fisher, 2011; Russak & Rigel, 2012; Springer & McClary, 2013).
- Medications that affect the immune system: Persons who take tumor necrosis factor-alpha blockers to treat rheumatoid arthritis and other autoimmune diseases are at increased risk for developing melanoma and other nonmelanoma skin cancers (Amari et al., 2011; Engkilde, Thyssen, Menne, & Johansen, 2011).
- Personal or family history of skin cancer: Individuals with a family history of melanoma, particularly in first-degree relatives, have twice the risk of developing melanoma as those without a family history (Berwick, et al., 2009; Russak & Rigel, 2012; Springer & McClary, 2013; Tucker, 2009). People who have had melanoma have an 11.4% risk for a second primary melanoma. This percentage is higher in older men and in those whose first melanomas appeared on the upper body and face (Hawryluk & Fisher, 2011; Russak & Rigel, 2012).
- UV radiation: UVA is a long wavelength (320–400 nm) and accounts for 95% of UV radiation. UVA penetrates deep into the skin. It is present during all daylight hours and can penetrate through clouds and glass year round. UVA causes more DNA damage than UVB. UVB is a shorter wavelength (290–320 nm) and penetrates the epidermal layer of the skin. It is to blame for burning, mild tanning, and speeding up of skin aging. UVC (100–290 nm) is the shortest wavelength and is filtered by the ozone layer; therefore, it does not reach the Earth's surface (Nolen et al., 2011; Russak & Rigel, 2012; Springer & McClary, 2013).

## WHEN TO REFER

Any abnormal lesion or biopsy-confirmed melanoma should be referred to a dermatologist and/or general surgeon for treatment and follow-up (Tan, 2013).

## PATIENT EDUCATION

A vital warning sign of melanoma is a new or rapidly changing skin lesion. Changes that occur over a short period of time (particularly over a few weeks) are most concerning. Despite great advances in the treatment of melanoma, the best prospect for patients is early diagnosis. Classic warning signs and symptoms include any cutaneous lesion that changes color, size, or shape. Persistent pruritus is also a common early symptom. More advanced lesions frequently become friable, tender, painful, crusted, or ulcerated (Herr, 2011).

The American Cancer Society developed the ABCDEs to serve as a simple guideline of early melanoma warning signs (Herr, 2011; Springer & McClary, 2013; Skin Cancer Foundation, 2013).

- Asymmetry: A lesion or nevus that is irregular and not equal on each half could be indicative of skin cancer.
- Border: Nevi with irregular or smudged borders could be a sign of a skin cancer.
- Color: A pigmented nevus with color variation is one of the earliest signs of melanoma.
- Diameter: A lesion or nevus with a diameter of 6 mm or larger should be evaluated.
- Evolution: A mole or lesion that has changed in size, color, or appearance should be biopsied.

## RESOURCES FOR PATIENTS

- American Academy of Dermatology: www.aad.org
- American Cancer Society: www.cancer.org
- American Society for Dermatologic Surgery:www.asds.net
- Melanoma Patients' Information Page: www.mpip.org
- National Cancer Institute: www.cancer.gov
- National Comprehensive Cancer Network: www.nccn.org
- Skin Cancer Foundation: www.skincancer.org
- UV index information: www.epa.gov/sunwise/uvindex.html

# SQUAMOUS CELL CARCINOMA

## OVERVIEW

SCC is the second most common form of skin cancer (Figure III.51). Most cases of SCC of the skin are induced by UV radiation (James et al., 2006). In the United States, approximately 700,000 cases of SCC are diagnosed each year, resulting in almost 2,500 deaths (Skin Cancer Foundation, 2013).

## EPIDEMIOLOGY

SCCs are at least twice as frequent in men as women and rarely appear before age 50; they are most common in individuals in their 70s (Nolen et al., 2011; Skin Cancer Foundation, 2013). The majority of cutaneous SCC (70%) occurs on the head and neck, with an additional 15% found on the upper extremities. Tumors of sun-protected skin are more prevalent in Blacks and Hispanics. These tumors carry a higher mortality

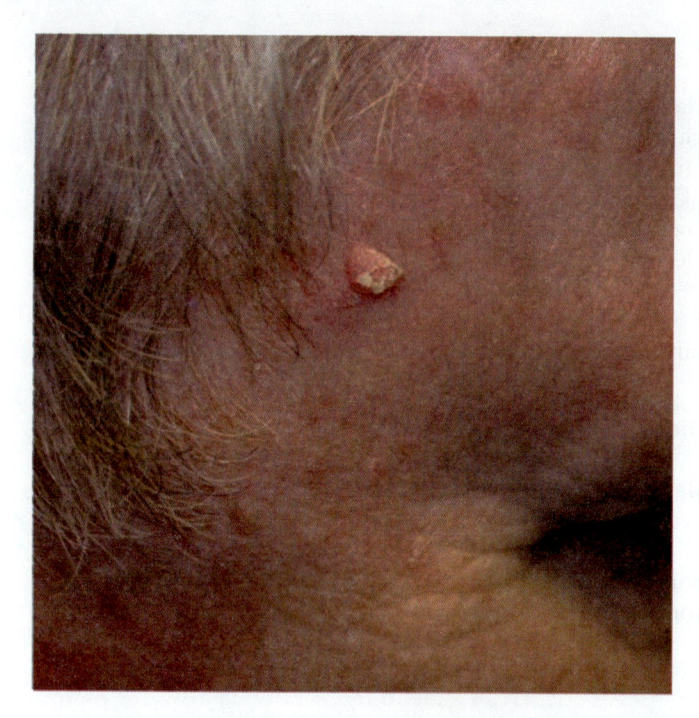

FIGURE III.51  Squamous cell carcinoma
Courtesy of Kelly Nelson, National Cancer Institute

risk, possibly resulting from delayed diagnosis. Bowen disease has a similar distribution, but this condition is also seen in subungual, periungual, palmar, genital, and perianal locations. Erythroplasia of Queyrat refers to Bowen disease on the glans penis (Khalyl-Mawad, 2011).

SCC represents 10% to 20% of cutaneous malignancies. Its incidence increases sharply with age, such that the occurrence rate of SCC for persons older than age 75 years is approximately tenfold greater than the overall incidence. SCCs are twice as frequent in men as in women and rarely appear before age 50 (Nolen et al., 2011). The prevalence of this condition varies inversely with geographic latitude and proportionally with skin fairness. In 1994 in the United States, the overall lifetime risk of developing SCC was 9% to 14% in men and 4% to 9% in women. The risk increases significantly in recipients of solid organ transplants (Khalyl-Mawad, 2011).

## PATHOLOGY/HISTOLOGY

Different pathologic classifications of SCC include (Khalyl-Mawad, 2011):

- *Bowen disease/SSC in situ* (SSCIS) is characterized by full-thickness epidermal replacement by crowded keratinocytes that demonstrate disordered dyspolarity, loss of maturation, and nuclear pleomorphism with hyperchromasia. The main feature distinguishing SCC from SSCIS is extension of malignant squamous epithelium in the dermis. Transgression of the basement membrane is easily identified in moderately or poorly differentiated cases, resulting in raggedy or angulated dermal protrusions that are associated with stromal reaction. However, in well-differentiated SCC, the neoplastic squamous epidermis advances in the dermis as broad, smooth-edged, keratinizing tongues that are difficult to accurately diagnose on superficial shave biopsies.

- *Verrucous carcinoma* (VC) is a slow-growing, low-grade, well-differentiated variant of SCC. This entity has a bland squamous cytology and a deceiving pattern of growth as bulbous, smooth-edged tongues pushing in the dermis without an associated stromal response (see Figure III.52). This neoplasm occurs in orolaryngeal mucosa (Ackerman tumor), anogenital areas (Buschke–Lowenstein tumor), plantar skin (epithelioma cuniculatum), and less commonly, other sites. In most locations, the association with various types of HPV is strong.
- *Warty SCC* typically occurs in anogenital locations and is distinguishable from VC by its higher grade morphology, including cytologic atypia and infiltrative growth pattern.
- *Spindle cell (sarcomatoid) carcinoma* is made up of spindle cells invading the dermis in a haphazardly arranged pattern. Evidence of keratinization is often absent. Differentiation of this entity from other cutaneous spindle cell neoplasms requires immunohistochemical profiling.
- *Keratoacanthoma* (KA) has a controversial status. Although stringent clinical, biologic, and cytogenetic criteria identify bona fide keratoacanthoma, many cases, including the metastatic keratoacanthoma represent well-differentiated SCC.

## CLINICAL PRESENTATION

SCC presents as a raised, firm, skin-colored or pink, often keratotic papule or plaque on a background of severely sun-damaged skin, with mottled pigmentary alteration, telangiectasia, and the presence of multiple actinic keratoses. SCC is typically slow growing, although some variants of SCC, such as the spindle cell type, enlarge rapidly. Bowen disease presents as a slow-growing, irregular, sharply circumscribed, erythematous, velvety or scaly plaque on sun-exposed or sun-protected skin (Khalyl-Mawad, 2011).

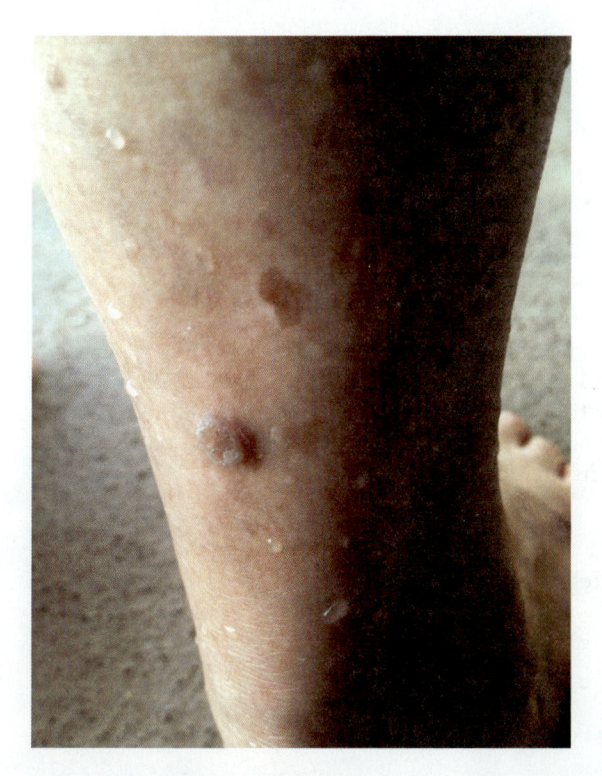

FIGURE III.52   Verrucous carcinoma

Common causes of SCC include sunlight, susceptible phenotype, compromised immunity, environmental conditions, and disease (Urist & Soong, 2007). SCC develops from flat, scale-like skin cells called keratinocytes, which lie under the top layer of the epidermis. Most SCCs occur on sun-exposed areas, especially on the head and upper extremities. SCCs typically present as enlarging bumps that may have an irregular or reddened surface. The classic appearance is a skin depression with raised edges that is typically more indurated and inflamed than BCC and often crusts or oozes (Arora & Attwood, 2009). There are two main types of SCC (Nolen et al., 2011):

1. *SCC in situ* is the earliest form of SCC. The cancer has not invaded the surrounding tissue. Cancers will appear as large reddish patches that are scaly and crusted.
2. *Invasive SCC* is highly likely to spread (metastasize). The skin cancer lesions can grow rapidly over a few months. Eventually they become ulcerated, which can increase likelihood of the cancer spreading.

Patients who have had SCC have a twofold increase in their risk for developing bladder cancer, breast cancer in women, leukemia, lung cancer, melanoma, non-Hodgkin lymphoma, and testicular and prostate cancer in men. Patients should be followed at 3- to 6-month intervals because there is a 35% risk of developing a second SCC within 3 years and 50% risk within 5 years (Leber, Perron, & Sinni-McKeehen, 1999).

## DIFFERENTIAL DIAGNOSIS

The following are considered in the differential diagnosis of SCC and Bowen disease.

- Atypical fibroxanthoma
- Epithelioid angiosarcoma
- Keratoacanthoma
- Merkel cell carcinoma
- Metastatic hepatic carcinoma
- Paget disease
- Sebaceous carcinoma
- Spindle cell melanoma (Khalyl-Mawad, 2011)

## TREATMENT/MANAGEMENT

SCC that is found in the early stages of development and removed quickly is usually curable and does not cause significant damage. However, if not treated, SCCs will penetrate the underlying tissues and can become disfiguring, metastasize, and even become fatal. There are several effective ways to clear SCC, and the treatment choice is based on the type, size, location, and depth of the tumor, as well as the patient's age and general health. Treatment options include:

- Mohs micrographic surgery
- Excisional surgery
- Curettage and electrodesiccation (electrosurgery)
- Cryosurgery
- Radiation
- PDT
- Laser surgery
- Topical medications (Skin Cancer Foundation, 2013)

## SPECIAL CONSIDERATIONS

Genetic disorders, including xeroderma pigmentosum and albinism, are associated with increased risk for many types of skin cancer. A history of chronic conditions of the skin such as burn scars (Marjolin ulcer), draining sinuses, infections, and ulcers often are associated with development of SCCs (Urist & Soong, 2007). More than two thirds of all SCCs that occur in African Americans are in preexisting inflammatory conditions (hidradenitis suppurativa, cutaneous lupus), burn injuries, or trauma, and these lesions are usually more aggressive (Leber et al., 1999).

Compared with BCC, SCC has overall significantly higher risks of metastasis (2%–6%) and tumor death (Khalyl-Mawad, 2011). The rate of SCC metastasis from all skin sites ranges from 0.5% to 5.2%. Careful attention should be paid to regional lymph nodes draining the site of the SCC. Risk factors for local recurrence and metastasis include:

- Treatment with a modality that does not check the margins of the specimen (such as curettage and desiccation, cryotherapy, or radiation)
- Recurrence after previous treatment
- Certain locations (temples, scalp, ear, or lip areas have a higher percentage of recurrence)
- Larger lesions (>2 cm in diameter)
- Skin lesions deeper than 4 mm and lip lesions deeper than 8 mm
- Histologic differentiation
- Histologic evidence of perineural invasion
- Histologic evidence of desmoplastic features
- Precipitating factors other than UV light
- Immunosuppression (James et al., 2006)

## WHEN TO REFER

Treatment options for the patient with advanced SCC tumors should be evaluated jointly with a surgeon, dermatologist, and radiotherapist (Baded, 2013).

## PATIENT EDUCATION

Baded (2013) suggests:

- Instruct patients to avoid possible risk factors (e.g., sun exposure, ionizing radiation, arsenic ingestion, tanning beds). Recommend sun-protective clothing and glasses when outdoors.
- If surgery is warranted, explain the procedure and the extent of surgery that is required.
- Teach self-skin examinations and the signs of skin cancer to look for.
- Follow the American Cancer Society's recommendations and advise a dermatologic examination every 3 years for people in the second to fourth decades of life and every year for people after the fourth decade of life.

## REFERENCES

Amari, W., Zeringue, A. L., McDonald, J. R., Caplan, L., Eisen, S. A., & Ranganathan, P. (2011). Risk of non-melanoma skin cancer in a national cohort of veterans with rheumatoid arthritis. *Rheumatology, 50,* 1431–1439.

Armstrong, A. W., Liu, V., & Mihm, M. C. (2013). *Pathologic characteristics of melanoma*. Retrieved from http://www.uptodate.com/contents/pathologic-characteristics-of-melanoma

Arora, A., & Attwood, J. (2009). Common skin cancers and their precursors. *Surgical Clinics of North America, 89*, 703–712.

Baded, R. S. (2013, March 11). *Basal cell carcinoma*. Retrieved from http://emedicine.medscape.com/article/276624-overview#aw2aab6b2b2

Berman, B., Bienstock, L., Kuritzky, L., Mayeaux, E. J., Jr., & Tyring, S. K. (2006). Actinic keratosis: Sequelae and treatments. Recommendations from a consensus panel. *Journal of Family Practice, 55*(Suppl.), 1–8.

Berwick, M., Erdei, E., & Hay, J. (2009). Melanoma epidemiology and public health. *Dermatology Clinics, 27*, 205–214.

Brodsky, J. (2009). Management of benign skin lesions commonly affecting the face: Actinic keratosis, seborrheic keratosis, and rosacea. *Current Opinion in Otolaryngology & Head and Neck Surgery, 17*, 315–320.

Buzaid, A. C., & Gershenwald, J. E. (2013). *Staging work-up and surveillance after treatment of melanoma*. Retrieved from http://www.uptodate.com/contents/staging-work-up-and-surveillance-after-treatment-of-melanoma

Chapman, P. B. (2011). How Zelboraf (vemurafenib), a new FDA-approved therapy, extends life for patients with metastatic melanoma. *Melanoma Letter. A Publication of the Skin Care Foundation, 29*(2), 5.

Chartier, T. K., & Aasi, S. Z. (2011). *Treatment and prognosis of basal cell carcinoma*. Retrieved from http://www.uptodate.com/content/treatment-and-prognosis-of-basel-cell-carcinoma

Chiarello, S. E. (2000). Cryopeeling (extensive cryosurgery) for treatment of actinic keratosis: An update and comparison. *Dermatologic Surgery, 26*(8), 728–732.

Cockerell, C. J., & Wharton, J. R. (2005). New histopathological classification of actinic keratosis (incipient intraepidermal squamous cell carcinoma). *Journal of Drugs in Dermatology, 4*(4), 462–467.

Doben, A. R., & MacGillivray, D. C. (2009). Current concepts in cutaneous melanoma: Malignant melanoma. *Surgical Clinics of North America, 89*, 713–725.

Engel, A., Johnson, M. L., & Haynes, S. G. (1988). Health effects of sunlight exposure in the United States. Results from the first National Health and Nutrition Examination Survey, 1971–1974. *Archives of Dermatology, 124*, 124–172.

Engkilde, K., Thyssen, J. P., Menne, T., & Johansen, J. D. (2011). Association between cancer and contact allergy: A linkage study. *BMJ Open, 1*, 1–5.

Englert, C., & Hughes, B. (2012). A review of actinic keratosis for the nurse practitioner: Diagnosis, treatment, and clinical pearls. *Journal of the American Academy of Nurse Practitioners, 24*, 290–296.

Fitzpatrick, J. E., & Morelli, J. G. (2011). *Dermatology secrets plus* (4th ed.). Philadelphia, PA: Elsevier/Saunders.

Gao, X., Simon, K. C., Han, J., Schwarzchild, M. A., & Ascherio, A. (2009). Family history of melanoma and Parkinson disease risk. *Neurology, 73*, 1286–1291.

Gemmill, J. A. (2010). Cancers, infections, and endocrine disease in women with endometriosis. *Fertility and Sterility, 94*(5), 1627–1631.

Habif, T. P. (2004). *A color guide to diagnosis and therapy: Clinical dermatology* (4th ed.). Philadelphia, PA: Elsevier/Mosby.

Habif, T. (2010). *Clinical dermatology: A color guide to diagnosis and therapy.* (5th ed.). China: Mosby.

Habif, T., Campbell, J., Chapman, M., Dinulos, J., & Zug, K. (2011). *Skin disease diagnosis and treatment* (3rd ed.). Philadelphia, PA: Elsevier, Saunders.

Hawryluk, E. B., & Fisher, D. E. (2011). Melanoma epidemiology, risk factors, and clinical phenotypes. In A. W. Armstrong (Ed.), *Advances in malignant melanoma-clinical and research perspectives* (pp. 3–28). Retrieved from http://www.intechopen.com/articles/show/title/melanoma-epidemiology-risk-factors-and-clinical-phenotypes

Herr, M. W. (2011, August 18). *Skin cancer—Melanoma*. Retrieved from http://emedicine.medscape.com/article/846566-overview

James, W. D., Berger, T. G., & Elston, D. M. (2006). *Andrews' diseases of the skin: Clinical dermatology* (10th ed.). Philadelphia, PA: Saunders/Elsevier.

Khalyl-Mawad, J. (2011, April 7). *Pathology of squamous cell carcinoma and Bowen disease*. Retrieved from http://emedicine.medscape.com/article/1960631-overview

Leber, K., Perron, V. D., & Sinni-McKeehen, B. (1999). Common skin cancers in the United States: A practical guide for diagnosis and treatment. *Nurse Practitioner Forum, 10*(2), 106–112.

Little, E. G., & Eide, M. J. (2012). Update on the current state of melanoma incidence. *Dermatology Clinics, 30,* 355–361.

Liu, R., Gao, X., Lu, Y., & Chen, H. (2011). Meta-analysis of the relationship between Parkinson's disease and melanoma. *Neurology, 76,* 2002–2009.

Marrot, L., & Meunier, J. R. (2008). Skin DNA photodamage and its biological consequences. *Journal of the American Academy of Dermatology, 58*(5, Suppl. 2), S139–S148.

MD Consult. (2010). *Melanoma and other skin cancers: Patient education.* Retrieved from http://www.mdconsult.com

Nolen, M. E., Beebe, V. R., King, J. M., Bryn, N., & Limaye, K. M. (2011). Nonmelanoma skin cancer part 1. *Journal of the Dermatology Nurses' Association, 3*(5), 260–283.

Padilla, R. S. (2012). *Epidemiology, natural history, and diagnosis of actinic keratosis.* Retrieved from http://www.uptodate.com/contents/epidemiology-natural-history-and-diagnosis-of-actinic-keratosis

Russak, J. E., & Rigel, D. S. (2012). Risk factors for the development of primary cutaneous melanoma. *Dermatology Clinics, 30,* 363–368.

Schwartz, R. A., Bridges, T. M., Butani, A. K., & Ehrlich, A. (2008). Actinic keratosis: An occupational and environmental disorder. *Journal of the European Academy of Dermatology Venereology, 22*(5), 606–615.

Skin Cancer Foundation. (2011). *Skin cancer facts.* Retrieved from http://www.skincancer.org/skin-cancer-facts

Skin Cancer Foundation. (2013). *Squamous cell carcinoma.* Retrieved from http://www.skincancer.org/skin-cancer-information/squamous-cell-carcinoma-(SCC)

Springer, L., & McClary, L. G. (2013). Early diagnosis of malignant melanoma. *Clinical Advisor, 16*(8), 36–46.

Swetter, S., & Geller, A. (2013). *Skin examination and clinical features of melanoma.* Retrieved from http://www.uptodate.com/contents/skin-examination-and-clinical-features-of melanoma

Tan, W. W. (2013, June 10). *Malignant melanoma.* Retrieved from http://emedicine.medscape.com/article/280245-overview

Tucker, M. A. (2009). Melanoma epidemiology. *Hematology/Oncology Clinics of North America, 23,* 383–395.

Urist, M. M., & Soong, S. (2007). Melanoma and cutaneous malignancies. In C. Townsend, D. Beauchamp, M. Evers, & K. Mattox (Eds.), *Sabiston textbook of surgery* (18th ed., pp. 767–785). Philadelphia, PA: Saunders.

# Tinea Infections

## TINEA CAPITIS

### OVERVIEW

*Tinea capitis* is a skin disorder that is the result of a fungal infection of the scalp, eyebrows, and eyelashes, with a propensity for infecting hair shafts and follicles. Children are most often affected with tinea capitis, and adults who are diagnosed with tinea capitis are frequently misdiagnosed and instead have seborrheic dermatitis or another inflammatory disease (Goldstein & Goldstein, 2013; Kao, 2013).

### EPIDEMIOLOGY

In the United States, the exact occurrence of the disease is no longer reported to public health agencies because of the frequency of the disease. Black male children have a higher incidence of tinea capitis, with 92.5% of all children younger than 10 years affected (Kao, 2013).

Tinea capitis is prevalent in some urban areas, particularly in children of Afro-Caribbean origin. In Southeast Asia, the occurrence has decreased in the past 50 years (from 14% to 1.2%) because of improved sanitary conditions and personal hygiene. In the United Kingdom and North America, *Trichophyton tonsurans* is responsible for more than 90% of cases of tinea capitis. In the nonurban communities, random infections (< 10%) acquired from small pets are caused by *Microsporum canis*, and in rural areas occasional infection (e.g., *Trichophyton verrucosum* from cattle) occurs (Kao, 2013).

The gender prevalence of tinea capitis depends on the causative fungal organism. *Microsporum audouinii* is more common in boys than in girls. However, after puberty, girls are affected more than boys. *M. canis* is usually higher in boys. *Trichophyton* infections on the scalp occur equally in boys and girls, but as adults, women are infected more frequently than men (James, Berger, & Elston, 2006; Kao, 2013).

### PATHOLOGY/HISTOLOGY

*Dermatophytes*, pathogenic fungi that grow on skin, are one of the most common infectious agents occurring in humans, causing various clinical disorders that are together termed *dermatophytosis*. At the site of the primary infection, the fungal hyphae grow into the stratum corneum. The fungus continues downward growth into the hair and infesting keratin. As the hair grows, the area of involvement extends upward (approximately 2 weeks), and it is visible above the skin surface. By the third week, the hair is brittle, and broken hairs are evident (Kao, 2013).

Three types of hair penetration are observed.

1. Ectothrix (gray-patch tinea capitis) infection is represented by the growth of arthroconidia on the surface of the hair shaft. The cuticle of the hair is damaged, and affected hairs will appear bright greenish yellow in color when fluoresced under a Wood's light ultraviolet light. Frequent causes include *M. canis*, *Microsporum gypseum*, *Trichophyton equinum*, and *T. verrucosum*.
2. Endothrix (black dot tinea capitis) is the most common form of tinea capitis in the United States. Endothrix hair infection is characterized by the growth of arthroconidia within the hair shaft. The cuticle of the hair remains intact, and the affected hair does not fluoresce under a Wood's ultraviolet light. In endothrix infection, spherical to box-like spores are found within the hair shaft. This particular infection is caused by *T. tonsurans* or *Trichophyton violaceum*.
3. Favus (tinea favosa) is caused by *Trichophyton schoenleinii* and generates favus-like crusts or scutula and resultant hair loss. (Goldstein & Goldstein, 2013; James et al., 2006; Kao, 2013)

## CLINICAL PRESENTATION

Various clinical findings of tinea capitis are recognized as being inflammatory or noninflammatory, and patchy alopecia may be present. Infection with inflammatory variants may have regional lymphadenopathy present. Relevant physical presentations are limited to the skin of scalp, eyebrows, and eyelashes. Principal skin lesions of tinea capitis present with the following:

- Lesions begin as red papules with progression to pale gray, ring-formed patches with perifollicular papules.
- Pustules have inflamed crusts, exudate, matted infected hairs, and debris.
- Black dot tinea capitis causes breakage of the hair and resultant infected dark stubs visible in the follicular orifices.
- Kerion celsi may result in asporadic distribution and severe hair loss with scarring alopecia.
- Dermatophyte idiosyncratic or id reactions are symptoms of the immune response to dermatophytosis. Id reactions do not occur at the infected site, and the lesions do not contain organisms. Id reactions may be caused by treatments with antifungal medications. The most common type of id reaction is an acute vesicular dermatitis of the hands and feet. The grouped vesicles are firm, pruritic, and painful. Such reactions are observed in patients with inflammatory ringworm of the feet, caused by an infection by *Trichophyton mentagrophytes*, and similar presentations may occur on the trunk.
- Vesicular lesions may develop into a scaly eczematoid reaction or a follicular papulovesicular eruption.
- Other unusual types of id reactions include annular erythema and erythema nodosum. These patients have a strong delayed-type hypersensitivity reaction to intradermal trichophytin.
- Cervical lymphadenopathy may be present in patients with kerion formation as a result of severe inflammation. (Goldstein & Goldstein, 2013; James et al., 2006; Kao, 2013)

## DIFFERENTIAL DIAGNOSIS

- Alopecia areata
- Atopic dermatitis
- Drug eruptions
- Id reaction (autoeczematization)
- Impetigo
- Lupus erythematosus, subacute cutaneous
- Psoriasis, plaque
- Psoriasis, pustular
- Seborrheic dermatitis
- Syphilis
- Trichotillomania

## TREATMENT/MANAGEMENT

Conclusive diagnosis is dependent on an adequate specimen submitted for examination by direct microscopy and culture. Selected hair samples are cultured or allowed to soften in 10% to 20% potassium hydroxide before examination under the microscope. Choice of treatment depends on the type of fungus present, the severity of inflammation, and the health status of the patient. Treatment for tinea capitis includes the following (Goldstein & Goldstein, 2013; James et al., 2006; Kao, 2013):

- Griseofulvin is the treatment of choice in all ringworm infections of the scalp. Griseofulvin makes the affected hair and nails resistant to infection by fungal organisms. Treatment is required for 4 to 6 weeks, which is the amount of time needed for infected keratin to be replaced by resistant keratin. In inflammatory tinea capitis, wet compresses are needed to aid in the removal of pus and infected scale. Treatment progress is evaluated by routine examinations with the Wood's lamp to check for fluorescent species such as *M. audouinii* and *M. canis*. Griseofulvin side effects include nausea and rashes. The drug is not used in pregnancy, and it is recommended that men do not father a child for 6 months after treatment. Griseofulvin treatment schedules for children are 20 to 25 mg/kg/d (microsize formulation) for 6 to 12 weeks or 10 to 15 mg/kg/d (ultramicrosize formulation) for 6 to 12 weeks.
- Itraconazole has been associated with heart failure; therefore, it is currently not recommended as a first-line therapy for tinea. However, for serious *M. canis* infections, itraconazole may be used because *M. canis* is resistant to terbinafine. Treatment doses for children are 3 to 5 mg/kg/d for 4 to 6 weeks or pulse therapy with itraconazole capsules at doses of 5 mg/kg/d for 1 week each month for 2 to 3 months.
- Terbinafine tablets at doses of 3 to 6 mg/kg/d for approximately 2 to 4 weeks have shown efficacy in *T. tonsurans* infections. Treatment is usually given for 2 to 4 weeks, and dosage is determined by body weight.
  - 10–20 kg: 62.5 mg/d
  - 20–40 kg: 125 mg/d
  - Greater than 40 kg: 250 mg/d
- Fluconazole tablets or oral suspension at 3 to 6 mg/kg/d is given for 6 weeks.
- Oral ketoconazole is also an acceptable alternative to griseofulvin; however, it is expensive, and liver enzymes need to be monitored. This is used to treat deep follicular infections seen with Majocchi granuloma.

- Oral steroids may be used for the treatment of kerion to prevent permanent alopecia. Topical steroids should be avoided during the treatment of dermatophyte infections.
- Shampoos containing povidone-iodine are more effective than those containing econazole and selenium sulfide. Shampoo hair twice weekly for 15 minutes for 4 consecutive weeks.

## SPECIAL CONSIDERATIONS

Tinea capitis destroys hair and pilosebaceous structures, resulting in severe hair loss and scarring alopecia. This can be physically and mentally damaging to those who are affected. Children and adolescents with itchy scalp and hair loss are often ridiculed, isolated, and bullied by peers (Kao, 2013).

Tinea capitis with unusual presentations or failure to respond to treatment should alert providers to the possibility of an underlying immunologic problem (Goldstein & Goldstein, 2013).

## WHEN TO REFER

If kerion celsi is present, the patient should be referred to a dermatologist.

## PATIENT EDUCATION

- Schools with young children should be evaluated for tinea capitis infection to reduce transmission of the disease.
- People who are infected should not share their toys and personal care objects (e.g., combs or hairbrushes).
- Household contacts should be treated for tinea capitis (Goldstein & Goldstein, 2013; Kao, 2013)

### CLINICAL PEARLS

- Tinea capitis: ICD-9, 110.0; ICD-10, B35.0
- Family members should be instructed to use the antifungal shampoo three to four times weekly (Habif et al., 2011).
- Griseofulvin is absorbed more effectively with a fatty meal; children can be given ice cream or whole milk with this medication (Habif, 2011).
- Topical antifungal agents have limited value (Goodheart, 2011).

# TINEA CORPORIS

## OVERVIEW

*Tinea corporis* is a dermatophyte infection that occurs anywhere on the skin with the exception of the scalp, groin, palms, and soles (Figure III.53). There are three types of dermatophytoses: *Trichophyton*, *Microsporum*, and *Epidermophyton* (James et al., 2006; Lesher, 2012).

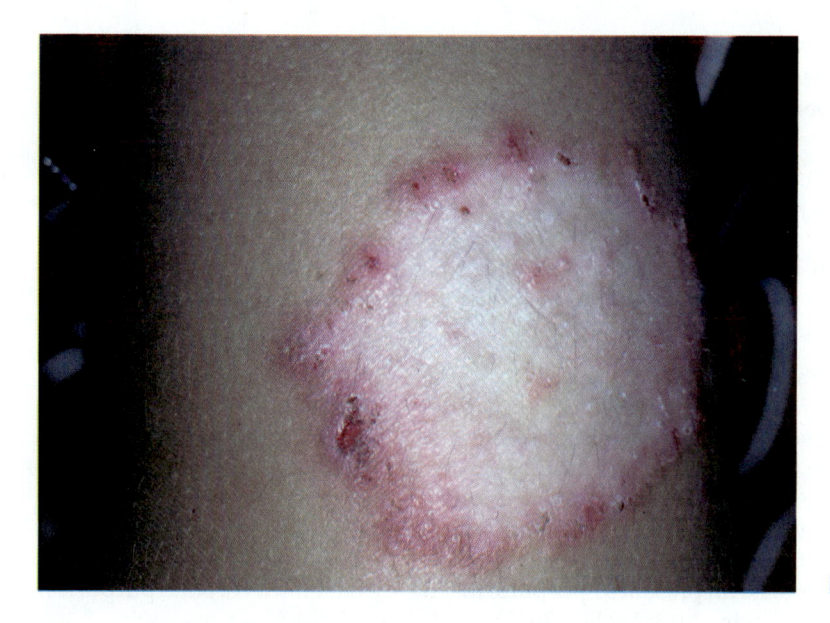

FIGURE III.53   Tinea corporis

## EPIDEMIOLOGY

Tinea corporis is not gender specific and occurs in all age groups, but prevalence is higher in children (Lesher, 2012).

## PATHOLOGY/HISTOLOGY

Tinea corporis can be caused by a variety of dermatophytes.

- Internationally, the most common cause is *Trichophyton rubrum.*
- *T. tonsurans, T. mentagrophytes, Trichophyton interdigitale, T. verrucosum, M. canis,* and *M. gypseum* are also sources of infection.
- Tinea imbricata is caused by *Trichophyton concentricum.*
- *T. verrucosum* is responsible for almost all the dermatophyte infections in cattle and is showing increased incidence of infection in humans who have contact with the infected cattle.
- *T. mentagrophytes* is spread by rabbits, guinea pigs, and small rodents.
- Infection with *M. gypseum*, a geophilic organism, can mimic tinea imbricata (Goldstein & Goldstein, 2013; Lesher, 2012)

Dermatophytes preferentially inhabit the dead, cornified layers of the skin, hair, and nail, because of the warm, moist environment that attracts fungal growth. Fungi typically do not invade deeply, but stay in the epidermis. This is caused by host defense mechanisms that may include the activation of serum inhibitory factor, complement, and polymorphonuclear leukocytes (Lesher, 2012).

One to three weeks after exposure, dermatophytes attack superficially in an annular pattern, which causes the active border to be raised and scaled. This creates a partial shield by shedding the infected skin and leaving new, healthy skin in the middle of the advancing lesion. Eradication of dermatophytes is accomplished by cell-mediated immunity. *T. rubrum* has a cell wall that is resistant to elimination. This defensive barrier contains mannan, which may block cell-mediated immunity, slow the proliferation of keratinocytes, and improve the organism's struggle to the skin's natural defenses (Lesher, 2012).

A skin biopsy of tinea corporis with a hematoxylin and eosin staining shows spongiosis, parakeratosis, and a superficial inflammatory infiltrate. A major diagnostic clue for tinea corporis is the presence of neutrophils in the stratum corneum (Lesher, 2012).

## CLINICAL PRESENTATION

Relevant clues in the history of a person with tinea corporis are symptoms, contact history, recent travel, and international residence. Infected patients may have variable symptoms.

- Patients can be asymptomatic.
- Patients may present with a pruritic, circular plaque. Occasionally one can experience a burning sensation. Inflammation, scale, crust, papules, vesicles, and even bullae can develop, especially in the advancing border.
- HIV-positive or immunocompromised patients may experience severe pruritus or pain and often will have atypical presentations, including deep abscesses or a disseminated skin infection.
- Rarely, tinea corporis can present as purpuric macules, called tinea corporis purpurica. (Goldstein & Goldstein, 2013; Lesher, 2012)

Tinea corporis may result from contact with infected humans, animals, or inanimate objects. The history may include occupational (e.g., farmworker, zookeeper, laboratory worker, veterinarian), environmental (e.g., gardening), or recreational (e.g., contact sports, contact with sports facilities) exposure.

Clinical variants of tinea corporis are:

- Majocchi granuloma, typically caused by *T. rubrum*, is a fungal infection in hair, hair follicles, and, often, the surrounding dermis, with an associated granulomatous reaction. Majocchi granuloma often occurs in females who shave their legs.
- Tinea corporis gladiatorum is a dermatophyte infection spread by skin-to-skin contact between wrestlers and is often seen on the head, neck, and arms.
- Tinea imbricata is a form of tinea corporis found mainly in Southeast Asia, the South Pacific, Central America, and South America. It is caused by *T. concentricum*. Tinea imbricata is recognized clinically by its distinct scaly plaques arranged in concentric rings.
- Tinea incognito is tinea corporis with an altered, nonclassic presentation caused by corticosteroid treatment.

## DIFFERENTIAL DIAGNOSIS

- Atopic dermatitis
- Candidiasis, cutaneous
- Erythema annulare centrifugum
- Erythema multiforme
- Erythrasma
- Granuloma annulare
- Granuloma faciale
- Impetigo
- Lupus erythematosus, subacute cutaneous
- Lymphocytic skin infiltration
- Nummular dermatitis

- Parapsoriasis
- Pityriasis rosea
- Psoriasis, annular
- Psoriasis, plaque
- Seborrheic dermatitis
- Syphilis
- Tinea versicolor

## TREATMENT/MANAGEMENT

Laboratory tests that aid in the diagnosis of tinea corporis are:

- A potassium hydroxide (KOH) examination of skin scrapings is used to diagnose tinea corporis. The skin sample should be taken from the scaled border of a lesion because this area contains the largest amount of fungal elements. A sample from a vesicular lesion should be taken from the roof of the vesicle. The KOH dissolves the keratin and leaves fungal components intact, revealing numerous septate, branching hyphae among epithelial cells.
- A fungal culture is more specific than KOH for detecting a dermatophyte infection; therefore, if the KOH result is negative, but clinical suspicion is high, a fungal culture should be obtained. (Goldstein & Goldstein, 2013; James et al., 2006; Lesher, 2012)

Treatment options include the following:

- The topical azoles (e.g., econazole, ketoconazole, clotrimazole, miconazole, oxiconazole, sulconazole, sertaconazole) inhibit the enzyme lanosterol 14-alpha-demethylase, a cytochrome P450-dependent enzyme that converts lanosterol to ergosterol. By blocking this enzyme, the fungal cell membranes are volatile, and this causes membrane leakage. The weakened dermatophyte is unable to reproduce and is slowly killed by the medication. Sertaconazole nitrate is one of the newest topical azoles. It has fungicidal and anti-inflammatory qualities and is used as a broad-spectrum agent.
- Allylamines (e.g., naftifine, terbinafine) and the related benzylamine butenafine inhibit squalene epoxidase, which converts squalene to ergosterol, are possible treatment agents. Blockage of this enzyme causes squalene, a substance toxic to fungal cells, to accumulate intracellularly and leads to rapid cell death. Allylamines bind effectively to the stratum corneum because of their lipophilic nature. They also penetrate deeply into hair follicles.
- Ciclopirox olamine is a topical fungicidal agent. It causes membrane volatility by collecting inside fungal cells and interfering with amino acid transport across the fungal cell membrane.
- A low to medium potency topical corticosteroid is used to provide rapid relief from the inflammatory component of the infection; however, this should only be applied for the first few days of treatment. Prolonged use of steroids can lead to persistent and recurrent infections, longer length of treatment regimens, and adverse effects of skin atrophy, striae, and telangiectasias.
- Systemic therapy may be indicated for tinea corporis in patients who have extensive skin infection, immunosuppression, resistance to topical antifungal therapy, and associated infections of tinea capitis or tinea unguium.
  - Griseofulvin at a dosage of 10 mg/kg/d for 4 weeks is effective. In addition, griseofulvin induces the cytochrome P450 enzyme system and can increase the metabolism of CYP450-dependent drugs. It is the systemic drug of choice for tinea corporis infections in children.

- Systemic azoles (e.g., fluconazole, itraconazole, ketoconazole) cause cell membrane destruction.
- Oral ketoconazole at 3 to 4 mg/kg/d may be given.
- Fluconazole at 50 to 100 mg/d or 150 mg once weekly for 2 to 4 weeks may be given.
- Oral itraconazole in doses of 100 mg/d for 2 weeks shows high efficacy. With an increased dose of 200 mg/d, the treatment duration can be reduced to 1 week. However, the cytochrome P450 activity of itraconazole allows for potential interactions with other commonly prescribed drugs.
- Oral terbinafine may be used at a dosage of 250 mg/d for 2 weeks; the potential exists for cytochrome P450, specifically CYP2D6, drug interactions with this agent. (Goldstein & Goldstein, 2013; James et al., 2006; Lesher, 2012)

## SPECIAL CONSIDERATIONS

Athletes with tinea corporis are generally not allowed to participate in matches or practice because of concerns about the spread of infection (Goldstein & Goldstein, 2013).

## WHEN TO REFER

Tinea corporis that is resistant to treatment should be referred to a dermatologist and/or an infectious disease specialist.

## PATIENT EDUCATION

- Stress the importance of preventing the spread of a dermatophyte infection by discouraging close contact between infected and noninfected individuals and the sharing of personal objects (e.g., towels, hats, clothing).
- Patients should not wear tight clothing and should choose fabrics that facilitate air flow to the skin. Also, completely dry the skin, especially skin folds, after bathing or swimming.

### CLINICAL PEARLS

- Tinea corporis: ICD-9, 110.9; ICD-10, B35.4
- It may be warranted to treat wrestlers throughout the season to prevent reinfection (Habif et al, 2011).
- Secondary, *Staphylococcus aureus* cutaneous infections do occur (Habif et al, 2011).

# TINEA FACIEI

## OVERVIEW

*Tinea faciei* is an exterior dermatophyte infection that occurs on areas of the face that lack hair. In children and women, the infection may appear on any surface of the face, to include the upper lip and chin. In men, if the infection occurs in the bearded areas it is known as *tinea barbae* (James et al., 2006; Szepietowski, 2012).

## EPIDEMIOLOGY

Tinea faciei occurs globally. However, as with other fungal skin infections, it occurs more frequently in tropical regions with high temperatures and humidity. Tinea faciei characterizes approximately 19% of all superficial fungal infections in children with dermatomycoses. Tinea faciei may appear in persons of any age; however, there are two common age occurrences: one involves children, and the other occurs in those aged 20 to 40 years (Szepietowski, 2012).

## PATHOLOGY/HISTOLOGY

Keratinophilic fungi are responsible for tinea faciei. Dermatophytes release multiple enzymes, including keratinases, which allow the fungus to invade the stratum corneum of the epidermis. Histologic examination may be useful for proving the diagnosis, but it is usually unnecessary. Its pattern is erratic, ranging from mild focal spongiosis to anchronic spongiotic psoriasi form dermatitis with a mixed dermal inflammatory infiltrate and fungi in the cornified layer. If using hematoxylin-eosin staining, cutaneous fungal elements will be present, but periodic acid–Schiff staining is recommended to aid visualization. Hyphae may be identified in the stratum corneum of the epidermis. Infections with *T. rubrum* or *T. verrucosum* may attack hairs and follicles. A mixed cellular inflammatory infiltrate is usually present in the papillary dermis, and neutrophils may extend into the horny layers above (James et al., 2006; Szepietowski, 2012).

## CLINICAL PRESENTATION

Tinea faciei of the face is frequently misdiagnosed. Typical annular rings are usually lacking, and the lesions are photosensitive. Frequently, the misdiagnosis of lupus erythematosus is made. Biopsies for direct immunofluorescence often demonstrate some reactants on sun-exposed skin, which also confuses the diagnosis (James et al., 2006).

The dermatophytes responsible for tinea faciei vary depending on geographic regions. Generally, animal reservoirs of zoophilic dermatophytes, especially *M. canis*, are global among pets and livestock. In Asia, *T. mentagrophytes* and *T. rubrum* are common. In contrast, in North America, *T. tonsurans* is the main isolated pathogen (James et al., 2006; Szepietowski, 2012).

Tinea faciei appears as annular or serpiginous erythematous scaled patches that have a border comprising papules, vesicles, and/or crusts. The cheeks are the most common area for occurrence, but the entire face can be affected. Some patients may have multiple lesions present in different areas of the face (James et al., 2006; Szepietowski, 2012).

## DIFFERENTIAL DIAGNOSIS

- Candidiasis, cutaneous
- Contact dermatitis, allergic
- Contact dermatitis, irritant
- Granuloma annulare
- Lupus erythematosus, acute
- Lupus erythematosus, bullous
- Lupus erythematosus, discoid
- Lupus erythematosus, drug induced

- Lupus erythematosus, subacute cutaneous
- Neonatal lupus erythematosus
- Perioral dermatitis
- Pityriasis alba
- Pityriasis rosea
- Rosacea
- Sarcoidosis
- Seborrheic dermatitis
- Syphilis

## TREATMENT/MANAGEMENT

Even in the best mycology laboratories, as many as 30% of culture results may be negative, particularly in chronic infections. Mycologic evaluation, which includes direct microscopic examination for hyphal elements and culturing, is vital in the diagnosis of tinea faciei. The surface scrapings should be obtained from the border of the lesions where the more severe inflammatory reaction occurs and where more fungal components are present (Szepietowski, 2012).

Scrapings are placed in 10% to 20% potassium hydroxide (KOH) solution, usually with the addition of dimethyl sulfoxide, which helps to dissolve background keratinocytes to enable visualization of the fungal elements. After drying the slide for a short period, the specimen is examined with a light microscope. Culturing allows the identification of the causative pathogen because the media changes from yellow to red with the growth of dermatophytes after a few days of incubation (James et al., 2006; Szepietowski, 2012).

Most cases of tinea faciei are treated successfully with topical antifungal agents. Fungal folliculitis may be present if a topical steroid has been used, and this requires systemic therapy. Topical treatment efficacy is dependent on the active ingredients within the preparation (James et al., 2006; Szepietowski, 2012). Topical ciclopirox and terbinafine also have anti-inflammatory properties, which are necessary for infections caused by zoophilic dermatophytes. If follicular papules are present, topical therapy will be insufficient. The two classes of antifungal medication used most frequently to treat tinea faciei are azoles and allylamines. Azoles block lanosterol 14-alpha-demethylase, an enzyme that changes lanosterol to ergosterol, a necessary component of the fungal cell wall. Membrane damage causes permeability problems and leaves the fungus unable to reproduce. Allylamines stop squalene epoxidase, an enzyme that changes squalene to ergosterol; this leads to the increase of toxic levels of squalene in the cell and then cell death. Reevaluation of the tinea diagnosis is important if clinical improvement is not observed after 4 weeks of therapy.

## SPECIAL CONSIDERATIONS

Tinea faciei causes facial lesions that can be embarrassing for patients. Children with tinea faciei can be ridiculed by peers for their appearance.

## WHEN TO REFER

Resistant cases of tinea faciei should be referred to a dermatologist.

## PATIENT EDUCATION

Patients should be taught that pets that are infected should be isolated and treated to prevent spread of dermatophytes.

### CLINICAL PEARLS

- Tinea faciei: ICD-9, 110.8; ICD-10, B35.0
- A positive bacterial culture of the lesion (usually staphylococcus) does not rule out tinea (Habif et al., 2011).

# TINEA PEDIS

## OVERVIEW

*Tinea pedis* refers to a dermatophyte infection on the soles of the feet and between the toes. This infection is the most common dermatophyte encountered in practice. Tinea pedis occurs when arthrospores shed from infected individuals on the floors of locker rooms, bathrooms, and swimming pools. The dermatophyte responsible for the infection is *T. rubrum* (Goldstein & Goldstein, 2013; Robbins, 2012).

## EPIDEMIOLOGY

Tinea pedis is the world's most common dermatophytosis, with 70% of the population becoming infected with tinea pedis at some point in their lifetime. Tinea pedis does not have any age or racial predilection. Tinea pedis occurs in males more than females. Childhood infection is rare. The risk for tinea pedis increases with age, with most cases occuring after puberty (Robbins, 2012).

## PATHOLOGY/HISTOLOGY

The dermatophytes *T. rubrum*, *T. mentagrophytes*, and *Epidermophyton floccosum* most commonly cause tinea pedis. *T. rubrum* is the most common, and *T. tonsurans* has been implicated in children. Nondermatophyte etiologies include *Scytalidium dimidiatum*, *Scytalidium hyalinum*, and, rarely, *Candida* species (Goldstein & Goldstein, 2013; Robbins, 2012).

Dermatophyte fungi invade the superficial keratin of the skin by using enzymes called keratinases. The fungal cell walls contain mannans, which block the immunity response of the infected person and reduce keratinocyte proliferation; this results in a decreased rate of skin shedding, aiding in sustaining the infection (Robbins, 2012).

A skin biopsy and histopathologic study are usually not needed to confirm the diagnosis of tinea pedis. A periodic acid–Schiff or Gomori methenamine-silver stain is used to visualize fungal components within the stratum corneum. Inflammation or tinea pedis affecting toe web spaces can make visualization of fungal components difficult, especially if the infection is also complicated by a secondary bacterial infection. If neutrophils are present within the stratum corneum, a dermatophyte infection should be considered. In vesicular tinea pedis, spongiotic intraepidermal vesicles are present; in the chronic hyperkeratotic (moccasin) type, hyperkeratosis and epidermal acanthosis usually are present (Robbins, 2012).

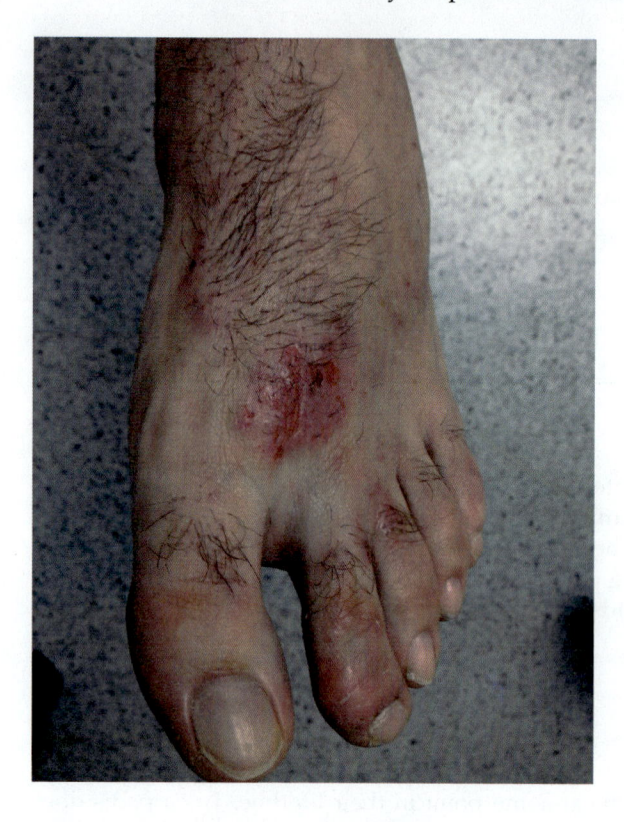

FIGURE III.54   Example of tinea pedis

## CLINICAL PRESENTATION

Commonly, patients who are infected with tinea pedis will describe pruritic, scaled feet with painful areas between the toes. Patients may have other associated dermatophyte infections, such as onychomycosis, tinea cruris, and tinea manuum. Tinea manuum is often unilateral and associated with moccasin-type tinea pedis (2-feet–1-hand syndrome). Typically, there are four types of clinical presentations of tinea pedis (Crawford, 2008; Goldstein & Goldstein, 2013; Robbins, 2012).

1. The interdigital type of tinea pedis is most often caused by *T. rubrum*. Other possible causative organisms in tinea pedis include *T. mentagrophytes* var. *interdigitale* and *E. floccosum*. This type appears as erythema, maceration, fissuring, and scaling, most often seen between the fourth and fifth toes. This type is often accompanied by pruritus.
2. The chronic hyperkeratotic type of tinea pedis is usually caused by *T. rubrum*, and is often referred to as moccasin tinea pedis. Other possible causative organisms include *T. mentagrophytes* var. *interdigitale*, *E. floccosum*, and the nondermatophyte molds *S. hyalinum* and *S. dimidiatum*. This type is characterized by chronic plantar erythema with slight scaling to diffuse hyperkeratosis. This type can be asymptomatic or pruritic. Both feet are usually affected. Typically, the dorsal surface of the foot is clear, but, in severe cases, the condition may extend onto the sides of the foot.
3. Both the inflammatory/vesicular type of tinea pedis are most commonly caused by the zoophilic fungus *T. mentagrophytes* var. *mentagrophytes*. This type is painful, with pruritic vesicles or bullae in the instep or anterior plantar surface. The lesion often

contains either clear or purulent fluid that will rupture, leaving a scaled, erythematous area. Cellulitis, lymphangitis, and adenopathy may also be present.
4. The ulcerative type of tinea pedis is most commonly caused by the zoophilic fungus *T. mentagrophytes* var. *mentagrophytes*. This type is characterized by rapidly spreading vesiculopustular lesions, ulcers, and erosions, typically in the web spaces, and is often accompanied by a secondary bacterial infection. Cellulitis, lymphangitis, pyrexia, and malaise can accompany this infection. Immunocompromised and diabetic patients often will have the entire sole peeled off from this type of infection.

## DIFFERENTIAL DIAGNOSIS

- Candidiasis, cutaneous
- Contact dermatitis, allergic
- Dyshidrotic eczema
- Erythema multiforme
- Erythrasma
- Friction blisters
- Pityriasis rubra pilaris
- Psoriasis, plaque
- Psoriasis, pustular
- Syphilis

## TREATMENT/MANAGEMENT

Tinea pedis can be treated with topical or oral antifungals or a combination of both. Topical agents are used for 1 to 6 weeks, depending on manufacturers' recommendations. A patient with chronic hyperkeratotic (moccasin) tinea pedis should be instructed to apply medication to the bottoms and sides of his or her feet. For interdigital tinea pedis, even though symptoms may not be present, a patient should apply the topical agent to the interdigital areas and to the soles because of the likelihood of plantar-surface infection (Robbins, 2012).

Clotrimazole, miconazole, sulconazole, oxiconazole, ciclopirox, econazole, ketoconazole, naftifine, terbinafine, flutrimazole, bifonazole, and butenafine are all effective topical antifungal agents (James et al., 2006). Crawford (2008) noted that creams containing allylamines are the most effective. When there is moderate maceration between the toes, the application of cotton between the toes in the evening can aid in treatment. Soaking feet for 20 minutes two to three times per day in aluminum chloride 10% or Burrow's solution can also be beneficial if vesicles or maceration are present. If secondary bacterial infection is present, the use of Bactroban or Gentamicin ointment is effective. Keratolytic agents with salicylic acid, resorcinol, lactic acid, and urea are useful if hyperkeratosis is present (James et al., 2006; Goldstein & Goldstein; 2013).

If systemic therapy is needed, griseofulvin at a dosage of 500 to 1,000 mg/d is effective. Other effective options for adults include terbinafine at 250 mg/d for 1 to 2 weeks; itraconazole at 200 mg twice daily for 1 week; and fluconazole at 150 mg once a week for 2 to 6 weeks (Bell-Syer et al., 2009; James et al., 2006; Goldstein & Goldstein, 2013).

Pediatric dosing options include the following:

- Terbinafine: 10–20 kg, 62.5 mg daily; 20–40 kg, 125 mg daily; > 40 kg, 250 mg daily
- Itraconazole: 5 mg/kg daily
- Fluconazole: 6 mg/kg weekly
- Griseofulvin: 10–15 mg/kg daily or in divided doses (Goldstein & Goldstein, 2013)

## SPECIAL CONSIDERATIONS

Patients with extensive chronic hyperkeratotic or inflammatory/vesicular tinea pedis usually require oral therapy, as do patients with coexistent onychomycosis, diabetes, peripheral vascular disease, or immunocompromising disorders (Robbins, 2012).

## WHEN TO REFER

Resistant tinea pedis should be referred to a dermatologist. Other conditions can mimic tinea pedis, or the patient may have more than one diagnosis.

## PATIENT EDUCATION

According to Robbins (2012), patients should be made aware of the following:

- Wearing protective footwear in public areas can help decrease the chance of acquiring tinea infection.
- Hyperhidrosis is a risk factor for tinea pedis. Keeping feet dry will help prevent tinea pedis.
- It is important to launder clothing, bath towels, and sheets frequently because fungal organisms can be present on these items.
- Wearing nonocclusive shoes and cotton socks and adding a drying powder with antifungal action in the shoes may be helpful.
- Reinfection can occur if one is re-exposed to dermatophytes. Old shoes are often sources of reinfection and should be disposed of or treated with antifungal powders.

### CLINICAL PEARLS

- Tinea pedis: ICD-9, 110.4; ICD-10, B35.3
- The feet are the most commonly affected skin site for a tinea infection (Habif, 2010).
- If in doubt about the rash on the feet use a topical antifungal cream (Habif et al., 2011).
- Advise patients to put socks on before putting on underwear. If patients pull up their underwear over exposed feet with tinea pedis, they may infect the groin area with fungal organisms from the feet.
- After bathing, completely dry feet and toe web spaces. Apply topical antifungal medication and put cotton balls between the toes to prevent moisture buildup.

# TINEA VERSICOLOR

## OVERVIEW

*Tinea versicolor* is a common, benign, superficial cutaneous fungal infection usually characterized by hypopigmented or hyperpigmented macules and patches on the chest and the back (Figure III.55). Unlike other tinea infections, tinea versicolor is not a dermatophyte infection. The organism responsible for tinea versicolor is *Malassezia furfur*, a saprophytic, lipid-dependent yeast (Burkhart, 2012; Goldstein & Goldstein, 2012).

Tinea Infections 317

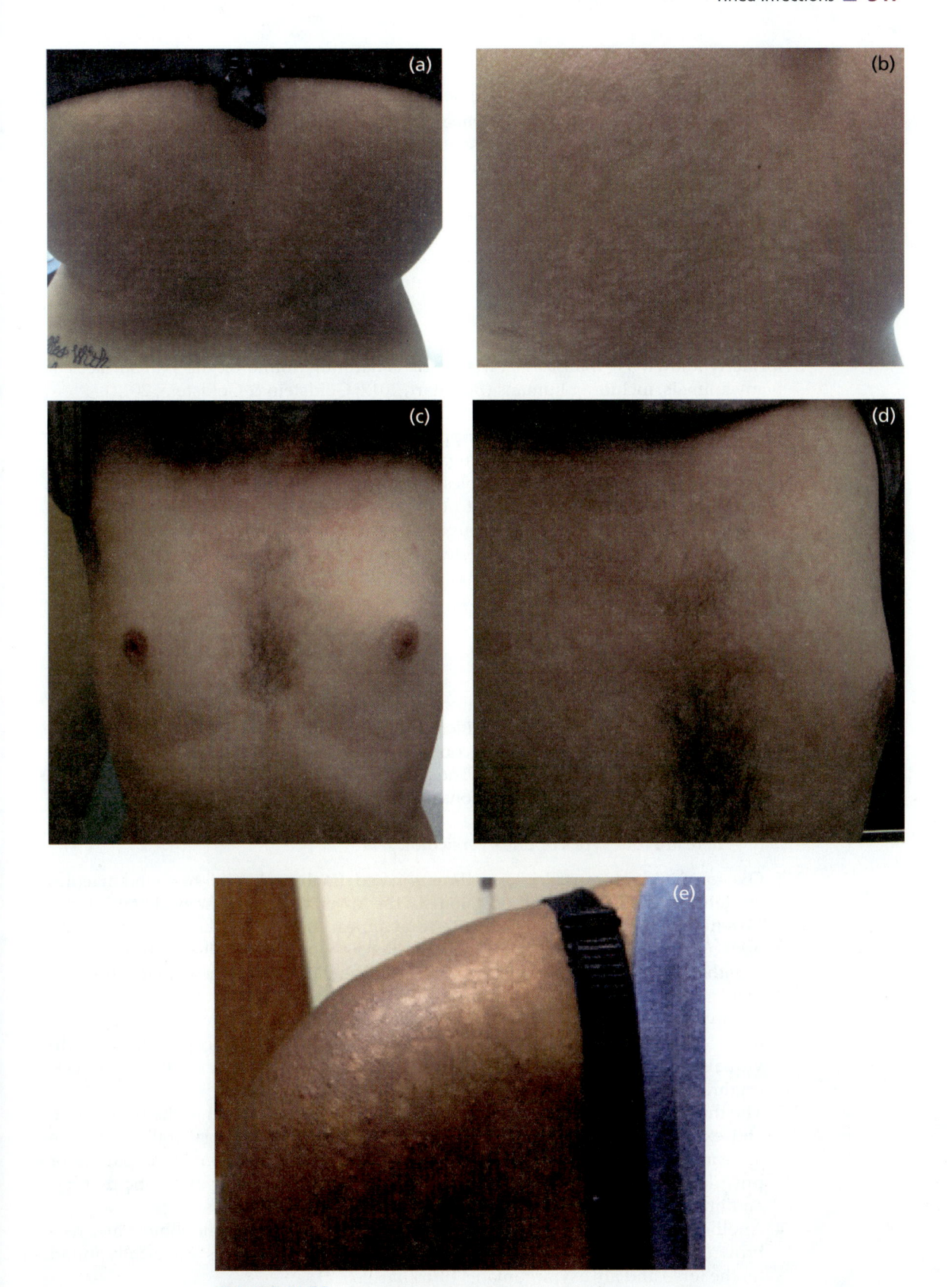

FIGURE III.55 (a–e) Examples of tinea versicolor

## EPIDEMIOLOGY

In the United States, tinea versicolor occurs more frequently in hot climates with high humidity. The national incidence of this condition is 2% to 8% of the population, although it is difficult to assess because those who are affected usually do not seek medical attention. The incidence of tinea versicolor is the same in all races and genders, it most commonly occurs in persons aged 15 to 24 years. This is attributed to the age when the sebaceous glands are most active. Tinea versicolor rarely affects individuals before puberty and the elderly aged 65 and older (Burkhart, 2012).

## PATHOLOGY/HISTOLOGY

Tinea versicolor is caused by the dimorphic, lipophilic organisms in the genus *Malassezia*, formerly known as *Pityrosporum*. *Malassezia* is naturally found on the skin surfaces of many animals, including humans (Burkhart, 2012; Goldstein & Goldstein, 2012).

The fungus is readily seen in skin scrapings of the lesions. Applying tape to the lesions and removing it (tape stripping) can also visualize the fungus. Under the microscope there are short, thick fungal hyphae and moderate numbers of various-sized spores. The appearance resembles "spaghetti and meatballs" (James et al., 2006).

*M. furfur* is usually localized to the stratum corneum and can be revealed by hematoxylin and eosin alone, although periodic acid–Schiff or methenamine-silver staining are more conclusive. The epidermis reveals mild hyperkeratosis and acanthosis, and a mild perivascular infiltrate is present in the dermis (Burkhart, 2012).

## CLINICAL PRESENTATION

Most individuals with tinea versicolor seek medical attention because of the abnormal pigmentation on their bodies. The affected skin areas are usually the trunk, the back, the abdomen, and the upper extremities. The face, the scalp, and the genitalia are not usually affected. The color of each lesion varies from off-white to a reddish brown, and a thin, mild scale covers the lesions. The lesions will not tan in the summer, and some patients report pruritus with the lesions (Burkhart, 2012; Goldstein & Goldstein, 2012; James et al., 2006).

There are four types of tinea versicolor.

1. One form presents as multiple, well-marginated, finely scaly, oval-to-round macules scattered over the trunk and occasionally the lower abdomen, the neck, and upper extremities. The macules tend to merge and appear as irregular shaped patches with various pigmentation changes. The condition is more visible during the summer months because of tanning. Light scraping of the lesion with a scalpel blade will yield a moderate amount of keratin.
2. An inverse form of tinea versicolor also exists that affects the flexural areas, the face, or isolated areas of the extremities and is often seen in immunocompromised individuals. This type can be mistaken for candidiasis, seborrheic dermatitis, psoriasis, erythrasma, and dermatophyte infections.
3. The third type involves the hair follicle and is typically localized to the back, chest, and extremities. This type is hard to differentiate from bacterial folliculitis. The appearance of *Pityrosporum* folliculitis is a perifollicular, erythematous papule or pustule. Risk factors include diabetes, high humidity, steroid or antibiotic therapy, and immunosuppressant therapy.
4. Another clinical presentation is multiple, firm, 2- to 3-mm, monomorphic, red-brown, inflammatory papules, with or without scale. The lesions are usually found on the torso and are asymptomatic. (Burkhart, 2012)

## DIFFERENTIAL DIAGNOSIS

- Erythrasma
- Mycosis fungoides
- Pityriasis alba
- Pityriasis rosea
- Psoriasis, guttate
- Seborrheic dermatitis
- Secondary syphilis
- Tinea corporis
- Vitiligo

## TREATMENT/MANAGEMENT

The reason *M. furfur* causes tinea versicolor in some individuals and not others remains a mystery. A person's nutritional health and immune response play an important role in prevention. The organism is lipophilic, and lipids are essential for growth. Oily skin, especially during puberty, creates a sebum-rich area for the organism to grow (Burkhart, 2012).

The clinical appearance of tinea versicolor is unique, and the diagnosis is often made without any laboratory studies. The ultraviolet black (Wood's) light can be used to reveal the yellow-green fluorescence of tinea versicolor, although sometimes the lesions appear darker than the unaffected skin and do not fluoresce (Burkhart, 2012; James et al., 2006).

Treatment is as follows.

- Topical antifungals: The shampoo form of ketoconazole has been studied for the treatment of tinea versicolor and appears to be effective with a relatively short duration of therapy. The shampoo is applied to affected areas and washed off after 5 minutes. Treatment with other topical antifungals can be successful. Topical terbinafine applied twice daily for 1 week and topical ciclopirox olamine both have shown efficacy. Selenium sulfide 2.5% lotion is often prescribed twice daily without rinsing. Other agents used are zinc pyrithione, propylene glycol, sulfur with salicylic acid, benzoyl peroxide, and Whitfield's ointment.
- Systemic therapy: Oral azole antifungals such as ketoconazole, itraconazole, and fluconazole are effective. Terbinafine and griseofulvin are not effective for tinea versicolor. Oral antifungals are typically reserved for patients with recalcitrant tinea versicolor or widespread disease that make application of topical medication difficult. Liver enzymes need to be monitored with azole medications. The following doses are appropriate for tinea versicolor: ketoconazole 200 mg daily for 5 days, itraconazole 200 mg daily for 7 days, fluconazole 300 mg once weekly for 2 weeks. (Goldstein & Goldstein, 2012; James et al., 2006)

## SPECIAL CONSIDERATIONS

Individuals who are immunocompromised or those with organ transplants are at greater risk for *Pityrosporum* folliculitis. These patients require systemic treatment with oral antifungal medications.

## WHEN TO REFER

Tinea versicolor often recurs, and prophylactic treatment with a topical or oral agent is usually needed. For resistant tinea pedis, consider dermatology referral.

## PATIENT EDUCATION

Explain to patients that tinea versicolor is caused by a natural fungus on the skin's surface and is not contagious. Pigmentation changes may take 1 to 2 months to resolve after treatment is started (Burkhart, 2012).

Patients who experience frequent recurrence of tinea versicolor (especially immunocompromised patients) can prevent recurrences with the use of topical or oral preventative therapy, particularly in warm weather. Topical selenium sulfide 2.5% or ketoconazole 2% shampoo applied to the entire body for 10 minutes once per month is effective therapy (Goldstein & Goldstein, 2012).

## CLINICAL PEARLS

- Tinea versicolor: ICD-9, 111.0; ICD-10, B36.0
- Tinea versicolor presents as hyper- or hypopigmented scaley lesions on the chest and back that are frequently exacerbated by heat and humidity (Fitzpatrick & Morelli, 2011).
- Tinea versicolor, also known as pityriasis versicolor, should be re-treated with topical anti-fungal cream or shampoo 1 week before the next exposure to a warm climate (Goodheart, 2011).

## REFERENCES

Bell-Syer, S., Hart, R., Crawford, F., Torgerson, D. J., Tyrell, W., & Russell, I. (2009). Oral treatments for fungal infections of the skin of the foot. Retrieved from the *Cochrane Database of Systemic Reviews, 10,* CD003584.

Burkhart, C. G. (2012, September 18). *Tinea versicolor.* Retrieved from http://emedicine.medscape.com/article/1091575-overview

Crawford, F. (2008). Athlete's foot. In H. Williams, M. Bigby, T. Diepgen, A. Herxeimer, L. Naldi, & B. Rzany (Eds.), *Evidence-based dermatology* (2nd ed., pp. 358–361). Malden, MA: Blackwell.

Goldstein, B. G., & Goldstein, A. O. (2012). *Tinea versicolor.* Retrieved from http://uptodate.com/contents/tinea-versicolor

Goldstein, A. O., & Goldstein, B. G. (2013). *Dermatophyte (tinea) infections.* Retrieved from http://www.uptodate.com/dermatophyte-tinea-infections

Goodheart, H. (2011). *Goodheart's same-site differential diagnosis: A rapid method of diagnosing and treating common skin disorders.* Philadelphia, PA: Lippincott Williams & Wilkins.

Habif, T. (2010). *Clinical dermatology: A color guide to diagnosis and therapy* (5th ed.). China: Mosby.

Habif, T., Campbell, J., Chapman, M., Dinulos, J., & Zug, K. (2011). *Skin disease diagnosis and treatment* (3rd ed.). Philadelphia, PA: Elsevier, Saunders.

James, W. D., Berger, T. G., & Elston, D. M. (2006). *Andrews' diseases of the skin: Clinical dermatology* (10th ed.). Philadelphia, PA: Elsevier/Saunders.

Kao, G. F. (2013, May 14). *Tinea capitis.* Retrieved from http://emedicine.medscape.com/article/1091351-overview

Lesher, J. L. (2012, January 24). *Tinea corporis.* Retrieved from http://emedicine.medscape.com/article/1091473-overview

Robbins, C. M. (2012, January 24). *Tinea pedis.* Retrieved from http://emedicine.medscape.com/article/1091084-overview

Szepietowski, J. C. (2012, January 25). *Tinea faciei.* Retrieved from http://emedicine.medscape.com/article/1118316-overview

# Urticaria

## OVERVIEW

Urticaria is the most frequent dermatologic disorder seen in urgent care centers and emergency departments; approximately 20% of people are affected at some point in their life (Bingham, 2013; Linscott, 2013). Chronic urticaria is a persistent condition characterized by red, pruritic, raised wheals that come and go for more than 6 weeks, whereas acute urticaria appears and is usually resolved within 24 hours (Figure III.56) (Stanway, Cohen, Chen, Hauser, & Binney, 2009).

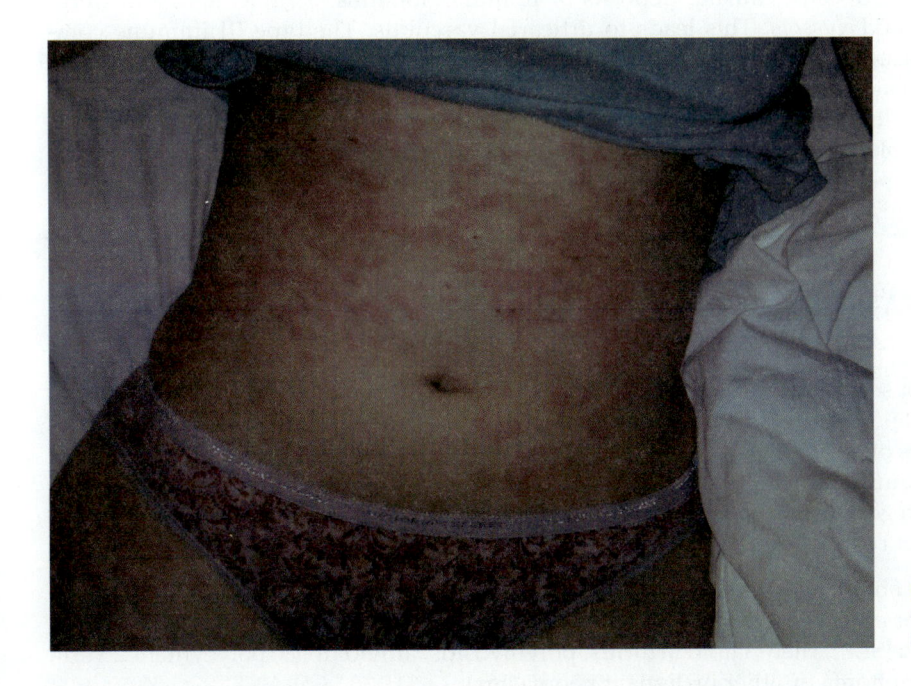

**FIGURE III.56** Urticaria
Courtesy of Heather Richardson, FNP

## EPIDEMIOLOGY

In the United States and internationally, acute urticaria affects 15% to 20% of the general population at some time during their lifetime (Peroni, Colato, Schena, & Girolomoni, 2010). Acute urticaria is usually self-limited and commonly resolves within 24 hours but may last up to 6 weeks. Chronic urticaria lasts more than 6 weeks and affects 0.5% to 3% of the general population (Peroni et al., 2010; Stanway et al., 2009). There is no racial preference noted, and incidence rates for acute urticaria are similar for men and women. Chronic urticaria, however, occurs more frequently in women (60%). Urticaria can occur in any age group, although chronic urticaria is more common in the fourth and fifth decades (Linscott, 2013; Peroni et al., 2010; Saini, 2013).

## PATHOLOGY/HISTOLOGY

Urticaria is the result of the release of histamine, bradykinin, leukotriene C4, prostaglandin $D_2$, and other vasoactive materials from mast cells and basophils in the dermis. This causes leakage of fluid into the dermis, and the result is an urticarial lesion. The severe itching of urticaria is a result of histamine released into the dermis. Histamine is the ligand for two membrane-bound receptors, the $H_1$ and $H_2$ receptors, which are present on many cell types. The activation of the $H_1$ histamine receptors on endothelial and smooth muscle cells leads to increased capillary permeability. The activation of the $H_2$ histamine receptors leads to arteriolar and venule vasodilation (Linscott, 2013).

The urticarial process is caused by several mechanisms. The type I allergic immunoglobulin E (IgE) response is initiated by antigen-mediated IgE immune complexes that bind and cross-link Fc receptors on the surface of mast cells and basophils, thus causing degranulation with histamine release. The type II allergic response is mediated by cytotoxic T cells, causing deposits of immunoglobulins, complement, and fibrin around blood vessels. This leads to urticarial vasculitis. The type III immune complex disease is associated with systemic lupus erythematosus and other autoimmune diseases that cause urticaria (Linscott, 2013).

Histologic examination of urticarial lesions reveals dermal edema and dilation of dermal blood vessels, without signs of wall damage or leukocytoclasis, and a small amount of perivascular infiltrate that is composed of macrophages, lymphocytes, and granulocytes (Peroni et al., 2010).

## CLINICAL PRESENTATION

Urticaria is characterized by blanching, raised, palpable wheals, which can be linear, annular, or serpiginous. These lesions occur on any skin area and are usually temporary and mobile. They are often separated by normal skin but may coalesce rapidly to form large areas of erythematous, raised lesions that blanch with pressure (Linscott, 2013).

Obtaining a history of previous urticaria and duration of rash and itching is useful for categorizing urticaria as acute, recurrent, or chronic (Bingham, 2013; Linscott, 2013; Peroni et al., 2010; Saini, 2013).

- Inquire about triggers, such as heat, cold, pressure, exercise, sunlight, emotional stress, or chronic medical conditions (e.g., hyperthyroidism, systemic lupus erythematosus [SLE], rheumatoid arthritis, polymyositis, amyloidosis, polycythemia vera, and lymphoma or other malignant neoplasms).
- Obtain medical history of health conditions that can cause pruritus (usually without rash), such as diabetes mellitus, chronic renal insufficiency, primary biliary cirrhosis, or other nonurticarial dermatologic disorders (e.g., eczema, contact dermatitis).

- Ask about family and personal medical history of angioedema, which is urticaria of the deeper tissues and can be life threatening if it involves the larynx and vocal cords. Causes specific to angioedema include hereditary angioedema (a deficiency in $C_1$-inhibitors) and acquired angioedema (associated with angiotensin-converting enzyme inhibitors and angiotensin receptor blockers).
- If acute urticaria is present, consider the following in subjective findings:
  - Recent illness (e.g., fever, sore throat, cough, rhinorrhea, vomiting, diarrhea, headache)
  - Medication use, including penicillins, cephalosporins, sulfas, diuretics, aspirin, nonsteroidal anti-inflammatory drugs (NSAIDs), iodides, bromides, quinidine, chloroquine, vancomycin, isoniazid, antiepileptic agents, and other agents
  - Intravenous radiocontrast media
  - Travel (could indicate amebiasis, ascariasis, strongyloidiasis, trichinosis, or malaria)
  - Foods (e.g., shellfish, fish, eggs, cheese, chocolate, nuts, berries, tomatoes)
  - New perfumes, hair dyes, detergents, lotions, creams, or clothes
  - Exposure to new pets (dander), dust, mold, chemicals, or plants
  - Pregnancy (usually occurs in last trimester and typically resolves spontaneously soon after delivery)
  - Contact with nickel (e.g., jewelry, stud buttons on jeans), rubber (e.g., gloves, elastic bands), latex, industrial chemicals, and nail polish
  - Sun or cold exposure
  - Exercise

The physical examination should focus on conditions that might cause urticaria or could be serious complications (Linscott, 2013).

- Angioedema of the lips, tongue, or larynx
- Dermographism (urticarial lesions resulting from light scratching on the skin)
- Individual urticarial lesions that are painful, long lasting (> 36–48 hours), or are ecchymotic; also, urticarial lesions that leave residual hyperpigmentation or ecchymosis after resolution (suggesting urticarial vasculitis)
- Systemic signs or symptoms, particularly fever, arthralgias, arthritis, weight changes, bone pain, or lymphadenopathy
- Scleral icterus, hepatic enlargement, or tenderness that suggests hepatitis or cholestatic liver disease
- Thyromegaly suggesting autoimmune thyroid disease, connective tissue disease, rheumatoid arthritis, or SLE
- Pneumonia or bronchospasm (asthma)
- Bacterial or fungal infection

Urticaria pigmentosa is a hereditary skin disorder illustrated by hyperpigmented (yellow, tan, or brown) papules or plaques that may be related to lymphoproliferative disorders. These lesions are composed of mast cells. When the lesion of urticaria pigmentosa is rubbed, a linear wheal will appear; this is a diagnostic sign known as the *Darier sign* (Linscott, 2013).

## DIFFERENTIAL DIAGNOSIS

The following should be considered for differential diagnosis (Bingham, 2013; Linscott, 2013; Peroni et al., 2010; Saini, 2013).

- Arthropod bite reactions
- Atopic dermatitis

- Auriculotemporal syndrome
- Autoimmune bullous diseases
- Autoimmune progesterone dermatitis
- Contact dermatitis, allergic
- Cryoglobulinemia
- Crypyrin-associated periodic syndromes
- Cutaneous small vessel vasculitis
- Drug eruptions
- Eosinophilic cellulitis (Wells syndrome)
- Erythema multiforme
- Henoch–Schönlein purpura (anaphylactoid purpura)
- Hypereosinophilic syndrome
- Mastocytosis
- Neutrophilic eccrine hidradenitis
- Pityriasis rosea
- Plant-induced reactions
- Pruritic urticarial papules and plaques of pregnancy
- Scabies
- Schnitzler syndrome
- Sweets syndrome
- Systemic lupus erythematosus
- Urticaria-like follicular mucinosis
- Urticaria pigmentosa
- Urticarial vasculitis
- Viral exanthems

## TREATMENT/MANAGEMENT

The treatment goal is to reduce the severity, occurrence, and symptoms of the urticarial attacks (Stanway et al., 2009). The cause of the lesions often is undetermined, but the most commonly identified causes are infections (~40% of cases). Known causes for acute urticaria include:

- Infections (e.g., pharyngitis, gastrointestinal infections, genitourinary infections, respiratory infections, fungal infections [e.g., dermatophytosis], malaria, amebiasis, hepatitis, mononucleosis, coxsackievirus, mycoplasmal infections, infestations [e.g., scabies], HIV, parasitic infections)
- Caterpillars and moths
- Foods (particularly shellfish, fish, eggs, cheese, chocolate, nuts, berries, tomatoes)
- Drugs (e.g., penicillins, sulfonamides, salicylates, NSAIDs, codeine, antihistamines)
- Environmental factors (e.g., pollens, chemicals, plants, danders, dust, mold)
- Exposure to latex
- Exposure to undue skin pressure, cold, or heat
- Emotional stress
- Exercise
- Pregnancy (i.e., pruritic urticarial papules and plaques of pregnancy) (Bingham, 2013; Linscott, 2013; Peroni et al., 2010)

Chronic urticaria can be related to all of these factors as well as to (Bingham, 2013; Peroni et al., 2010):

- Autoimmune disorders (e.g., SLE, rheumatoid arthritis, polymyositis, thyroid autoimmunity, and other connective tissue diseases; approximately 50% of chronic urticaria is autoimmune)

- Cholinergic urticaria, induced by emotional stress, heat, or exercise (examine for other signs of cholinergic stimulation, including lacrimation, salivation, and diarrhea)
- Chronic medical illness, such as hyperthyroidism, amyloidosis, polycythemia vera, malignant neoplasms, lupus, lymphoma, and many others
- Cold urticaria, cryoglobulinemia, cryofibrinogenemia, or syphilis
- Mastocytosis
- Inherited autoinflammatory syndromes

Recurrent urticaria can be related to:

- Sun exposure (solar urticaria), occurring only on skin exposed to the sun
- Exercise (cholinergic urticaria)
- Emotional or physical stress
- Water (aquagenic urticaria)

Laboratory tests are usually not needed for acute urticaria. The patient's history and physical examination should guide the need for diagnostic testing. For chronic or recurrent urticaria, basic laboratory studies should include a complete blood count, erythrocyte sedimentation rate, thyroid-stimulating hormone, C-reactive protein, and an antinuclear antibodies. Imaging studies are recommended if patient history or clinical examination suggest an underlying problem that would warrant further testing (Bingham, 2013; Linscott, 2013; Peroni et al., 2010; Saini, 2013).

Resistant cases of chronic urticaria may improve with glucocorticosteroids, topical therapy with 5% doxepin cream (Zonalon) or capsaicin; cyclosporine and omalizumab have also been shown to be effective. Chronic urticaria may benefit from doxepin, a tricyclic antidepressant with potent antihistamine properties (Linscott, 2013).

Most patients with urticaria can be treated at home on $H_1$ antihistamines (i.e., diphenhydramine 50 mg every 6 hours or hydroxyzine 50 mg every 6 hours for 24–48 hours) or, in refractory cases, use a combination of $H_1$ and $H_2$ antihistamines plus oral glucocorticoids. Pregnant patients may be treated with chlorpheniramine, 4 mg orally every 4 to 6 hours. Lactating women can be treated with loratadine (Bingham, 2013; Stanway et al., 2009).

If the patient has angioedema that is treated successfully in the emergency department, the patient should be sent home with an EpiPen prescription and told to keep it with him or her at all times; it should be used if swelling of the lips, tongue, or face develops or if his or her voice becomes acutely hoarse (Bingham, 2013; Linscott, 2013).

## SPECIAL CONSIDERATIONS

Associated conditions that may be present with chronic urticaria include:

- Autoimmune disorders such as thyroid disorders, celiac disease, Sjögren syndrome, systemic lupus erythematosus, rheumatoid arthritis, and type 1 diabetes mellitus have been associated with urticaria.
- Patients with noncutaneous malignancies can develop associated dermatologic disorders, and urticarial vasculitis has been associated with malignancy. (Saini, 2013)

Affected individuals with chronic urticaria may have several attacks each day for several months in a row. This can become a debilitating problem that affects employment and quality of life. The symptoms associated with urticarial lesions can also affect sleep. Patients with urticaria are often frustrated and depressed because of lack of response to treatment and/or the unknown cause (Peroni et al., 2010; Stanway et al., 2009).

## WHEN TO REFER

Consultation with or referral to a dermatologist, allergist, immunologist, or rheumatologist may be appropriate in selected cases, particularly in cases of complicated, recurrent, refractory, severe, or chronic urticaria. Dermatology referral is mandatory if vasculitic urticaria is suspected (Linscott, 2013).

## PATIENT EDUCATION

- Patients with urticaria should avoid any medication, food, or other allergen that has previously precipitated urticaria or other serious allergic reaction.
- Some patients with urticaria will have flares that worsen with physical activity and heat. Avoidance of activities that induce sweating would be beneficial. Cool showers may help.
- If stress is a trigger, avoidance of activities or situations that cause increased stress is advised.
- Anti-inflammatory medications and alcohol may worsen symptoms in some patients.

## CLINICAL PEARLS

- Urticaria: ICD-9, 708.0; ICD-10, L50
- Antihistamines blocking the $H_1$ receptor are the main medications used to control urticaria (Katila, 2011).
- Allergens such as food, drugs, insect stings, and infection are the typical secondary causes of acute urticaria (Katila, 2011).
- Chronic urticaria is usually idiopathic (Katila, 2011). Some cases of chronic urticaria recur and do not resolve after months and years (Habif, Campbell, Chapman, Dinulos, & Zug, 2013).
- Individual hive or urticarial lesions migrate, change in shape, and typically resolve within 24 hours (Habif et al., 2013, p. 87).

## REFERENCES

Bingham, C. O. (2013). *New onset urticaria: Diagnosis and treatment*. Retrieved from http://www.uptodate.com/contents/new-onset-urticaria-diagnosis-and-treatment

Habif, T., Campbell, J., Chapman, M., Dinulos, J., & Zug, K. (2011). *Skin disease diagnosis and treatment* (3rd ed.). Philadelphia, PA: Elsevier/Saunders.

Katila, R. (2011). Urticaria and angioedema. In J. E. Fitzpatrick & J. G. Morelli, *Dermatology secrets plus* (4th ed., pp. 166–170). Philadelphia, PA: Elsevier/Mosby.

Linscott, M. S. (2013, April 1). *Urticaria*. Retrieved from http://emedicine.medscape.com/article/762917-overveiw#a0101

Peroni, A., Colato, C., Schena, D., & Girolomoni, G. (2010). Urticarial lesions: If not urticaria, what else? The differential diagnosis of urticaria. *Journal of the American Academy of Dermatology, 62*, 541–555.

Saini, S. (2013). *Chronic urticaria: Clinical manifestations, diagnosis, pathogenesis, and natural history*. Retrieved from http://www.uptodate.com/contents/chronic-manifestations-diagnosis-pathogenesis-and-natural-history

Stanway, A. D., Cohen, S. N., Chen, C.-M., Hauser, C., & Binney, L. (2006). H1-antihistamines for chronic urticaria. *Cochrane Database of Systematic Reviews* (3). Art. No.: CD006137. doi: 10.1002/14651858.CD006137

# Vasculitis

## LEUKOCYTOCLASTIC VASCULITIS

### OVERVIEW

Leukocytoclastic vasculitis (LCV) is a hypersensitivity vasculitis that is also known as small-vessel vasculitis (Figure III.57). LCV has many causes, but in 50% of cases, no cause can be identified. LCV may be isolated on the skin or manifest in other organs. The internal organs commonly affected include the joints, the gastrointestinal tract, and the kidneys. If no internal involvement is present, the prognosis of LCV is good (Callen, 2012).

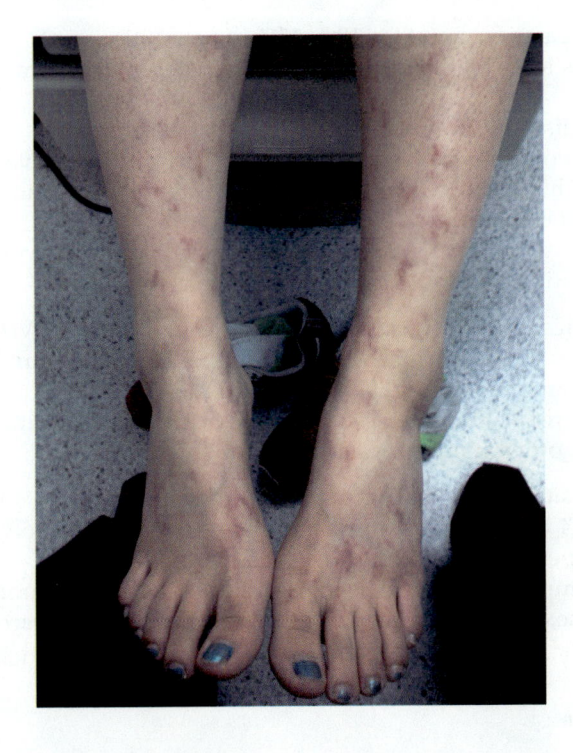

FIGURE III.57  Leukocytoclastic vasculitis

## EPIDEMIOLOGY

As noted, the prognosis of LCV is good, but if there is internal organ involvement, mortality is possible. LCV occurs more often in Whites than in other races. LCV affects men and women equally and is not age specific. In children, it is referred to as Henoch–Schönle in purpura (Callen, 2012).

## PATHOLOGY/HISTOLOGY

Circulating immune complexes are involved in the pathogenesis of LCV, as well as autoantibodies, such as antineutrophil cytoplasmic antibody (ANCA), inflammatory mediators, and local factors that involve the endothelial cells and adhesion molecules (Callen, 2012). The adhesion molecules adhere to activated endothelial cells and infiltrate into vessel walls, which causes the release of lytic enzymes (James, Berger, & Elston, 2006; Sais et al., 1998).

## CLINICAL PRESENTATION

Between 0.3% and 0.5% of the cases of cutaneous vasculitis are idiopathic. Although all drugs have the potential to cause LCV, the most common drugs that can cause cutaneous vasculitis are antibiotics, nonsteroidal anti-inflammatory drugs, and diuretics. Other causes of LCV include:

- Various infections, such as upper respiratory tract infections, particularly with beta-hemolytic streptococci, and viral hepatitis
- HIV infection
- Bacterial endocarditis
- Foods or food additives
- Hepatitis C
- Collagen-vascular diseases (account for 10%–15% of vasculitis cases)
- Autoimmune diseases such as rheumatoid arthritis, Sjögren syndrome, and lupus erythematosus
- Inflammatory bowel disease, ulcerative colitis, and Crohn's disease
- Malignancy is rare, accounting for less than 1% of cases of cutaneous vasculitis
- Tumors at any site (however, lymphoproliferative diseases are more common, particularly hairy cell leukemia)
- Larger-vessel vasculitis, such as Wegener granulomatosis, polyarteritisnodosa, microscopic polyarteritis, or Churg–Strauss syndrome (Callen, 2012)

Three characteristics are significant in making the diagnosis of LCV: (1) palpable purpura is nonblanching; (2) the purpuric patches are 1 to 3 mm and found on dependent areas of the body, such as the thighs, legs, and buttocks; and (3) each macule is regular and circular (Blereau, 2013; James et al., 2006). Although purpura is the most common manifestation, other symptoms may develop, including:

- Urticarial vasculitis lesions differ from acute in that they are present for longer periods of time (often > 24 hours), are less pruritic, and will possibly resolve with skin changes (bruise or hyperpigmentation).
- Patients with hypocomplementemic urticarial vasculitis may form chronic obstructive pulmonary disease; careful examination of the heart and lungs is recommended.

- Livedoreticularis is a rare occurrence of small-vessel vasculitis. It is frequently seen in patients with occlusive or inflammatory disease of medium-sized vessels.
- Nodular lesions can occur in a few patients with small-vessel vasculitis.
- Ulceration is commonly observed in vasculitis that affects large vessels; physical examination is warranted and should include specific observation of the cardiopulmonary, musculoskeletal, and gastrointestinal systems. (Callen, 2012)

## DIFFERENTIAL DIAGNOSIS

- Amyloidosis, AA (inflammatory)
- Antiphospholipid syndrome
- Atrial myxoma
- Behçet disease
- Immune thrombocytopenic purpura
- Meningococcemia
- Scurvy
- Wegener granulomatosis

## TREATMENT/MANAGEMENT

Subjective inquiry should include evaluation for fever, arthritis, myalgia, abdominal pain, diarrhea, hematochezia, cough, hemoptysis, joint pain, sinus congestion, paresthesia, weakness, hematuria, and symptoms of an associated disorder. Determine whether there is a history of intravenous drug use, hepatitis, blood transfusion, or recent travel, as well as symptoms or a previous episode of inflammatory bowel disease and history or symptoms of a collagen vascular disorder, particularly rheumatoid arthritis, lupus erythematosus, or Sjögren syndrome. The following workup is recommended to rule out causes of LCV (Callen, 2012; Blereau, 2013; James et al., 2006).

- Laboratory tests that are indicated are a complete blood count, erythrocyte sedimentation rate, urinalysis, and blood chemistry panel.
- Although stool guaiac testing and Hematest are variable, these tests are recommended in patients with cutaneous vasculitis.
- Serologic studies, such as antinuclear antibody, ANCA (cytoplasmic ANCA [cANCA], perinuclear ANCA [pANCA], atypical ANCA), and rheumatoid factor should be performed in patients with no clear etiology for cause of LCV. Immunoglobulin A (IgA)-type antiphospholipid antibodies have been linked with Henoch–Schönle in purpura in adult patients.
- In patients with suspected lupus erythematosus or with urticarial vasculitis, it is recommended to obtain complement levels, including total hemolytic complement (CH100 or CH50), C3 levels, and C4 levels.
- In patients without identified disease, testing for serum protein electrophoresis, cryoglobulins, and hepatitis C antibody are recommended.
- Patients with malaise and/or a cardiac murmur should have a cardiac ultrasonography and blood cultures.
- If patient is high risk for HIV infection, testing should be performed.
- If the peripheral smear on the complete blood count result is abnormal, consider a bone marrow biopsy.

- Chest radiography should be included in a routine evaluation for LCV.
- Visceral angiography is considered for patients with a severe vasculitic syndrome.
- Pulmonary function tests are needed in patients with hypocomplementemic urticarial vasculitis.
- LCV should be confirmed with a skin biopsy.
- If severe vasculitic syndromes are present, a muscle or nerve biopsy or biopsy of visceral organs may be performed.
- Direct immunofluorescence microscopy may be warranted. IgA results are positive in patients with Henoch–Schönle in purpura.

The initial treatment for most cases of LCV in patients who are well and have normal urinalysis should be conservative. Rest and elevation of the legs are recommended. If symptomatic, other treatment options to consider are as follows:

- LCV often affects dependent areas; therefore, elevation of the legs or compression stockings are recommended.
- Treat the cause of LCV.
- Discontinue the drug that is suspected to be the cause for vasculitis. LCV clears quickly once a drug is stopped.
- In patients with cutaneous vasculitis, with or without joint manifestations, colchicine (0.6 mg two to three times a day) or dapsone (50–200 mg/day) for 2 to 3 weeks may be administered.
- Antihistamines are used for pruritis.
- Nonsteroidal anti-inflammatory agents may be used.
- Corticosteroids (60–80 mg/day) alone or in conjunction with an immunosuppressive agent (e.g., cyclophosphamide, azathioprine, methotrexate) are used to treat those affected with severe visceral involvement.
- Severe or debilitating disease can also be treated with biologic agents such as Rituximab or intravenous immunoglobulin. (Callen, 2012; James et al., 2006)

## SPECIAL CONSIDERATIONS

LCV is usually acute and self-limited. LCV may affect employment if patients are required to stand for long periods of time, which can worsen LCV. With a diagnosis of LCV patients should be referred to the following specialists as appropriate.

- Rheumatologist
- Dermatologist
- Nephrologist
- Gastroenterologist or hepatologist
- Immunologist or allergist
- Pulmonologist

## PATIENT EDUCATION

Patients should be encouraged to rest and elevate legs when possible. Compliance with compression stockings is helpful.

## CLINICAL PEARLS

- LCV: ICD-9, 709.1; ICD-10, L95
- Leukocytoclastic vasculitis is the most common form of vasculitis of the skin (Sunderkotter, Bonsmann, Sindrilaru, & Luger, 2005).
- LCV may manifest in organs other than the skin (Callen, 2012).
- Hypersensitivity vasculitis, cutaneous vasculitis, urticarial vasculitis are stated as synonyms of LCV (Patient.co.uk, 2013).
- LCV is created by deposits of immune complexes at the vessel wall (Sunderkotter, Bonsmann, Sindrilaru, & Luger, 2005).

# SPIDER VEINS AND VARICOSE VEINS

## OVERVIEW

Varicose veins and telangiectasia (spider veins) are indicators of an underlying problem with reverse venous flow, which is also termed *venous insufficiency syndrome* (Figure III.58). Varicose veins affect 10% to 30% of men and women, with increasing rates as a person ages (Allen, 2009; Armstrong, 2013). The annual medical cost of venous

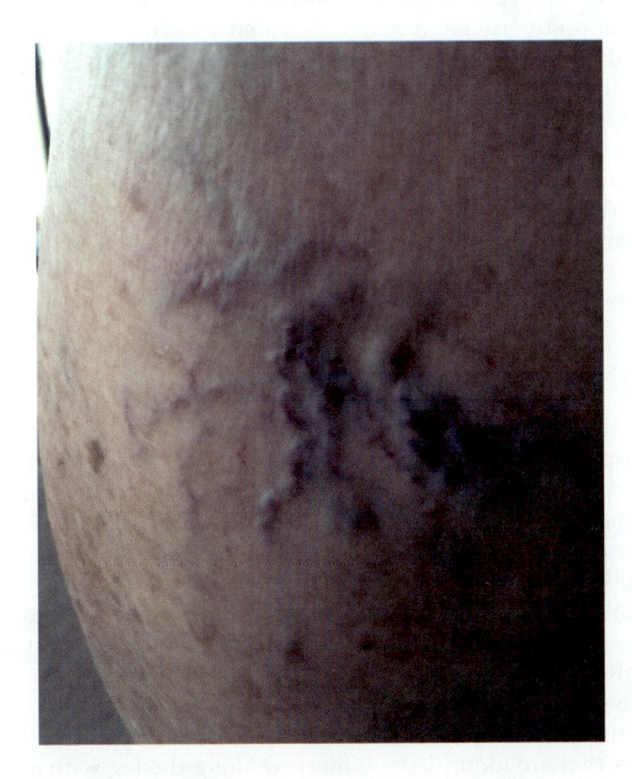

FIGURE III.58　Varicose veins

disease in the United States could potentially reach $1 billion (Hamdan, 2012). Mild forms of venous insufficiency are simply uncomfortable and considered unattractive, but severe venous disease can produce significant systemic effects (Weiss, 2012).

## EPIDEMIOLOGY

In the United States, the age and the gender of the population determines the incidence and prevalence of venous insufficiency disease. Approximately 22 million women and 11 million men between the ages of 40 and 80 years have varicose veins (Hamdan, 2012). The occurrence of venous disease is higher in Westernized and developed countries; this is attributed to alterations in lifestyle and activity (Weiss, 2012).

## PATHOLOGY/HISTOLOGY

Varicose veins and spider veins are healthy veins that have dilated under the effect of increased venous pressure. Within the veins, one-way valves direct the flow of venous blood upward and inward. Blood is gathered in superficial venous capillaries, transfers into larger superficial veins, and finally passes through valves into the deep veins and then travels to the heart and lungs. Superficial veins are closer to the skin surface, whereas deep veins are within the muscle fascia. Perforating veins allow blood to pass from the superficial veins to the deep veins (Allen, 2009; Armstrong, 2013; James et al., 2006; Weiss, 2012).

Frequently, a solitary venous valve weakens and results in a high-pressure leak between the deep and superficial systems. Elevated pressure within the superficial system causes local dilatation, and with the increased stretching, the valves within the veins will eventually fail. After multiple valves have failed, the affected veins can no longer direct blood upward and inward. This causes the venous blood to flow in the direction of the pressure gradient: outward and downward into a congested leg. Over time, large numbers of poorly functioning superficial veins will appear dilated and convoluted (Weiss, 2012). Advanced disease causes excessive venous bulging, pruritus, pain, edema, and fatigue in legs. Pigmentation changes will occur in lower legs and ankles as a result of hemosiderin deposits from leakage of red blood cells (Allen, 2009; Armstrong, 2013).

## CLINICAL PRESENTATION

Risk factors for varicose veins include being a female, advanced age, prolonged standing, taller height, congenital valvular dysfunction, venous hypertension of obesity, and multiple pregnancies (Hamdan, 2012; James et al., 2006; Weiss, 2012). Heredity also affects the occurrence of varicosities; if both parents have varicose veins, their offspring have a 90% chance of having them (Hamdan, 2012).

Patients often present with complaints of lower extremity edema, restless leg syndrome, limb heaviness and fatigue, aching in the legs, burning and tingling, pruritus, pain, and nighttime leg cramping (Hamdan, 2012).

It is recommended that veins and their pathways are thoroughly evaluated and a venous map completed that will aid in selecting treatment options. The courses of all the dilated veins that are identified are marked along the leg with a pen and transcribed into the medical record as a diagram of all known areas of venous insufficiency (Weiss, 2012). Varicose veins are often classified by practitioners by the use of a clinical classification that illustrates the current physical findings on examination: 0 indicates no visible or palpable signs of venous disease; a 1 indicates spider veins or telangiectasias; a 2 indicates varicose veins; a 3 indicates the presence of edema; a 4 indicates skin changes; a 5 indicates a healed ulcer; and a 6 is for an active ulceration (Armstrong, 2013; Hamdan, 2012).

## DIFFERENTIAL DIAGNOSIS

- Cellulitis
- Osler–Weber–Rendu syndrome
- Stasis dermatitis

## TREATMENT/MANAGEMENT

Laboratory testing is not indicated for varicose veins unless there is suspicion of underlying etiology. Imaging studies may be needed to assess the venous system. The most useful modalities available for venous imaging are contrast venography, magnetic resonance imaging, and color-flow duplex ultrasonography (Allen, 2009; Weiss, 2012).

Patients with varicose veins may present with serious varicose complications, including variceal bleeding, new-onset dermatitis, thrombophlebitis, cellulitis, and ulceration. A history of the venous system should include inquiring about the following.

- Previous venous insufficiency
- Presence or lack of predisposing factors (e.g., heredity, trauma to the legs, occupational prolonged standing, sports participation)
- History of edema
- History of any prior evaluation of or treatment for venous disease
- History of superficial or deep thrombophlebitis
- History of any other vascular disease
- Family history of vascular disease of any type (Weiss, 2012)

The goal of treatment for varicose veins is to improve and maintain the best venous return to the heart, prevent sign and symptoms, and prevent disease progression. Daily conservative management of varicosities and spider veins should include exercise, leg elevation, and compression stockings (Armstrong, 2013; Hamdan, 2012).

Sclerotherapy, laser and intense pulsed-light therapy, radiofrequency or laser ablation, and ambulatory phlebectomy are the modern techniques used to ablate varicosities. Numerous reports describe success rates of greater than 90% for less invasive techniques, which are associated with fewer complications, with comparable efficacy (Armstrong, 2013; Hamdan, 2012; James et al., 2006; Weiss, 2012).

The primary aim of surgical therapy is to improve venous circulation by fixing venous insufficiency through the elimination of major reflux pathways. The most common invasive procedures to treat significant varicose disease include ligation of the saphenofemoral junction with vein stripping, phlebectomy performed through microincisions, endovenous radiofrequency thermal ablation, and endovenous laser thermal ablation. The principal surgical approach to small-vein disease is by microincision alphlebectomy followed by sclerotherapy (Allen, 2009; Armstrong, 2013; Weiss, 2012).

## SPECIAL CONSIDERATIONS

Varicose veins of pregnancy are commonly caused by hormonal changes that reduce the strength of venous walls. The sudden appearance of new dilated varicosities during pregnancy should be evaluated to rule out acute deep vein thrombosis

(Weiss, 2012). Varicose veins may cause discomfort, skin changes, employment issues for missed work, and medical and emotional disabilities (Hamdan, 2012).

## WHEN TO REFER

If ultrasound imaging demonstrates isolated spider veins without underlying reflux, the problem may be treated in the office without difficulty. Patients with identifiable underlying reflux or other signs of significant venous disease must be referred for consultation with a phlebologist (a physician or surgeon with specialized training in venous diagnosis and therapeutics) (Weiss, 2012).

## PATIENT EDUCATION

Patients should be informed of the following (Allen, 2009; Weiss, 2012):

- Prolonged standing is a risk factor for venous insufficiency syndromes. Exercise is recommended.
- Elevating legs whenever possible may help.
- Wearing 30 to 40 mm Hg gradient compression hose whenever standing is helpful.
- Weight loss is recommended in cases of obesity.

Hamdan, Livingston, and Lynm (2013) recommend the following resource sites for patient information:

- Healthy Veins: www.healthyveins.org
- American Venous Forum: www.veinforum.org
- National Heart, Lung, and Blood Institute: www.nhlbi.gov/health/health-topics/topics/vv/

## CLINICAL PEARLS

- Spider veins/Telangietasia: ICD-9, 362.15; ICD-10, 178.1
- Varicose veins: ICD-9, 454.9; ICD-10, I86
- Approximately 30% to 60% of adults develop varicose veins or spider veins (WebMD, 2012).
- Stasis dermatitis is associated with varicose veins (Habif et al., 2011).
- Avoiding sun exposure and using sunscreen can reduce spider vein formation to the skin, especially the face.

## REFERENCES

Allen, L. (2009). Assessment and management of patients with varicose veins. *Nursing Standard*, 23(23), 49–57.
Armstrong, K. E. (2013). The reflux: An update on treatment for symptomatic varicose veins. *Nursing*, 27–33.
Blereau, R. P. (2013). Leukocytoclastic vasculitis. *Consultant*, 250–251.
Callen, J. P. (2012). *Leukocytoclastic vasculitis*. Retrieved from http://emedicine.medscape.com/article/333891-overview

Habif, T., Campbell, J., Chapman, M., Dinulos, J., & Zug, K. (2011). *Skin disease diagnosis and treatment* (3rd ed.). Philadelphia, PA: Elsevier/Saunders.

Hamdan, A. (2012). Management of varicose veins and venous insufficiency. *Journal of the American Medical Association, 308*(24), 2612–2621.

Hamdan, A., Livingston, E. H., & Lynm, C. (2013). Treatment of varicose veins. *Journal of the American Medical Association, 309*(12), 1306.

James, W. K., Berger, T. G., & Elston, D. M. (2006). *Andrews' diseases of the skin. Clinical dermatology* (10th ed.). Philadelphia, PA: Saunders/Elsevier.

Patient.co.uk. (2013). *Hypersensitivity vasculitis.* Retrieved from www.patient.co.uk/pdf/2288.pdf

Sais, G., Vidaller, A., Jucgla, A., Servitje, O., Condom, E., & Peyri, J. (1998). Prognostic factors in leukocytoclasticvasculitis. *Archives of Dermatology, 134*, 309–314.

Sunderkotter, C., Bonsmann, G., Sindrilaru, A. & Luger, T. (2005). Management of leukocytoclasticvasculitis. *Journal of Dermatological Treatment. 16*(4), 193-206.

WebMD. (2012). *Varicose veins and spider veins.* Retrieved from http://www.webmd.com/skin-problems-and-treatments/cosmetic-procedures-spider-veins

Weiss, R. (2012, November 14). *Varicose veins and spider veins.* Retrieved from http://emedicine.medscape.com/article/1085530-overview

# Verruca Vulgaris

## OVERVIEW

Verruca vulgaris, commonly called warts, is caused by human papillomavirus (HPV) and consists of benign growths confined to the epidermis (Goodheart, 2011). There are more than 100 strains of HPV, and warts caused by this virus can occur anywhere on the epidermal surface; however, some warts have an affinity to infect specific body sites (Figure III.58). If the skin's protective barrier is compromised from trauma or other reasons, the HPV can be transmitted by either direct or indirect contact. Most warts are transmitted primarily through skin-to-skin contact (Goodheart, 2011). Warts tend to be resistant to treatment, and treatment failure is common. However, warts do resolve spontaneously without treatment (Mulhem & Pinelis, 2011; Shenefelt, 2012).

## EPIDEMIOLOGY

Warts are widespread throughout the world. The actual occurrence of warts is unknown but is estimated at 7% to 12% of the population. The rate of infection for school-age children is higher, estimated at 10% to 20%. Pregnant women, immunocompromised individuals, and meat and fish handlers (butchers and fishmongers) are all at increased risk for developing warts (Goodheart, 2011; James, Berger, & Elston, 2006; Lipke, 2006; Shenefelt, 2012).

Common warts are generally asymptomatic but some may be tender. Warts can create cosmetic disfigurement. Plantar warts are usually painful and, if located on the sole of the foot, can impair walking (Figure III.59). Although rare, nongenital warts can undergo malignant changes. This type of lesion is mistaken for a wart but is actually a verrucous carcinoma, a slow-growing, locally invasive, well-differentiated squamous cell carcinoma. This type of skin cancer rarely metastasizes but can be locally destructive (Shenefelt, 2012).

**338** ■ III. Common Dermatologic Conditions

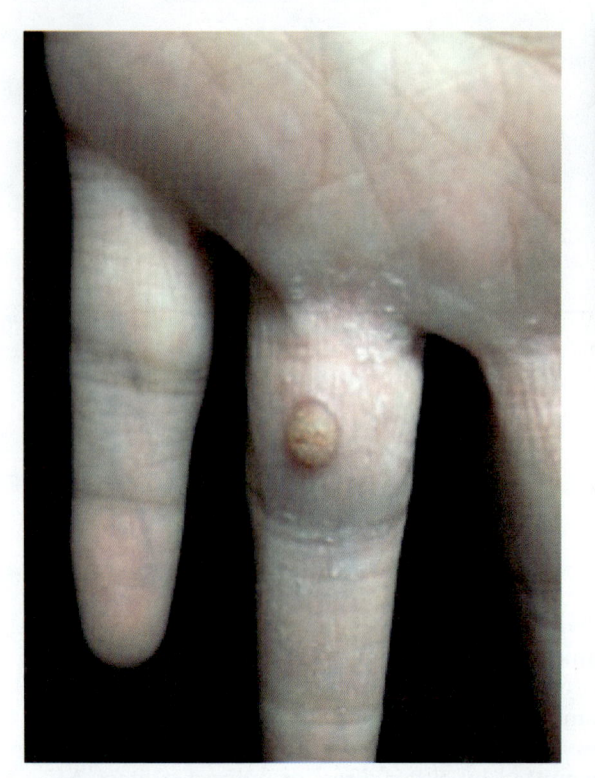

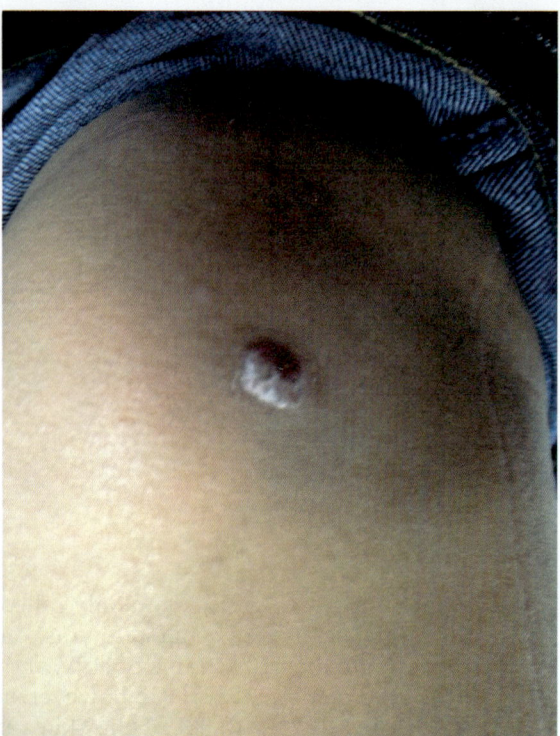

FIGURE III.59  Examples of verruca vulgaris (warts) on the hand and knee

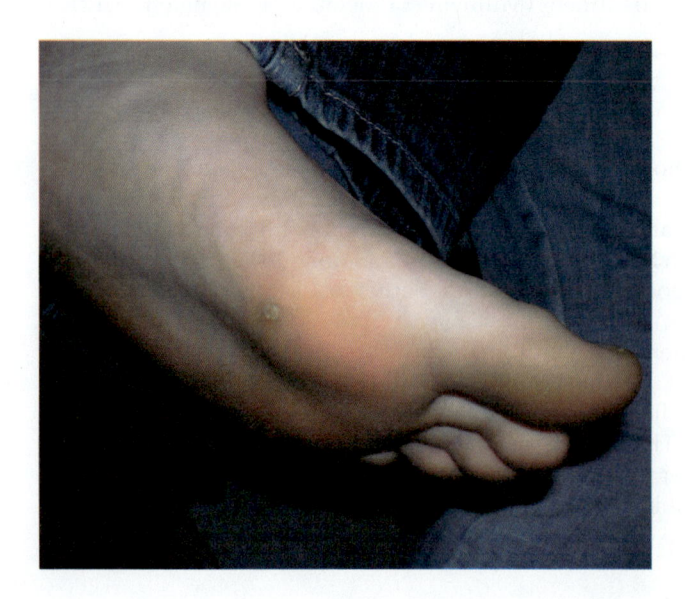

FIGURE III.60  A plantar wart

Warts affect all races, but common warts occur twice as frequently in Whites than in the Black or Asian populations. Warts also occur at any age but occur more frequently in school-age children and young adults (peaking between 12 and 16 years)

and are unusual in infants and young children (Shenefelt, 2012). The occurrences of warts in females and males are equal.

## PATHOLOGY/HISTOLOGY

Warts, confined to the epidermis, can affect any area of the skin and mucous membranes. The HPV infects the epithelium without any systemic distribution of the virus. Viral replication occurs in the upper portion or the epidermis, within differentiated epithelial cells; however, viral particles can be located in the basal layer or the skin (Shenefelt, 2012).

All warts are caused by HPV, a double-stranded, circular, supercoiled DNA virus. More than 150 types of HPV have been identified. Goldstein and Goldstein (2103), James et al. (2006), Lipke (2006), and Shenefelt (2012) noted the following wart types and histologic findings of nongenital warts:

- Common warts: Caused by HPV types 2 and 4, followed by 1, 3, 27, 29, and 57, these warts have elongated rete ridges that are directed toward the center of the lesion. In the granular layer, infected cells can contain keratohyaline granules and vacuoles surrounded by wrinkle-appearing nuclei.
- Deep palmoplantar warts (myrmecia): Caused by HPV type 1, followed by 2, 3, 4, 27, 29, and 57, these warts differ from common warts because of location. The majority of the lesion lies deep in the plane of the skin's surface. The endophytic epidermal growth is polygonal andretractile. Eosinophilic, cytoplasmic inclusions made of keratin filaments form in ring-like structures.
- Flat warts: Caused by HPV types 3, 10, and 28, these lesions tend to have muted features under microscopy of a common wart. Prominent perinuclear vacuolization cells surrounding pyknotic, basophilic cells, with central nuclei features are present and may be referred to as *owl's eye cells*.
- Butcher's warts: Caused by HPV type 7, these warts have prominent acanthosis, hyperkeratosis, and papillomatosis. They consist of small vacuolized cells in the center with reduced nuclei in clusters in the rete ridges of the granular layer.
- Focal epithelial hyperplasia (Heck disease): Caused by HPV types 13 and 32, this displays hyperplastic mucosa with thin parakeratotic stratum corneum, and acanthosis. Blunting of rete ridges and pale epidermal cells resulting in intracellular edema are noted.
- Cystic warts: Caused by HPV type 60, these are cysts filled with horny material. The walls are composed of basal, squamous, or granular cells.

## CLINICAL PRESENTATION

The majority of HPV transmission is direct skin-to-skin contact; however, indirect contact is also a mode or transmission, as is autoinoculation. The HPV incubation period ranges from 1 to 6 months. Latency periods of up to 3 years have been reported (Goldstein & Goldstein, 2013; Shenefelt, 2012).

Physical findings for types of nongenital warts are as follows (James et al., 2006; Lipke, 2006; Shenefelt, 2012).

- Common warts, or verruca vulgaris, are hyperkeratotic papules with rough irregular surfaces most commonly occurring on the hands and knees. They can grow from 1 mm to 1 cm in size.
- Filiform warts are long thin lesions, generally found on the face around the lips, eyelids, or nares.

- Deep palmoplantar warts grow as small shiny papules and progress to deep endophytic, sharply defined, round lesions with a rough keratotic surface, surrounded by a smooth collar of thickened skin. The warts are painful because they grow deep. Myrmecia warts on the plantar surface are typically found on the weight-bearing areas (metatarsal head and heel).
- Flat warts, also called plane warts or verruca plana, are characterized as flat or slightly elevated skin-colored papules that can be smooth or barely keratotic. Their size ranges from 1 to 5 mm or more, and there can be a few or hundreds of warts that are grouped or confluent. The face, hands, and shins are the most common skin surfaces for flat warts. Sites of trauma may create a linear distribution as the result of scratching (Koebner phenomenon). These warts may regress.
- Butcher's warts, seen most commonly on the hand, are identified in meat handlers. They have a morphology similar to common warts, with an increased likelihood of hyperproliferative cauliflower growths.
- A mosaic wart is a plaque of grouped warts typically seen on the palms and soles.
- Focal epithelial hyperplasia (Heck disease) is a HPV infection in the oral cavity. Typically found on the lower labial mucosa, it also grows on the buccal or gingival mucosa, and rarely on the tongue. Their size range is 1 to 5 mm. Multiple confluent lesions can become plaques. They are most common in American Indian or Inuit children.
- Cystic warts are nodules on the weight-bearing surface of the sole. Typically they are smooth but can become hyperkeratotic.

## DIFFERENTIAL DIAGNOSIS

- Acquired digital fibrokeratoma
- Actinic keratosis
- Arsenical keratosis
- Cutaneous horn
- Lichen nitidus
- Lichen planus
- Molluscum contagiosum
- Prurigo nodularis
- Seborrheic keratosis
- Squamous cell carcinoma

## TREATMENT/MANAGEMENT

Warts can generally be diagnosed based on clinical assessment. The tiny black dots seen in the wart, often thought by lay people as "seeds," are actually thrombosed capillaries. A biopsy should be collected if the diagnosis is unclear (Goldstein & Goldstein, 2013; Shenefelt, 2012).

Multiple treatment options exist for warts; however, none are consistently effective. It is practical and appropriate to begin with the least painful, least expensive, and least time-consuming methods of treatment. The expensive and invasive treatments for warts should be reserved for refractory warts. Immunosuppressed patients' warts are most often resistant to treatments. Some of the various treatment methods available include (Goldstein & Goldstein, 2013; James et al., 2006; Lipke, 2006; Mulhem & Pinelis, 2011; Shenefelt, 2012; Treat cutaneous warts on a case-by-case basis, 2012):

Verruca Vulgaris ■ 341

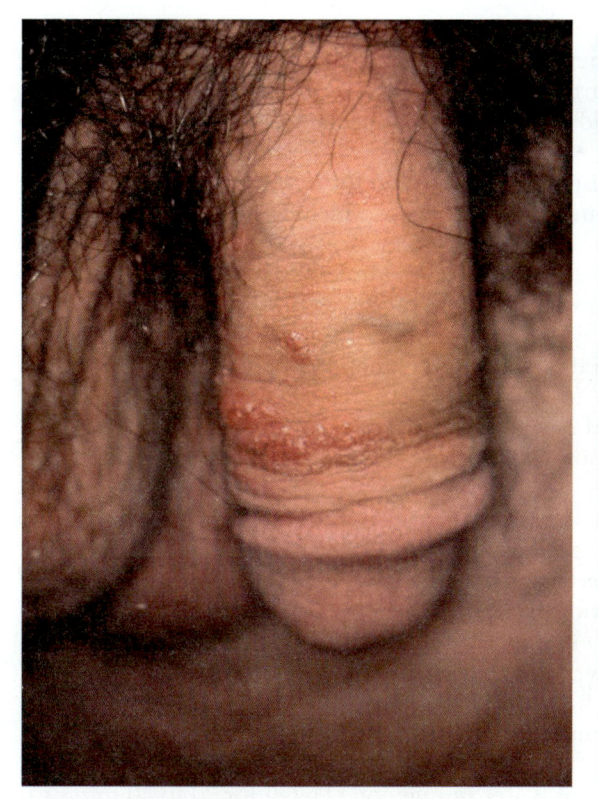

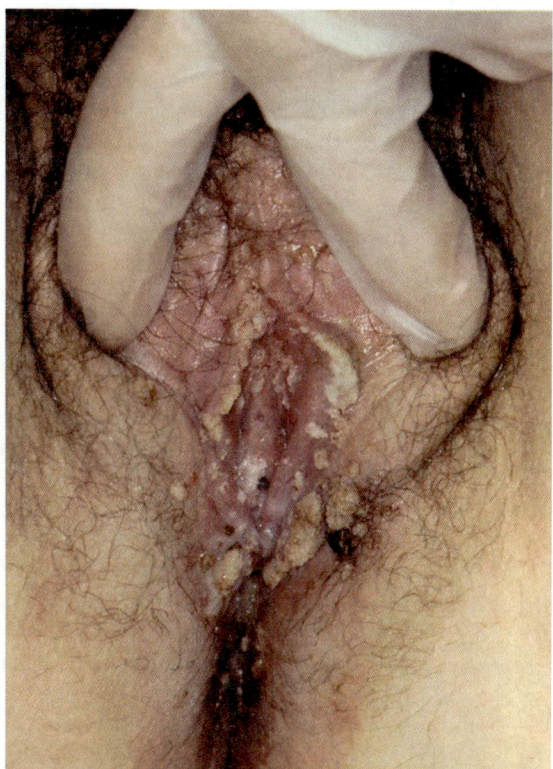

**FIGURE III.61**  Genital warts
Courtesy of Joe Miller, CDC

- Benign neglect is both safe and cost-effective. Approximately 65% of warts regress spontaneously within 2 years, so this is a viable option. Consider, however, that without treatment warts can enlarge and spread. Treatment should be recommended if warts are widespread and spreading, symptomatic, or have been present for more than 2 years.
- Topical salicylic acid is the first-line common wart therapy. It is over the counter, is patient applied, and has a high resolution rate that ranges between 70% and 80%.
- Topical agents available in a provider's office include the following:
  - Cantharidin, an extract of the blister beetle, creates epidermal necrosis and blistering.
  - Dibutyl squaric acid is a contact sensitizer.
  - Trichloroacetic acid is caustic and causes tissue necrosis.
  - Podophyllin, typically used to treat genital warts, is cytotoxic.
  - Aminolevulinic acid, a photosensitizer, is used in combination with a blue light to treat flat warts.
- Prescription medications that the patient can apply to treat warts include the following:
  - Imiquimod, an immune response modifier, treats genital and common warts.
  - Cidofovir, an antiviral typically used to treat cytomegalovirus in HIV patients, treats warts.
  - Podophyllotoxin is used to treat genital warts (Figure III.60) because of its effect on mucosal surfaces.

- 5-Fluorouracil (5-FU), a topical chemotherapeutic, used specifically to treat actinic keratosis, is an effective treatment when used under occlusion daily for 1 month. 5-FU has been used to treat warts on children.
- Tretinoin, a topical retinoic acid used primarily in acne treatment, has success in the treatment of flat warts.
- Intralesional injections are a treatment consideration for warts that are refractory to topical treatments. Intralesional injection choices can include injections of *Candida*, mumps, trichophyton, bleomycin, or interferon-alfa.
- Photodynamic therapy using a topical 5-aminolevulinic acid applied to the lesions then followed by photoactivation with red-light diodes at 2- to 3-week intervals can be used.
- Systemic agents that are used to treat warts are cimetidine, retinoids, and intravenous cidofovir.
  - Cimetidine, an antihistamine II receptor antagonist normally used to treat peptic ulcer disease, works by its immunomodulatory effects to treat warts. The response rates vary.
  - Retinoid, a synthetic vitamin A analog, assists with extensive hyperkeratotic warts in immunocompromised patients. It is thought to reduce pain and aid other treatment responses. Side effects are limiting and include liver abnormalities, increased serum lipid levels, and teratogenicity.
- Alternative treatments have been successful in treating warts. Some of these treatments include adhesiotherapy, hypnosis, hyperthermia, garlic, and vaccines.
  - Adhesiotherapy is the use of duct tape applied to the wart daily. The therapy is cheap, painless, and has been reported as successful.
  - Hypnosis has been used to treat refractory cases of warts.
  - Hyperthermia treatment uses hot water immersion (113°F) for 30 to 40 minutes, two to three times weekly.
  - Propolis, a resin, has immunomodulating treatment for common and plantar warts.
  - Garlic cloves (raw) have antiviral effects and should be rubbed on warts nightly then occluded.
  - Tea tree oil generally has been successful for its antimicrobial properties but has also been successful in treating warts.
- Surgical treatment has a place in wart therapy.
  - Cryotherapy is the use of liquid nitrogen at −196°C. Application of liquid nitrogen to the 1- to 2-mm rim of normal tissue every 1 to 4 weeks for up to 3 months offers the best resolution of warts. Following treatment, the skin can blister and be painful. Caution of underlying structures and nerves must be taken. Side effects can include scarring, ulceration, and pigment changes. Cryotherapy can cause a central clearing of the wart with an annular recurrence of the wart surrounding the treated area. This is called a doughnut wart (Figure III.61).
  - Electrodessication and curettage is painful, likely to scar, and HPV can be isolated in the plume. This treatment is typically avoided because of its risks.
- Laser treatment is expensive and requires multiple treatments, so it is generally reserved for extensive or refractory warts. Anesthesia may be required before the therapy. Health care workers are at risk for infection caused by HPV isolation in the plume and the chance of inhalation. Types of laser treatments include the following:
  - Carbon dioxide lasers treat resistant warts with success. These lasers can leave scarring and be painful during the procedure.
  - A flash-pumped pulse dye laser targets the blood vessels that supply the lesions. This laser has less risk of scarring or transmitting the HPV.
  - Nd:YAG laser is used to treat large, deep warts.

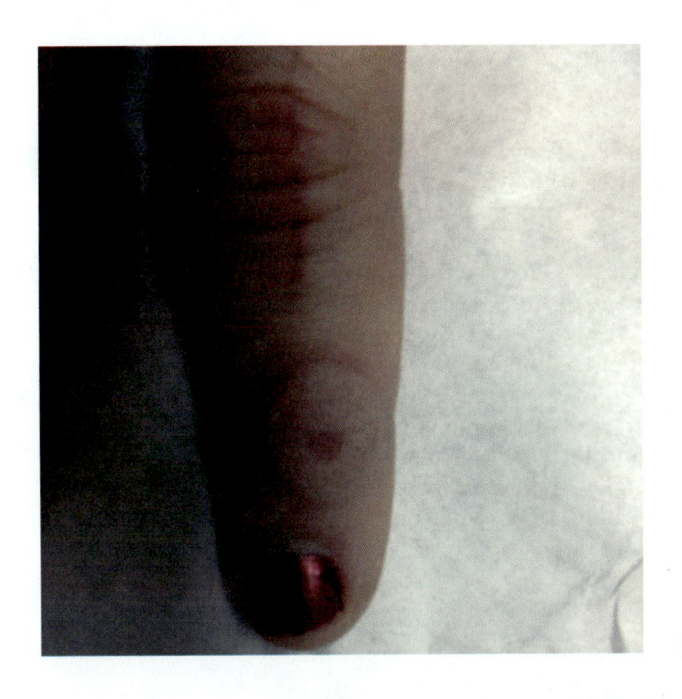

FIGURE III.62  Doughnut wart

The majority of warts (65%) resolve within 2 years without any form of treatment. When they resolve on their own, there is no scarring. Treatment methods described here can lead to scarring. Treatment failures are common, as are reoccurrences, especially in immunocompromised patients. The skin may appear normal but in fact harbors HPV, which can explain reoccurrences (Shenefelt, 2012).

## SPECIAL CONSIDERATIONS

Predisposing factors and conditions that can promote verruca include atopic dermatitis or any disease that creates decreased cell-mediated immunity (e.g., AIDS or organ transplantation; Goldstein & Goldstein, 2013). Verruca affects a patient's quality of life by creating embarrassment, fear of ridicule, and persistent refractory lesions (Lipke, 2006).

## WHEN TO REFER

Resistant and extensive warts require referral to a dermatologist for assessment and treatment.

## PATIENT EDUCATION

Patient education must emphasize risk factors for transmission of lesions. Risk factors include trauma or maceration of the skin, hands working in wet conditions for a large period of time, hyperhidrosis of the feet, swimming pools, and nail biting. Butchers and slaughterhouse employees are also at risk for developing warts (Shenefelt, 2012). Educate patients that picking or biting warts off can facilitate spread. Patients and parents need to understand the options for treatment, as well as the risks and costs of the various treatments.

## CLINICAL PEARLS

- Verruca vulgaris: ICD-9, 078.1; ICD-10, B07
- Practicing benign neglect for warts in children is a viable option; the majority of children's warts resolve spontaneously (Goodheart, 2011).
- Occlusion is the easiest and least costly treatment for warts. Cover the lesion in duct tape for 6 days and then soak, reduce the lesion with an emery board, leave uncovered overnight, then reapply the duct tape and repeat this cycle for 8 weeks (Goodheart, 2011). Studies have suggested that this is a more effective treatment for common warts than cryotherapy (Habif, 2004).
- Wart severity and duration may be explained by individual variations in cell-mediated immunity (Habif, Campbell, Chapman, Dinulos, & Zug, 2011).
- Warts grow in the epidermis and interrupt normal skin lines, so warts can be considered resolved when normal skin lines reappear (Habif et al., 2011).
- Warts are spread by biting, picking, or shaving of their surface (Habif et al., 2011).

## REFERENCES

Goldstein, B. G., & Goldstein, A. O. (2013). *Cutaneous warts*. Retrieved from http://www.uptodate.com/contents/cutaneous-warts

Goodheart, H. (2011). *Same-site differential diagnosis*. Philadelphia, PA: Lippincott Williams &Wilkin.

Habif, T. (2004). *Clinical dermatology: A color guide to diagnosis and therapy* (4th ed.). Philadelphia, PA: Mosby.

Habif, T., Campbell, J., Chapman, M., Dinulos, J., & Zug, K. (2011). *Skin disease diagnosis and treatment* (3rd ed.). Philadelphia, PA: Elsevier/Saunders.

James, W. D., Berger, T. G., & Elston, D. M. (2006). *Andrews' diseases of the skin: Clinical dermatology* (10th ed.). Philadelphia, PA: Saunders/Elsevier.

Lipke, M. M. (2006). An armamentarium of wart treatments. *Clinical Medicine & Research*, 4(4), 273–293.

Mulhem, E., & Pinelis, S. (2011). Treatment of nongenital cutaneous warts. *American Family Physician*, 84(3), 288–293.

Shenefelt, P. D. (2012, October 30). *Nongenital warts*. Retrieved from http://emedicine.medscape.com/article/1133317-overview

(2012). Treat cutaneous warts on a case-by-case basis, taking into account patient factors and the available clinical evidence. *Drugs & Therapy Perspectives*, 28(8), 15–19.

# Vitiligo

## OVERVIEW

Vitiligo is an acquired pigment disorder of the skin and mucous membranes characterized by circumscribed depigmented macules and patches (Figure III.63). Vitiligo is a progressive disorder in which some or all of the melanocytes in the affected skin are selectively destroyed. Vitiligo affects 0.5% to 2% of the world population, and the average age of onset is 20 years (Groysman, 2011; James, Berger, & Elston, 2006; Silverberg, 2010; Wheeland, 2006).

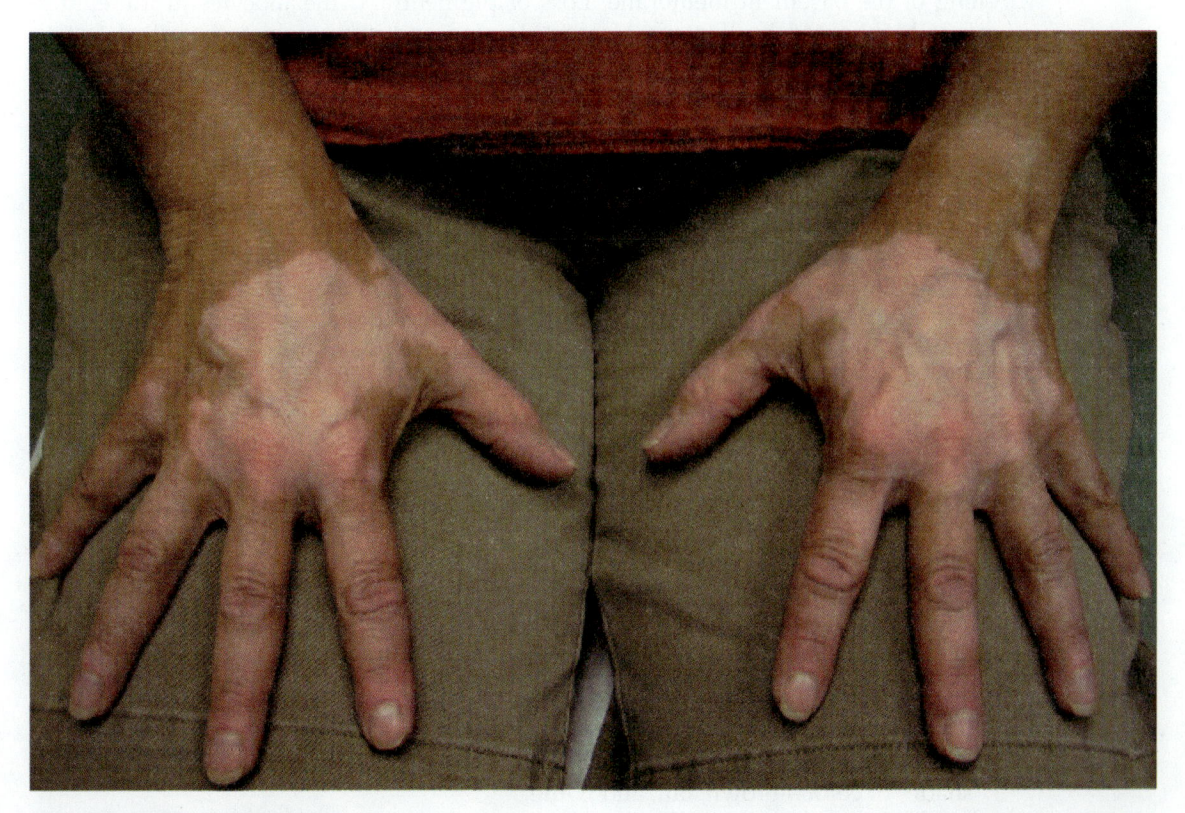

FIGURE III.63.   Vitiligo

## EPIDEMIOLOGY

In the United States, the rate of vitiligo is 1% to 2%; specific countries, such as India, report prevalence rates of 4.0% to 8.8%. Females have been reported to be more frequently affected; however, the discrepancy has been attributed to an increase in reporting of cosmetic concerns by female patients. Vitiligo may appear at any age, although the onset is most commonly observed in persons aged 10 to 30 years. A positive family history is present in 30% of patients (Bhandarkar, 2012; Chan & Chua, 2012; Groysman, 2011; James et al., 2006; Wheeland, 2006).

## PATHOLOGY/HISTOLOGY

There are several proposed theories about the pathogenesis of vitiligo; however, the specific cause remains unknown. The generally agreed–upon theory supported by medical data is autoimmune pigment cell attack or destruction. This destruction is most likely a slow process, resulting in a progressive decrease of melanocytes. Other theories regarding destruction of melanocytes include cytotoxic mechanisms, an intrinsic defect of melanocytes, oxidant-antioxidant mechanisms, and neural mechanisms (Groysman, 2011; James et al., 2006; Silverberg, 2010).

Microscopic examination of involved skin shows a complete absence of melanocytes in association with a total loss of epidermal pigmentation. Superficial perivascular and perifollicular lymphocytic infiltrates are seen at the margin of the vitiligo patches, consistent with a cell-mediated process destroying melanocytes. Other changes noted include increased numbers of Langerhans cells, epidermal vacuolization, and thickening of the basement membrane. Loss of pigment and melanocytes in the epidermis is highlighted by Fontana-Masson staining and immunohistochemistry testing (Groysman, 2011).

## CLINICAL PRESENTATION

The most common form of vitiligo is an amelanotic macule surrounded by healthy skin. The macules are chalk or milk-white in color and well demarcated, and the borders may be convex. Lesions enlarge from the center over a period of time at an unpredictable rate. The size of lesions may range from millimeters to centimeters. Initial lesions occur most frequently on the hands, forearms, feet, and face, favoring a perioral and periocular distribution. Involvement of the mucous membranes is frequently observed in the setting of generalized vitiligo. Vitiligo often occurs around body orifices such as the lips, genitals, gingiva, areolas, and nipples (Groysman, 2011; James et al., 2006; Wheeland, 2006).

Body hair (leukotrichia) dispersed in vitiligo macules may be depigmented. Vitiligo of the scalp usually appears as a localized patch of white or gray hair, but total depigmentation of all scalp hair may occur. Scalp involvement is the most frequent, followed by involvement of the eyebrows, pubic hair, and axillary hair, respectively (Groysman, 2011).

Clinical variations of vitiligo are (Groysman, 2011):

- Trichrome vitiligo has an intermediate zone of hypochromia located between the achromic center and the peripheral unaffected skin. The natural evolution of the hypopigmented areas is progression to full depigmentation. This results in three shades of color—brown, tan, and white.

- Marginal inflammatory vitiligo results in a red, raised border, which is present from the onset of vitiligo (in rare cases) or may appear several months or years after the initial onset.
- Quadrichrome vitiligo is another variant of vitiligo that reflects the presence of a fourth color (i.e., dark brown) at sites of perifollicular repigmentation.
- Blue vitiligo results in blue coloration of vitiligo macules. This type has been observed in patients with postinflammatory hyperpigmentation who then develop vitiligo.
- Koebner phenomenon is defined as the development of vitiligo in sites of specific trauma, such as a cut, burn, or abrasion. Minimum injury is required for Koebner phenomenon to occur. Many of the most common sites of occurrence are areas subjected to repeated trauma, including the following:
  - Bony prominences
  - Extensor forearm
  - Ventral wrists
  - Dorsal hands
  - Digital phalanges

The most widely used classification system for vitiligo is based on distribution and describes localized, generalized, and universal types (Chan & Chua, 2012; Groysman, 2011; James et al., 2006; Wheeland, 2006).

- Localized vitiligo
  - Focal: This type is characterized by one or more macules in one area, most commonly in the distribution of the trigeminal nerve.
  - Segmental: This type manifests as one or more macules in a dermatomal pattern. It occurs most commonly in children. More than half the patients with segmental vitiligo have patches of white hair or poliosis. This type of vitiligo is not associated with thyroid or other autoimmune disorders. Segmental vitiligo has one or more macules along a defined dermatome. It is most common in children, and more than 50% of patients have patches of white hair called poliosis.
  - Mucosal: Mucous membranes alone are affected.
- Generalized vitiligo
  - Acrofacial: Depigmentation occurs on the distal fingers and periorificial areas.
  - Vulgaris: This is characterized by scattered patches that are widely distributed.
  - Mixed: Acrofacial and vulgaris vitiligo occur in combination, or segmental and acrofacial vitiligo and/or vulgaris involvement are noted in combination.
- Universal vitiligo: This is complete or nearly complete depigmentation. It is often associated with multiple endocrinopathy syndromes.

## DIFFERENTIAL DIAGNOSIS

- Addison disease
- Alezzandrini syndrome
- Chemical leukoderma
- Halo nevus
- Idiopathic guttate hypomelanosis
- Leprosy
- Malignant melanoma
- Mycosis fungoides mimicking vitiligo
- Nevus anemicus
- Onchocerciasis (river blindness)
- Piebaldism

- Pityriasis alba
- Postinflammatory depigmentation
- Prior treatment with corticosteroids
- Scleroderma
- Tinea versicolor
- Treponematosis
- Tuberous sclerosis
- Vogt–Koyanagi–Harada syndrome
- Waardenburg syndrome

## TREATMENT/MANAGEMENT

Although the diagnosis of vitiligo is generally made on the basis of clinical findings, biopsy is occasionally helpful for differentiating vitiligo from other hypopigmentary disorders. Vitiligo may be associated with autoimmune diseases, especially thyroid disease and diabetes mellitus, pernicious anemia, Addison disease, and alopecia areata. Patients should be made aware of signs and symptoms that suggest the onset of hypothyroidism, diabetes, or other autoimmune diseases. If signs or symptoms occur, appropriate tests should be performed (Groysman, 2011; James et al., 2006; Silverberg, 2010; Wheeland, 2006).

- Thyrotropin testing is the most cost-effective screening test for thyroid disease. Clinicians should also consider investigating for serum antithyroglobulin and antithyroid peroxidase antibodies. Antithyroid peroxidase antibodies are regarded as a sensitive and specific marker of autoimmune thyroid antibodies.
- A complete blood count with indices helps rule out macrocytic anemia.
- Screening for diabetes can be accomplished with fasting blood glucose or glycosylated hemoglobin testing.
- Vitamin D levels that are lower than 15 ng/mL may indicate possible autoimmune disorders.
- Antinuclear antibody (ANA) testing is ordered to screen for autoimmune disorders.
- Homocysteine levels should be evaluated in South American, Middle Eastern, and Indian patients because of restricted diets.
- Folic acid, vitamin $B_6$, and vitamin $B_{12}$ levels should be done if macrocytic anemia or homocysteine levels are elevated.

   Types of therapy include:

- Systemic phototherapy induces cosmetically satisfactory repigmentation in up to 70% of patients with early or localized disease. Narrow-band ultraviolet (UV)-B phototherapy is widely used and produces good clinical results. This treatment can be safely used in children, pregnant women, and lactating women. Short-term adverse effects include pruritus and xerosis.
- Psoralen photochemotherapy involves the use of psoralens combined with UVA light. Treatment with 8-methoxypsoralen, 5-methoxypsoralen, and psoralen plus UVA (PUVA) has often been the most practical choice for treatment, especially in patients with skin types IV to VI who have widespread vitiligo. Psoralens can be applied either topically or orally, followed by exposure to artificial UV light or natural sunlight. Vitiligo on the back of the hands and feet is highly resistant to therapy. The best results from PUVA can be obtained on the face, trunk, and proximal parts of the extremities. However, two to three treatments per week for many months are required before repigmentation from perifollicular openings merges to

produce confluent repigmentation. The total number of PUVA treatments required is 50 to 300. Repigmentation occurs in a perifollicular pattern.
- Another innovation is therapy with an excimer laser, which produces monochromatic rays at 308 nm to treat limited, stable patches of vitiligo. This new treatment is an efficacious, safe, and well-tolerated treatment for vitiligo when limited to less than 30% of the body surface. However, therapy is expensive. Localized lesions of vitiligo are treated twice weekly for an average of 24 to 48 sessions.
- Systemic steroids (prednisone) have been used, although prolonged use is undesirable owing to their toxicity. Steroids have been reported anecdotally to achieve success when given in pulse doses or small doses to minimize adverse effects.
- A topical steroid preparation is often chosen first to treat localized vitiligo because it is easy and convenient for both doctors and patients to maintain the treatment. The results of therapy have been reported as moderately successful, particularly in patients with localized vitiligo and/or an inflammatory component to their vitiligo, even if the inflammation is subclinical.
- Topical tacrolimus ointment (0.03% or 0.1%) is an effective alternative therapy for vitiligo, particularly when the disease involves the head and neck. Combination treatment with topical tacrolimus 0.1% plus the 308-nm excimer laser is superior to monotherapy with the 308-nm excimer laser for UV-resistant vitiliginous lesions. On the face, narrow-band UVB works better if combined with pimecrolimus 1% cream rather than used alone.
- Vitamin D analogs, particularly calcipotriol and tacalcitol, have been used as topical therapeutic agents in vitiligo. The combination of topical calcipotriene and narrow-band UVB or PUVA results in appreciably better improvement than that achieved with monotherapy.
- If vitiligo is widespread and attempts at repigmentation do not produce a satisfactory result, depigmentation may be attempted in selected patients. The long-term social and emotional consequences of depigmentation must be considered. Depigmentation should not be attempted unless the patient fully understands that the procedure generally results in permanent depigmentation. A 20% cream of monobenzylether of hydroquinone is applied twice daily for 3 to 12 months. Burning or itching may occur. Allergic contact dermatitis may be seen. (Chan & Chua, 2012; Groysman, 2011; James et al., 2006; Silverberg, 2010; Wheeland, 2006)

## SPECIAL CONSIDERATIONS

Skin color plays a major role in an individual's perception of health and wealth. Vitiligo can decrease one's chances of obtaining certain occupations because of an undesirable appearance and vitiligo can influence social interactions and affect self-esteem. Many patients find their disfigurement intolerable and may suffer from embarrassment and depression. Childhood, especially adolescence, is characterized by rapid psychological and social development, coupled with emotional vulnerability. Negative experiences as a result of disfiguring diseases such as vitiligo can affect childhood psychological and emotional development (Bhandarkar, 2012; Chan & Chua, 2012; James et al., 2006).

Vitiligo affects men and women equally, although studies suggest that women have more adverse effects on quality of life than men. Women tend to be more psychosocially affected by skin diseases. In some geographic regions, such as India and Saudi Arabia, vitiligo in women can have severe social consequences that affect their ability to find a partner (Bhandarkar, 2012; Chan & Chua, 2012).

## WHEN TO REFER

Consultation with a dermatologist and ophthalmologist is warranted. Additionally, psychological needs must be addressed on a continual basis with appropriate referrals to mental health specialists (Chan & Chua, 2012; Groysman, 2011).

## PATIENT EDUCATION

Patients should be advised about the risk of sunburn at areas of vitiligo. Application of sunscreen with UVA/UVB block SPF 30 is recommended.

### CLINICAL PEARLS

- Vitiligo: ICD-9, 709.1; ICD-10, L80
- A helpful resource is the National Vitiligo Foundation (www.nvfi.org).
- Vitiligo is characterized by enlarging depigmented "starkwhite" lesions on the periorbital, perioral, anogenital, elbows, knees, axillae, inguinal folds, and forearms (Yohn, 2011).
- When assessing vitiligo, using a Wood's light to examine lesions differentiates depigmentation from hypopigmentation (Wolff, Johnson & Saavedra, 2013).
- A Wood's light examination of vitiligo should expose a "milk-white" fluorescence (Goodheart, 2011).
- A skin biopsy identifies normal skin without melanocytes (Wolff et al., 2013).
- Appropriate treatment requires an honest discussion of the patient's goals and expectations and the benefits and risks of treatment choices (Habif, Campbell, Chapman, Dinulos, & Zug, 2011).

## REFERENCES

Bhandarkar, S. S. (2012). Quality-of-life issues in vitiligo. *Dermatology Clinics, 30,* 255–268.

Chan, M. F., & Chua, T. L. (2012). The effectiveness of therapeutic interventions on quality of life for vitiligo patients: A systematic review. *International Journal of Nursing Practice, 18,* 396–405.

Habif, T., Campbell, J., Chapman, M., Dinulos, J., & Zug, K. (2011). *Skin disease diagnosis and treatment* (3rd ed.). Philadelphia, PA: Elsevier/Saunders.

Goodheart, H. (2011). *Goodheart's same-site differential diagnosis: A rapid method of diagnosing and treating common skin disorders.* Philadelphia, PA: Lippincott Williams & Wilkins.

Groysman, V. (2011, September 29). *Vitiligo.* Retrieved from http://emedicine.medscape.com/article/1068962-overview

James, W. D., Berger, T. G., & Elston, D. M. (2006). *Andrew's diseases of the skin: Clinical dermatology* (10th ed.). Philadelphia, PA: Saunders/Elsevier.

Silverberg, N. B. (2010). Update on childhood vitiligo. *Current Opinion in Pediatrics, 22,* 445–452.

Wheeland, R. G. (2006, December). What are those white patches? *Patient Care,* 47–50.

Wolff, K., Johnson, R. A., & Saavedra, A. (2013). *Fitzpatrick's color atlas and synopsis of clinical dermatology* (7th ed.). Philadelphia, PA: McGraw-Hill Medical.

Yohn, J. (2011). Disorders of pigmentation. In J. E. Fitzpatrick & J. G. Morelli (Eds.). *Dermatology secrets plus* (4th ed., pp. 126–134). Philadelphia, PA: Elsevier Mosby.

# Glossary

**Abrasion.** A breakage in the upper layers of the skin due to trauma from friction, typically in the epidermal layer of the skin. *See also* Skin tear.

**Abscess** (also called a boil or furuncle). A deep infection of a hair follicle.

**Acanthosis nigricans.** A skin condition that causes darkening and thickening of skin, mainly in the skinfolds of the neck, axillae, under breasts, and groin. This disorder is typically seen in obese patients, and although not curable, it may improve with weight loss. In most people, acanthosis nigricans precedes diabetes and is a skin manifestation of insulin resistance.

**Acne.** A common skin condition that affects all ages and both sexes. In acne, hyperkeratinization blocks the hair follicle, trapping the sebum. This entrapment results in inflammation of the hair follicle and the production of a comedone, which is the precursor of acne lesions.

**Acneform lesions.** Follicular eruptions that consist of papules and pustules that appear to be similar to acne; the dermatoses include acne vulgaris, rosacea, folliculitis, and perioral dermatitis.

**Actinic keratosis.** A cutaneous lesion that results from chronic ultraviolet (UV) exposure from the sun and tanning beds/booths, or UV therapy, causing abnormal production of atypical epidermal keratinocytes. Also known as a solar keratosis.

**Allergic contact dermatitis.** An acquired skin sensitivity to numerous substances that produce inflammatory reactions in persons who have been previously sensitized to the allergen.

**Alopecia.** Hair loss.

**Alopecia areata.** A common nonscarring disorder that causes hair loss.

**Androgenic alopecia.** A hair-loss disorder in which hair follicles contain androgen receptors, which stimulate genes that shorten the anagen (or growth) phase of hair follicles.

**Angular cheilitis.** An acute or chronic inflammation of the oral commissures caused by mechanical trauma and/or fungal (e.g., *Candida* species) or bacterial infection. Also called *perleche*.

**Annular lesions.** Lesions that occur in a ring shape with central clearing. Examples include tinea corporis, granuloma annulare, erythema migrans (the lesion associated with lyme disease), some dermatophyte infections (ringworm), and drug eruptions and secondary syphilis.

**Aphthous stomatitis.** A painful oral mucosal condition that is not contagious and is not related to any viral, bacterial, or fungal infections. It is considered an unusual type of autoimmune reaction.

**Apocrine glands.** Specialized structures found only in the axillae, nipples, areolae, anogenital area, eyelids, and external ears. These glands are larger and located more deeply than the eccrine glands. In response to stimuli, these glands secrete a white fluid containing protein, carbohydrate, and other substances.

**Atopic dermatitis.** A skin disease of unknown origin that usually starts in early infancy and is characterized by pruritus, eczematous lesions, xerosis, and lichenification; also known as eczema.

**Atrophy.** A thinning of epidermis or dermis, or subcutaneous fat, creating a depression in the skin.

**Auspitz sign.** The appearance of bleeding points when scale from a rash is removed from psoriatic lesions.

**Basal cell carcinoma.** The most common skin cancer in the United States, Australia, New Zealand, and multiple other countries that have a large White, fair-skinned population. It is more common on sun-exposed skin. Lesions are slow growing and do not normally metastasize.

**Biopsy.** A procedure used to remove the skin cells or obtain skin samples to aid in diagnosis.

**Black hairy tongue (lingua villosa nigra).** A benign condition associated with antibiotic use, *Candida albicans*, or poor hygiene.

**Blackhead.** An open comedo. *See also* Acne; Comedo.

**Blanching.** A lesion whitens with a small amount of downward pressure, indicating that the erythema is the result of vasodilation rather than dermal bleeding. Blanching is often seen with drug eruptions, viral exanthems, Kawasaki disease, roseola, and scarlet fever.

**Blister.** *See* Bulla.

**Boil.** *See* Abscess.

**Bruise.** Discoloration of the skin resulting from injury to the underlying structures causing bleeding from ruptured blood vessels.

**Bulla.** A raised fluid-filled or pus-filled lesion 0.5 cm or larger.

**Bullosis diabeticorum.** Blisters that occur in diabetic patients with severe disease who have diabetic neuropathy. Also called diabetic blisters; they resemble burn blisters.

They occur on the fingers, hands, toes, feet, legs, or forearms. These painless blisters typically heal without treatment.

**Burns.** Skin injuries that result from heat (thermal), chemical exposure, or radiation (e.g., sunburn). Burns are classified as *first-degree (superficial)*, which involve the epidermis; *second-degree (superficial partial-thickness)*, which involve the epidermis and parts of the dermis; and *third-degree (full-thickness)*, which affect the epidermis and all of the dermis.

**Burrow.** A narrow, raised, twisting canal formed by a parasite.

***Candida.*** A genus of yeast that is currently the most common cause of fungal infections worldwide. The variations of infection with *Candida* species range from local mucous membrane infections to widespread dissemination and multisystem organ failure. *Candida albicans* causes a large number of fungal infections in diabetic patients.

**Cellular stratum.** The skin layer where keratin cells are synthesized.

**Cellulitis.** An acute, dispersing infection of dermal and subcutaneous tissues, distinguished by a red, hot, tender area of skin, often at the site of bacterial entry.

**Chemical cautery.** The selective destruction of skin tissues using chemical agents. Also called chemotherapy or chemosurgery.

**Clustered lesions.** Lesions that are grouped together. They are seen in herpes simplex or with insect bites.

**Comedo.** Entrapped sebum and dead cells that plug and inflame a hair follicle, often covered with a black (blackhead) or white (whitehead) dot. Comedones (pl.) are precursors of acne lesions.

**Confluent lesions.** Lesions that run together.

**Contact dermatitis.** A dermatoses caused by an external agent. The major types are irritant contact dermatitis and allergic contact dermatitis.

**Contusion.** *See* Bruise.

**Crust.** An accumulation of serum, blood, or purulent exudate that results from drying of plasma or exudate on the skin; also called a scab.

**Cryotherapy.** The controlled application of a cold substance, usually liquid nitrogen, used with the intent of causing tissue damage to treat a skin lesion.

**Culture.** A sensitivity test used to diagnose the etiology (bacterial or viral) of an infection in a sore, burn, surgical wound, or injury.

**Curettage.** A scraping or scooping technique performed with a dermal curette.

**Cyst.** A sac containing liquid or semisolid material usually in the dermis. *See also* Epidermoid/sebaceous cyst.

**Dermatitis.** A group of diseases that involve inflammation, erythema, and papulovesicular lesions of the skin with acute disease and scaling of the skin in chronic disease. The most common dermatitis presentations are atopic dermatitis, seborrheic dermatitis, and allergic/contact dermatitis.

**Dermatitis herpetiformis.** An autoimmune blistering disorder caused by a gluten-sensitive enteropathy and characterized by grouped excoriations due to severe pruritus; erythematous, urticarial plaques; and papules with vesicles. Areas commonly affected with lesions are the extensor surfaces of the elbows, knees, buttocks, and back. It is a lifelong disease, although periods of exacerbation and remission are common.

**Dermatomal lesions.** Zosteriform lesions follow a dermatome. The lesions of varicella-zoster (also known as shingles) are the classic example, but other lesions assume the same pattern.

**Dermatomes.** The portion of the skin surface that forms connective tissue, including the dermis.

**Dermatophytes.** Pathogenic fungi that grow on skin; one of the most common infectious agents occurring in humans, causing various clinical disorders that are together termed *dermatophytosis*.

**Dermatoscopy.** A noninvasive diagnostic technique used for evaluation of skin lesions by magnification.

**Dermatosis.** Skin disease.

**Dermis.** The layer of skin connected to underlying organs by the hypodermis; a subcutaneous layer that consists of loose connective tissue filled with fatty cells.

**Desquamation.** Shedding of stratum corneum or keratin; also called scaling, exfoliation, or peeling.

**Diaper dermatitis.** A form of irritant contact dermatitis that can affect anyone who is incontinent and wears diapers or disposable briefs. Diaper dermatitis can be caused by *Candida* species.

**Digital sclerosis.** A condition in diabetic persons that causes the skin on the toes, fingers, and hands to become thick, waxy, and tight. Stiffness of the finger joints can also occur.

**Discrete lesions.** Lesions that tend to remain separate.

**Disseminated granuloma annulare.** A condition in diabetic persons that causes sharply defined, ring- or arc-shaped areas on the skin. These lesions occur most often on the fingers and ears, but they can occur on the chest and abdomen.

**Distribution.** How the skin lesions are scattered or spread out.

**Ecchymosis.** Extravasation of blood into the skin that is greater than 0.5 cm in diameter and appearing as a purplish patch.

**Eccrine glands.** Glands that open directly to the skin and regulate body temperature through water secretion. These glands are all over the body except the lip margins, eardrums, nailbeds, inner surface of the prepuce, and the glans penis.

**Eczema.** *See* Atopic dermatitis.

**Electrocautery.** A cauterization technique that uses a low-voltage, high-amperage electric current to heat a filament tip. The tip transfers the heat to the patient's tissue, inducing coagulation.

**Electrodessication and curettage.** A treatment method to remove or destroy benign superficial skin lesions.

**Ephelides.** An increase in pigment content in the basal cell layer of skin from sun exposure that results in a small brownish spot; also called a freckle.

**Epidermis.** The outermost portion of the skin, consisting of two major layers: the stratum corneum and the cellular stratum.

**Epidermoid/sebaceous cyst.** The most common cutaneous cysts, epidermoid cysts are typically benign lesions with rare cases of malignancy. Also called *follicular infundibular cysts*, *epidermal cysts*, *epidermal inclusion cysts*, and *sebaceous cysts*.

**Erosion.** A loss of epidermis above the basal layer, leaving a denuded surface; due to location, erosions do not leave a scar.

**Eruptive xanthomatosis.** A skin lesion that occurs in diabetic persons with uncontrolled blood glucose and extremely elevated serum triglycerides. The lesions form as firm, yellow, pea-like papules on the skin of the feet, arms, legs, buttocks, and backs of the hands.

**Erysipelas.** An acute beta-hemolytic Group A streptococcal infection of the skin involving the superficial dermal lymphatics; also known as *St. Anthony's fire* or *ignis sacer*.

**Erythema multiforme.** An acute, immune-mediated condition characterized by the appearance of unique target-like lesions on the skin.

**Erythema nodosum.** The most commonly diagnosed form of inflammatory panniculitis, characterized by an acute, nodular, erythematous eruption that usually affects the extensor parts of the lower legs.

**Escar.** A hard, usually darkened, plaque covering an ulcer implying extensive tissue necrosis, infarct, or gangrene.

**Excisional biopsy.** A biopsy requiring a scalpel to remove an entire area or mass of abnormal skin (generally larger and deeper), including a portion of normal skin down to or through the fatty layer of skin.

**Excoriation.** Linear crust and erosion due to scratching or rubbing; traumatized or abraded skin caused by scratching or rubbing.

**Fibroblasts.** Cells in connective tissue that produce the skin's collagen and elastin fibers.

**Fissure.** A linear crack in the skin with sharply defined walls; created by a loss of the dermis and epidermis (e.g., cracked lips, cracks caused by fungal infection such as athlete's foot).

**Full-thickness wound.** A skin tear separating both the epidermis and the dermis from underlying structures.

**Furuncle.** *See* Abscess.

**Granuloma annulare.** A self-limited benign inflammatory skin condition that is fairly common and occurs in all age groups, although it is rare in infancy.

**Grouped lesions.** Lesions that group together (herpetic, zosteriform, agminate, and reticular).

**Hair follicles.** The hair root, hair shaft, and pilomotor or arrector pili muscles. Hair goes through cyclic changes: anagen (growth), catagen (atrophy), and telogen (rest), after which the hair is shed. Males and females have the same number of hair follicles, which are stimulated to differential growth by hormones.

**Herpes simplex virus.** A human pathogenic DNA virus that causes a variety of disease presentations, ranging from a localized skin and mucous membrane lesion to severe distributed infections. *Herpes simplex virus type 1* (HSV-1) infections are oral lesions that are also called *cold sores*. HSV-1 can occur in other areas such as the genitalia, liver, lung, eye, and central nervous system. *Herpes simplex virus type 2* (HSV-2), or genital herpes simplex virus, is a recurrent lifelong viral infection. HSV-1 and HSV-2 can cause genital herpes infections. The clinical symptoms and course of genital herpes caused by both types are impossible to distinguish, but recurrences are more common with HSV-2.

**Herpes zoster.** A cutaneous viral infection caused by the reactivation of varicella-zoster virus (VZV), a herpesvirus that also causes varicella (chickenpox). Herpes zoster is also known as *shingles*. The response to varicella and herpes zoster depends on an individual's immune status; those with no previous exposure to VZV, most commonly children, develop varicella, whereas those with previous exposure to varicella develop a localized recurrence, zoster.

**Herpetic whitlow.** A herpes simplex virus infection of the fingers that can occur as a complication of primary oral or genital herpes by inoculation of the virus through a break in the skin barrier.

**Herpetiform lesions.** Grouped umbilicated vesicles as arise in herpes simplex and herpes zoster infections.

**Hidradenitis suppurativa.** A chronic, follicular, occlusive disease characterized by recurrent boils or abscesses (cysts) primarily affecting the intertriginous skin of the axillae, groin, genital, perianal, and inframammary areas.

**Hirsutism.** Abnormal growth of hair.

**Hypodermis.** The adipose layer of skin that generates heat and provides insulation, shock absorption, and calorie reserve.

**Impetigo.** An acute, contagious Gram-positive bacterial infection of the upper layers of the epidermis that arises near the site of *Staphylococcus aureus* colonization, for example, in the nares.

**Incision and drainage.** The primary management for cutaneous abscess formation.

**Ingrown toenail (onychocryptosis).** A condition in which the lateral nail plate pierces the lateral nail fold and enters the dermis; the great toenail is primarily affected.

**Iris-target lesions.** Lesions that form a series of concentric rings and have a dark or blistered center. These lesions are frequently seen with erythema multiforme.

**Irritant contact dermatitis.** A type of contact dermatitis that occurs when the skin comes in contact with a substance that is harsh to the skin. The severity of the inflammation is dependent on the concentration of the irritant and the exposure time.

**Keloid.** An exaggerated connective tissue response of injured skin that extends beyond the edges of the original wound.

**Keratosis pilaris.** A common, autosomal dominant skin condition manifested by the appearance of rough, white or red bumps on the skin. It generally appears on the back and outer sides of the arm (although the forearm can be affected) and can also occur on the thighs, hands, and tops of legs, sides, buttocks, or any body part except the palms or soles of feet.

**Koebner phenomenon.** The development of typical lesions at the site of a trauma characteristic of psoriasis and lichen planus.

**Koebnerization.** Development of new psoriatic lesions at sites of trauma.

**Langerhans cells.** Originating in the bone marrow, these cells break down foreign material such as bacteria that enter our bodies through breaks in the skin and travel to the lymph nodes, which triggers an immune response.

**Lentigo.** A benign, small, sharply circumscribed, pigmented macule surrounded by normal-appearing skin that results from increased activity of the epidermal melanocytes and does not fade with lack of sun exposure.

**Lesion.** Any single area of skin or an organ that has suffered damage through injury or disease; this can include wounds, bruises, abscesses, tumors, for example.

**Leukocytoclastic vasculitis.** A hypersensitivity vasculitis, also known as small-vessel vasculitis, that may be isolated on the skin or manifest in other organs. The internal organs commonly affected include the joints, the gastrointestinal tract, and the kidneys.

**Lichen planus.** A rare, pruritic, inflammatory disease of the skin, mucous membranes, and hair follicles. The skin lesions are characteristically purple shiny, flat-topped papules.

**Lichen simplex chronicus.** Thickening of the skin that arises secondary to vigorous scratching, rubbing, or picking beyond the normal tolerable pain threshold; also known as neurodermatitis.

**Lichenification.** (1) An accentuation of skin markings commonly associated with thickening of epidermis usually caused by scratching or rubbing. (2) Skin marked by the presence of fine papules.

**Linear lesions.** Lesions that occur in a straight line or bandlike configuration. This descriptive term may apply to a wide variety of disorders and can be suggestive of some forms of contact dermatitis, linear epidermal nevi, and lichen striatus.

**Macule.** A circumscribed change in skin color without elevation or depression; may be brown, blue, red, or hypopigmented.

**Malignant melanoma.** A type of skin cancer that arises from the melanocytes in the skin, which may be abnormal or healthy. Melanoma can occur anywhere on the body. It is responsible for only about 5% of skin cancers; however, it accounts for three times as many deaths each year compared with nonmelanoma skin cancers.

**Melanin.** A protein that gives human skin color. Both heredity and exposure to UV light contribute to melanin production. Additionally, the color of one's hair and eyes is derived from melanin.

**Melanocytes.** Cells found in the lower epidermis that produce protein, a pigment called melanin.

**Melanonychia.** A brown or black pigmentation of the nail due to the presence of melanin in the nail plate.

**Melasma.** Hyperpigmentation of the skin.

**Milia.** A small superficial keratin cyst that has no evident opening.

**Mohs micrographic surgery.** A precise, microscopically controlled serial method of skin cancer removal that allows excision and maximum preservation of the normal tissue surrounding the lesion. The goal of the surgery is to completely excise the tumor and maximize tissue conservation.

**Molluscum contagiosum virus.** A large DNA-containing benign viral infection that affects humans and is caused by four closely related types of poxvirus. The virus causes characteristic skin lesions consisting of multiple, rounded, dome-shaped, pink, and waxy papules 2 to 5 mm in diameter.

**Morbilliform.** A rash consists of macular lesions that are red and are usually 2 to 10 mm in diameter but may be confluent in places.

**Multiform lesions.** Lesions that include a variety of shapes.

**Nails.** Epidermal cells converted to hard plates of keratin.

**Necrobiosis lipoidica diabeticorum.** A common condition that occurs in diabetes and is caused by changes in the blood vessels and the collagen and fat content underneath the skin. The overlaying skin area becomes thinned, raised, waxy in appearance, and reddened. Most lesions are found on the lower parts of the legs and have fairly well-defined borders between normal skin.

**Neurodermatitis.** *See* Lichen simplex chronicus.

**Nevi.** Sharply circumscribed intradermal benign skin lesions; commonly referred to as *moles* or *birthmarks*.

**Nikolsky sign.** The easy separation of the epidermis from the dermis with lateral pressure; associated with staphylococcal scalded skin syndrome and toxic epidermal necrolysis.

**Nodule.** A palpable solid lesion of varying size, greater than 0.5 cm and less than 2 cm in diameter, which may be present in the epidermis, dermis, or subcutis; a large nodule is called a tumor.

**Nummular lesions.** Round or coin-shaped lesions also known as discoid; an example is nummular eczema.

**Onychomycosis.** A fungal infection that can affect any part of the nails, causing pain, discomfort, and deformity of the nail that may produce serious physical and occupational limitations.

**Oropharyngeal candidiasis (thrush).** A common local fungal infection of the mouth.

**Palmar erythema.** Superficial reddening of the skin in pregnancy that usually appears within the first trimester, attributed to venous capillary engorgement.

**Papule.** A solid raised lesion usually 0.5 cm or less in diameter; color varies; may become confluent or form plaques.

**Parakeratosis.** A condition seen in psoriasis in which cells that normally shed their nuclei in the stratum granulosum keep their nuclei.

**Paronychia.** A superficial painful infection of the epithelium lateral and proximal to the nail plate. The purulent infection is most frequently caused by trauma to the nail fold and staphylococci infection but usually has mixed aerobic and anaerobic flora.

**Partial-thickness wound.** Tissue destruction that extends through the epidermis but not through the dermis.

**Pemphigus.** A group of autoimmune blistering diseases on the skin and mucous membranes. There are three types of pemphigus: pemphigus vulgaris, pemphigus foliaceus, and paraneoplastic pemphigus.

**Perioral dermatitis.** A common inflammatory disorder of facial skin that is more frequent in patients with rosacea.

**Petechiae.** A confined deposit of blood less than 0.5 cm in diameter.

**Pityriasis rosea.** A benign rash seen in healthy children and adults manifested by an acute papular eruption that usually lasts 1 to 2 months. It has a sudden onset, with a primary lesion called a *herald patch*.

**Plaque.** A raised superficial solid lesion more than 0.5 cm in diameter; can be formed by the confluence of papules.

**Polycystic.** Having or containing many cysts.

**Primary skin lesion.** A lesion that appears in reaction to the external or internal environment leading to physical changes in the skin caused by a disease process.

*Propionibacterium acnes.* A bacterium that is part of normal skin-surface flora that populates acne lesions.

**Psoriasis.** A persistent, noncommunicable, systemic, inflammatory disease typically characterized by scaled erythematous macules, papules, and plaques. Patients with psoriasis have a genetic susceptibility for the disorder. Lesions will typically appear on the scalp, torso, elbows, and knees.

**Punch biopsy.** A biopsy using a circular punch tool to remove a small section of skin including the epidermis, dermis, and superficial fat.

**Purpura.** A confined deposit of blood greater than 0.5 cm in diameter.

**Pustule.** A circumscribed elevated lesion filled with leukocytes and free fluid that varies in size, is smaller in size and more superficial than an abscess.

**Rash.** A widespread eruption of skin lesions.

**Recurrent aphthous stomatitis.** *See* Aphthous stomatitis.

**Rosacea.** A common chronic and relapsing inflammatory skin condition characterized by symptoms of facial flushing and clinical signs, including erythema, telangiectasia, roughness of skin, and inflammatory acne-like eruptions. Persistent erythema on the central face for greater than 3 months is the definition of rosacea.

**Scab.** *See* Crust.

**Scabies.** A contagious disease caused by the mite *Sarcoptes scabiei*.

**Scale.** Flakes or plates that represent compacted desquamated layers of stratum corneum; desquamation occurs when there are peeling sheets of scale following acute injury to the skin.

**Scar.** A dermal and epidermal change associated with wound healing. Scars are permanent fibrotic changes that occur on the skin after damage to the dermis. They can have secondary pigment characteristics. They may be hypertrophic (raised), atrophic (depressed), or icepack (stablike).

**Scleredema diabeticorum.** A rare condition that most often affects people with type 2 diabetes and causes a thickening of the skin on the back of the neck and upper back.

**Scrapings.** A procedure to diagnosis skin diseases. To evaluate a scaly lesion of suspected fungal etiology, a scalpel is used to gently scrape the superficial surface or active border of the lesion edge. The sample is then viewed under a microscope.

**Sebaceous cyst.** *See* Epidermoid/sebaceous cyst.

**Sebaceous glands.** Glands that secrete sebum, a lipid-rich substance that keeps the skin and hair from drying out.

**Seborrheic dermatitis.** A disorder that occurs on the sebum-rich areas of the scalp, face, and trunk; also linked to *Malassezia*, immunologic abnormalities, and activation of complement. Severity varies from mild dandruff to exfoliative erythroderma.

**Sebum.** A lipid-rich, oily, waxy substance produced by the sebaceous glands that lubricates the skin and keeps it from drying out.

**Secondary skin lesion.** A lesion resulting from changes over time caused by disease progression, manipulation (scratching, picking, rubbing), or treatment. Secondary lesions may evolve from primary lesions or may be caused by external forces such as scratching, trauma, infection, or the healing process.

**Serpiginous.** Lesions that appear wavy or serpentlike.

**Shave biopsy.** A biopsy using a scalpel to remove a small section of the epidermis and a portion of the dermis.

**Skin tear.** A breakage in the upper layers of the skin due to trauma from friction, separating the epidermis from the dermis (partial-thickness wound) or both the epidermis and the dermis from underlying structures (full-thickness wound).

**Skin Tear Audit Research (STAR) Classification System.** *See* STAR Classification System.

**Squamous cell carcinoma.** The second most common form of skin cancer. Most cases are induced by UV radiation. In the United States, approximately 700,000 cases are diagnosed each year, resulting in almost 2,500 deaths.

**STAR Classification System.** A method for classifying skin tears, organized into five categories.

**Stasis dermatitis.** An inflammatory skin disease that occurs on the lower extremities and is usually the earliest sign of chronic venous insufficiency with venous hypertension.

**Stratum corneum.** The outermost layer of the epidermis that protects the body against harmful environmental substances and restricts water loss. It has a waterproof keratin that lets water out but not in and protects the body from bacteria.

**Stratum germinativum.** The innermost layer of the epidermis. It is here that mitosis (growth of new cells) takes place, and new cells push old cells to the surface. Merkel cells, the receptors responsible for the sense of touch, are located in this layer.

**Striae distensae.** Linear dermal scars accompanied by epidermal atrophy, often forming during pregnancy; commonly referred to as stretch marks.

**Target lesions.** Appear as rings with central duskiness; common in erythema multiforme. Also called bull's-eye or iris lesions.

**Telangiectasia.** Small superficial dilated blood vessels.

**Telogen effluvium.** A hair-loss disorder marked by an increase in the percentage of terminal catagen/telogen hairs.

**Terminal hair follicles.** One of two types of hair follicles; terminal hair follicles are larger than vellus hair follicles, grow into the subcutaneous fat during hair growth, and produce hair that is 0.06 mm in diameter.

**Tinea barbae.** *See* Tinea faciei.

**Tinea capitis.** A skin disorder that is the result of a fungal infection of the scalp, eyebrows, and eyelashes, with a propensity for infecting hair shafts and follicles.

**Tinea faciei.** An exterior dermatophyte infection that occurs on areas of the face that lack hair. In children and women, the infection may appear on any surface of the face, to include the upper lip and chin. In men, if the infection occurs in the bearded areas it is known as *tinea barbae*.

**Tinea versicolor.** A common, benign, superficial cutaneous fungal infection usually characterized by hypopigmented or hyperpigmented macules and patches on the chest and the back. Unlike other tinea infections, tinea versicolor is not a dermatophyte infection. The organism responsible for tinea versicolor is *Malassezia furfur*, a saprophytic, lipid-dependent yeast.

**Topical medication.** A medication applied directly to the surface of the skin for treatment of a skin disease.

**Tzanck smear.** A method used to assist in the rapid diagnosis of HSV and VZV. The base of the blister is scraped with a scalpel blade, and then the adhering cells and material are spread onto a microscope slide.

**Ulcer.** A loss of epidermis through necrosis of the epidermis and part or all of dermis, leaving a depressed moist lesion.

**Urticaria.** A common dermatologic disorder characterized by blanching, raised, palpable wheals, which can be linear, annular, or serpiginous; it can be chronic (on and off for more than 6 weeks), or acute (usually resolves within 24 hours but can last up to 6 weeks). Urticaria lesions can occur on any skin area and are usually temporary and mobile.

**Vellus hair follicles.** One of two types of hair follicles; vellus hair follicles generally only extend into the reticular dermis and are usually less than 0.03 mm in diameter.

**Verruca vulgaris.** A benign growth confined to the epidermis that is caused by human papillomavirus (HPV); commonly called a wart.

**Vesicle.** A circumscribed elevated lesion that contains free fluid; vesicles are 0.5 cm or less in diameter.

**Vitiligo.** An acquired pigment disorder of the skin and mucous membranes characterized by circumscribed depigmented macules and patches.

**Vulvovaginal candidiasis.** A disorder characterized by signs and symptoms of vulvovaginal inflammation in the presence of *Candida* species.

**Wart.** *See* Verruca vulgaris.

**Wheal.** A rounded or flat-topped elevated firm plaque formed by local dermal edema, also called a hive. Wheals are generally transient and may last only a few hours.

**Whitehead.** A closed comedo. *See also* Acne; Comedo.

**Wood's light.** A hand-held black light that produces invisible long-wave (360 nm) UV radiation and can be used for diagnosis of skin diseases.

# Index

AA. *See* alopecia areata
abrasions/skin tears
   clinical presentation, 61–62
   overview, 61
   patient education, 63
   special considerations, 62–63
   treatment/management, 62
abrasives, 67
abscess, 19
acantholysis, 250
acanthosis nigricans, 30, 55
ACD. *See* allergic contact dermatitis
acid, chemical cautery, 46
acne
   classifications, 66
   clinical presentation, 66
   diagnostic tests, 66
   differential diagnosis, 67
   education and treatment plan, 69
   epidemiology, 66
   overview, 65
   pathology/histology, 66
   patient education, 69–70
   special considerations, 69
   treatment/management, 67–69
acneiform, 21
acquired diseases, 24
acquired pigment disorder of skin, 345
acral lentiginous melanoma, 290
actinic cheilitis, 281
actinic keratosis (AK)
   clinical presentation, 281
   differential diagnosis, 281–282
   epidemiology, 279–281
   overview, 279
   pathology/histology, 281
   patient education, 283
   special considerations, 282–283
   treatment/management, 282
   types of, 281
acute herpetic gingivostomatitis, 170
acute herpetic pharyngotonsillitis, 171
acute postinfectious cerebellar ataxia, 188
acute toxicity, vitamin A excess, 56
acute urticaria, 322, 323
acyclovir, 190
AD. *See* atopic dermatitis
adhesion molecules, 328
adhesiotherapy, 342
adolescence, KP, 125
aerobic bacterial cultures, 39
AGA. *See* androgenic alopecia
albinism, 299
Aldara, 45
allergic contact dermatitis (ACD)
   clinical presentation, 131
   differential diagnosis, 131–132
   epidemiology, 131
   ICD versus, 131
   overview, 129
   pathology/histology, 131
   patient education, 134
   special considerations, 133
   treatment/management, 132–133
allylamines, 309
alopecia
   alopecia areata, 72–73
   androgenic alopecia, 74–77
   overview, 71
   telogen effluvium, 73
alopecia areata (AA)
   AGA. *See* androgenic alopecia (AGA)
   autoimmune conditions, 72
   clinical presentations, 72
   epidemiology, 72
   hair-pull test aids, 75

alopecia areata (*cont.*)
  nutrition imbalance, cause of, 77
  overview, 71
  pathology/histology, 72
  T-cell-mediated autoimmune disease, 72
  treatment for, 76
alopecia universalis, 72
*Alphaherpesvirinae*, 170, 173
amelanotic macule, 346
American Cancer Society, 284, 289, 295
ANA. *See* antinuclear antibodies
anaerobic bacterial cultures, 39
anagen phase, 71
androgenic alopecia (AGA)
  clinical presentation, 74
  differential diagnosis, 74
  pathology/histology, 74
  patient education, 77
  special considerations, 76–77
  treatment/management, 74–76
anemias, 81
anesthesia, 342
angioedema, 323
angular cheilitis
  causes of, 96
  clinical presentation, 96
  differential diagnosis, 96
  epidemiology, 95
  overview, 95
  pathology/histology, 96
  patient education, 97
  special considerations, 97
  treatment/management, 97
annular, 21
anoplura, 205
antiandrogens, 121
antibacterial, topical treatment, 45
antibiotics, 68, 121, 154
antifungal agents
  SD, 145
  topical treatment, 45
antihistamines, 141
  atopic dermatitis/eczema, 137
anti-inflammatory medication, 257
antinuclear antibodies (ANA), 76
  testing, 348
antithyroid peroxidase antibodies, 348
antitumor-necrosis-factor, 252
antitumor-necrosis-factor alpha agents, 260
antiviral therapy, 154
  for erythema multiforme, 154
  for HIV, nail, 237
  for varicella-zoster virus, 183
anxiety, 69
aphthous stomatitis
  clinical presentation, 80
  consultation, 82

  differential diagnosis, 80–81
  epidemiology, 80
  overview, 79
  pathology/histology, 80
  patient education, 82
  special considerations, 82
  treatment/management, 81–82
apocrine glands, 16
arcuate dermal erythema, 165
areolas, in pregnancy, 29
arthralgia, 158
arthropoda, 205
Asboe–Hansen sign, 251
asymmetrical lesions, 22
atopic dermatitis (AD), 230
  causes of, 136
  clinical presentation, 135–136
  differential diagnosis, 135
  effects on childhood, 138
  epidemiology, 135
  overview, 134
  pathology/histology, 135
  patient education, 138
  scabies, 201
  special considerations, 138
  theories to development, 135
  treatment/management, 136–137
atrophy, 20
Auspitz sign, 37
autoantibodies, binding of, 250
autoimmune diseases, 250
autoimmune disorders, 77, 324, 325
axillae, 203


bacterial cultures, diagnostics, 39
bacterial infections, 159, 203
basal cell carcinoma (BCC)
  clinical presentation, 285–286
  differential diagnosis, 286–287
  epidemiology, 284
  overview, 283
  pathology/histology, 284–285
  patient education, 288
  special considerations, 288
  treatment/management, 287
  types of, 284
basic lesion. *See* primary lesion
basosquamous type BCC, 285
BCC. *See* basal cell carcinoma
Behçet disease, 159
Benadryl, 82
beta-hemolytic streptococci, 203
bilateral hilar lymphadenopathy, 158
bilateral lesions, 22
biologic immune modifying agents, 270
biologics, 93
biopsy, 39

biosynthetics, 93
biting insects. *See* insect bites
black hairy tongue
    clinical presentation, 98
    differential diagnosis, 98
    epidemiology, 98
    overview, 98
    pathology/histology, 98
    patient education, 99
    special considerations, 99
    treatment/management, 98–99
blanching of erythematous lesions, 37
bleeding disorders, 86
blister cells, 250
blood urea nitrogen, 153
blue nevi, 218, 219
blue vitiligo, 347
body hair (leukotrichia), vitiligo, 346
botulinum toxin, 121
Bowen disease, 296
Breslow thickness classification system, 291
bruise
    clinical presentation, 86
    differential diagnosis, 86
    epidemiology, 85
    overview, 85
    pathology/histology, 85
    patient education, 87
    special considerations, 87
    treatment/management, 86–87
bulla, 19
bullosis diabeticorum, 30
bullous diseases, 56
bullous impetigo, 194
burns
    classification of, 91
    clinical presentation, 91
    differential diagnosis, 91
    epidemiology, 90
    overview, 89
    pathology/histology, 90–91
    patient education, 94
    special considerations, 93
    treatment/management, 91–93
burrow, 20
butcher's warts, 339, 340

calcineurin inhibitors, 269
    psoriasis, 269
    seborrheic dermatitis, 145
*Candida*, 241, 242
    infection, 96
*Candida albicans*, 31, 95, 100, 105
    risk factors for development, 107
candidiasis
    angular cheilitis, 95–97
    black hairy tongue, 98–99
    diaper dermatitis, 99–102
    oral candidiasis, 102–104
    vulvovaginal candidiasis, 104–107
carbon dioxide lasers, 342
casal necklace, 56
catagen phase, 71
cauterization of lesions, 46
CD. *See* contact dermatitis
cell-mediated hypersensitivity, 131
cellular stratum, 15
cellulitis/erysipelas, 39
    antibiotics, 112
    assessment of, 111
    clinical presentation, 110
    differential diagnosis, 110–111
    epidemiology, 110
    nonantibiotic therapy, 112
    overview, 109
    pathology/histology, 110
    patient education, 114
    special considerations, 113
    treatment/management, 111–113
chemical cautery, 46
chemoresistant tumor, 293
chemosurgery. *See* chemical cautery
chemotherapeutics, 45
chemotherapy. *See* chemical cautery
chest radiography, 330
chickenpox, 181
children
    keratosis pilaris, 124, 125
    special considerations, 27
cholinergic urticaria, 325
chronic rashes, 35
chronic toxicity, vitamin A excess, 56
chronic urticaria, 321, 322, 324, 325
ciclopirox olamine, 309
Cidofovir, 341
cimetidine, 342
Clark method, 291
classic actinic keratosis, 281
cleansers, 67
climate, atopic dermatitis, 136
clinical management
    appropriate referrals, 56–57
    genetic counseling referrals, 58
    moisturizer, 54–55
    nutritional counseling, 55–56
    preventive care, 52
    protection from sun, 53–54
    routine skin care, 51–52
    skin self-examination, 52–53
clothing, protection from sun, 53
clotrimazole troche, 103
clustered, lesions, 21
coin rubbing, 28
cold-cap treatment, 76
cold sores, 169, 170, 172

comedo, 20, 66
common warts, 337, 339
compound melanocytic nevus, 217
compound nevi, 219
compresses, dressings, 92
compression, stasis dermatitis, 148
confluent, arrangement, 21
congenital/genetic diseases, 23
congenital ichthyosis, 23
congenital melanocytic nevi, 217, 219
contact dermatitis (CD)
    clinical presentation, 131
    differential diagnosis, 131–132
    epidemiology, 131
    overview, 129
    pathology/histology, 131
    patient education, 134
    treatment/management, 132–133
continuous erythema multiforme, 155
contusion. *See* bruise
conventional (acquired) melanocytic nevi, 217
corticosteroids, 154, 160
    interlesional injection of, 47
creatinine tests, 153
crust, 20
crusted scabies, 200
cryotherapy, 46–47, 121, 282, 342
cultural practices, 28–29
cupping, cultural practice, 28
curettage, 46, 282, 342
cyclosporin, 179, 269
cysts, 20
    epidermal inclusion cysts/sebacceous cyst. *See* epidermal inclusion cysts/sebacceous cyst
    HS. *See* hidradenitis suppurativa (HS)
    KP. *See* keratosis pilaris (KP)
    milia cyst. *See* milia cyst
cystic basal cell carcinoma, 285, 286
cystic warts, 339, 340

dandruff, 143
dapsone (diaminodiphenylsulfone), 179, 252
decision trees
    differential diagnoses and, 8–12
    evidence-based practice and, 6
deep palmoplantar warts (myrmecia), 339, 340
deep skin incisional biopsies, 160
dehydroepiandrosterone (DHEA), 66
*Demodex folliculorum*, 274
depression, 69
dermabrasion, 282
dermatitis, 129
    allergic/contact, 129–134
    atopic dermatitis/eczema, 134–138
    lichen simplex chronicus/neurodermatitis, 138–142
    seborrheic dermatitis, 142–146
    stasis dermatitis, 146–149

dermatitis herpetiformis (DH)
    clinical presentation, 178
    differential diagnosis, 178
    epidemiology, 178
    overview, 177–178
    pathology/histology, 178
    patient education, 179
    special considerations, 179
    treatment/management, 179
dermatologic disorder, urticaria, 321
dermatology
    diagnostic evaluations, 21
    distribution, type, characteristics, and pattern of lesions, 22
    patterns of intentional or unintentional injury, 22–25
    skin anatomy and physiology, 15–18
    skin terminology, 19–20
    vascular lesions, 21
dermatology education, 3, 4
    annual economic burden, 5
    conceptual framework, 6–8
    epidemiology and statistics of skin disorders, 4–5
    evidence-based practice and decision trees, 6
    quality of life implications, 5
dermatomes, 17, 18, 21
dermatophytes, 303
    onychomycosis, 241
    tinea corporis, 307
    tinea faciei, 311
    tinea infections, 303–304
dermatophytosis, 303
dermatoscopy, 41
dermatosis, 19
dermis, 15
desmoplastic melanoma, 290
desquamation, 20
DFA. *See* direct fluorescent antibody
DH. *See* dermatitis herpetiformis
DHEA. *See* dehydroepiandrosterone
diabetes
    in pregnancy, 30–31
    screening for, 348
diabetic dermopathy, 30
diagnostics
    mycology, 40–41
    specimens collection, 39–40
    use of mechanical devices, 41
diaminodiphenylsulfone (dapsone), 179
diaper dermatitis
    clinical presentation, 100
    differential diagnosis, 100
    epidemiology, 99
    overview, 99
    pathology/histology, 100
    patient education, 101–102
    special considerations, 101
    treatment/management, 100–101

diclofenac sodium, 282
diet, atopic dermatitis/eczema, 137
differential diagnoses, decision trees and, 8–12
digital sclerosis, 30
direct fluorescent antibody (DFA), to Tzanck smear, 183
direct immunofluorescence (DIF)
    specimen, 252
    staining and examination, 154
discoid, 21
discrete lesions, 21
disseminated granuloma annulare, 30
distal lateral subungualonychomycosis (DLSO), 241, 242
distribution, 22
DLSO. *See* distal lateral subungualonychomycosis
doughnut wart, 342, 343
dressings for burn management, 92
drug-induced pityriasis rosea, 261
dust mites control, atopic dermatitis/eczema, 137
dysplastic nevi, 219

ear impetigo, children, 193
EBP. *See* evidence-based practice
ecchymosis, 21
eccrine glands, 16
ecthyma, 194
ectothrix (gray-patch tinea capitis) infection, 304
eczema
    clinical presentation, 135
    differential diagnosis, 135
    epidemiology, 135
    overview, 134
    pathology/histology, 135
    patient education, 138
    special considerations, 138
    treatment/management, 136
edema, 158
elderly person, 27
electrocautery, 46
electrodessication, 46, 342
electrolyte values, 154
electrosurgery, 282
EN. *See* erythema nodosum
encephalitis, 188
endocrine disorder, 77
endocrinologic testing (androgen), 68
endothrix (black dot tinea capitis), 304
enteropathies, 159
environmental factors, psoriasis, 267
epidermal cysts, 115
epidermal growth factor, 252
epidermal inclusion cysts
    clinical presentation, 116
    differential diagnosis, 116
    epidemiology, 116
    overview, 115

pathology/histology, 116
patient education, 117
special considerations, treatment/management, 117
epidermal transglutaminase (e-TG), 178
epidermis, 15
epidermoid cysts, causes of, 117
epidermolysis bullosa, 24
erosion, 20
eruptive phase of erythema nodosum, 158
eruptive psoriasis, 268
eruptive xanthomatosis, 30
erysipelas, 110
    clinical presentation, 110
    differential diagnosis, 110–111
    epidemiology, 110
    overview, 109
    pathology/histology, 110
    patient education, 114
    special considerations, 113
    treatment/management, 111–113
erythema multiforme (EM)
    clinical presentation, 152–153
    differential diagnosis, 153
    epidemiology, 151–152
    overview, 151
    patient education, 155
    special considerations, 155
    treatment/management, 153–154
erythema nodosum (EN)
    clinical presentation, 158
    differential diagnosis, 158–159
    epidemiology, 158
    overview, 157
    pathology/histology, 158
    patient education, 160
    special considerations, 160
    treatment/management, 159–160
erythematotelangiectatic rosacea, 274
erythrocyte sedimentation rate, 154
erythrodermic psoriasis, 267
erythromycin, 113
eschar, 20
esophageal candidiasis, 103
e-TG. *See* epidermal transglutaminase
evidence-based practice (EBP), 6
exanthem, viral of leg, 38
excision of skin lesions, 47
excisional biopsy, 39
excoriation, 20


facial dermatitis, 130
family history
    of asthma, eczema, or allergies, 7
    skin assessment, 36

fat-soluble vitamins deficiencies, skin
    manifestations, 56
favus (tinea favosa), 304
fibroblasts, 16
fibroepithelioma, 285
filiform warts, 339
fire ant stings, 40
fissure, 20
fixed immobile psoriasis, 267
flash-pumped pulse dye laser, 342
flat warts, 339, 340
fleas inflict bites, reactions, 208
fluconazole, 305, 310
5-fluorouracil (5-FU), 45, 342
focal epithelial hyperplasia (Heck disease), 339, 340
follicular infundibular cysts, 115
food allergies, 81
food antigens, atopic dermatitis, 136
fungal folliculitis, 312
fungal infections, 159
    diabetes, 31
    seborrheic dermatitis, 143

GA. *See* granuloma annulare
gabapentin for varicella-zoster virus, 184
garlic cloves (raw), 342
gastrointestinal diseases, 81
generalized granuloma annulare, 165, 166
generalized lesions, 22
generalized vitiligo, 347
genetic counseling, 58
genetic diseases, 23
genetic factors, psoriasis, 267
genetics, 81
genital herpes infections, 173
genital herpes simplex virus, 172
genital warts, 341
geriatric patients, abrasions/skin tears, 62
gingivostomatitis, 172
gluten-sensitive enteropathy (GSE), 177
gluten-tissue transglutaminase (t-TG), 178
granuloma annulare (GA)
    clinical presentation, 164–165
    differential diagnosis, 165
    epidemiology, 163
    overview, 163–164
    pathology/histology, 164
    patient education, 166
    special considerations, 166
    treatment/management, 165–166
gridding, cultural practices, 28
griseofulvin, 305, 309, 319
Group A *streptococci*, 188
grouped lesions, 21
GSE. *See* gluten-sensitive enteropathy
guttate psoriasis, 267

hair, in pregnancy, 30
hair follicles, 16
    growth, continuous cycle of, 71
    T-cell-mediated autoimmune
        disease, 72
    types of, 71
hair loss disorders
hair-pull test aids, 75
harlequin ichthyosis, 24
head lice infestation, 204
Heck disease, 339, 340
hepatitis, 189
herald patch, 259, 260
herbal therapies, atopic dermatitis/eczema, 137
heredity, 332
    nails, special considerations, 237
herpes labialis, 171
herpes simplex virus (HSV)
    dermatitis herpetiformis, 177–179
    herpes zoster, 180–186
    *Herpetic Whitlow*, 175–177
    HSV-1, 169–172
    HSV-2, 172–175
    varicella, 186–191
herpes simplex virus type 1
    (HSV-1)
    clinical presentation, 170–171
    differential diagnosis, 171
    epidemiology, 170
    overview, 169–170
    pathology/histology, 170
    patient education, 172
    special considerations, 171–172
    treatment/management, 171
herpes simplex virus type 2 (HSV-2)
    clinical presentation, 173–174
    differential diagnosis, 174
    epidemiology, 172–173
    genital herpes, 175
    overview, 172
    in pregnancy, 174
    pathology/histology, 173
    patient education, 175
    seropositivity of, 172
    special considerations, 174
    treatment/management, 174
*Herpesviridae*, 170, 173
herpes zoster
    clinical presentation, 181–182
    conditions, 182
    differential diagnosis, 182–183
    epidemiology, 181
    overview, 180
    pathology/histology, 181
    patient education, 185–186
    signs and symptoms, 181
    special considerations, 184–185
    treatment/management, 183–184

herpes zoster ophthalmicus (Hutchinson sign), 185
herpes zoster oticus (Ramsay Hunt syndrome), 185
herpes zoster vaccine (Zostavax), 186
herpetic gingivostomatitis, 170
  acute, 170
herpetic pharyngotonsillitis, acute, 171
herpetic urethritis, 173
herpetic vesicles
  in men, 173
  in women, 173
*Herpetic Whitlow*
  clinical presentation, 176
  differential diagnosis, 176
  epidemiology, 176
  overview, 175–176
  pathology/histology, 176
  patient education, 177
  special considerations, 177
  treatment/management, 176–177
herpetiform, 21
herpetiform ulceration, 80
hidradenitis suppurativa (HS)
  axilla, 118
  clinical presentation, 119–120
  diabetics, 121
  differential diagnosis, 120
  epidemiology, 119
  genetic factors, 121
  growth, continuous cycle of, 71
  hormonal factors, 121
  hypercholesterolemia, 122
  immune factors, 121
  infection, 121
  lithium, 122
  overview, 118
  pathology/histology, 119
  patient education, 122
  sirolimus, 122
  smoking, 122
  special considerations, 121–122
  treatment/management, 120–121
hilar adenopathy, 158
histamine, 322
Hodgkin's disease, 159
homocysteine levels, 348
$H_1$ histamine receptors, 322
hormonal changes, 81
hormonal therapy, 68
hormone levels, seborrheic dermatitis, 143
HPV. *See* human papillomavirus
HS. *See* hidradenitis suppurativa
HSV. *See* herpes simplex virus
HSV-1. *See* herpes simplex virus type 1
HSV-2. *See* herpes simplex virus type 2
$H_2$-blocking drugs, 211
$H_2$ histamine receptors, 322

human lice
  differential diagnosis of, 206
  types of, 205
human papillomavirus (HPV), 281, 337
  transmission, 339
Hutchinson sign (herpes zoster ophthalmicus), 185
hygiene factor of atopic dermatitis, 136
hyperthermia treatment, 342
hypnosis, for warts, 342
hypocomplementemic urticarial vasculitis, 328
hypodermis, 15


I&D. *See* incision and drainage
ICD. *See* irritant contact dermatitis
IgA. *See* immunoglobulin A
IgG autoantibodies, 250
imiquimod (Aldara), 45, 282, 287, 341
immune disorders, 81
immunocompromised patients (HIV), 252
immunoglobulin A (IgA), 178
immunologic factors, psoriasis, 267
immunosuppressed patients' warts, 340
immunosuppression, 283
immunosuppressive drugs, 252
impetigo
  categories, 194
  children, 193
  clinical presentation, 194
  differential diagnosis, 195
  epidemiology, 193
  pathology/histology, 194
  patient education, 196
  special considerations, 196
  treatment/management, 195–196
incision and drainage (I&D), 47
indirect immunofluorescence (IDIF), 252
infants, 27
  abrasions/skin tears, 63
  scabies, characteristic sign of, 203
infections
  of atopic dermatitis, 136
  tinea. *See* tinea infections
infiltrative basal cell carcinoma, 285, 286
inflammatory acne, 65
infundibulocystic type basal cell carcinoma, 285
ingrown toenail
  clinical presentation, 236
  differential diagnosis, 236
  overview, 235
  epidemiology, 236
  pathology/histology, 236
  patient education, 238
  special considerations, 237
  treatment/management, 48–49, 236–237
ingrown toenails, treatment of, 48–49
ink-spot lentigines, 214

insect bites
   lice. *See* lice
   scabies. *See* scabies
   stings. *See* stings
intense pulsed light therapy, 276
intentional injury, patterns of, 22–25
interferon alfa-2b, 287
interlesional injection of corticosteroids, 47
intertriginous lesions, 22
intradermal melanocytic nevus, 217
intradermal nevi, 219
intralesional injections, 342
intravenous acyclovir, 190
invasive squamous cell carcinoma, 298
inverse psoriasis, 267
iPLEDGE program, 68
iris-target lesions, 21
irritant contact dermatitis (ICD), 129
   ACD versus, 131
isotretinoin, 68, 237
itching, 202
itraconazole, 305
ivermectin, 203

jellyfish sting, 40
junctional nevi, 218

KA. *See* keratoacanthoma
keloid, 20
keratinases, 313
keratinocyte cell membrane, 250
keratinophilic fungi, 311
keratoacanthoma (KA), 297
keratosis pilaris (KP)
   clinical presentation, 124
   differential diagnosis, 124
   epidemiology, 124
   overview, 123
   pathology/histology, 124
   patient education, 125
   risk factors for, 124
   special considerations, 125
   treatment/management, 124–125
keratotic basal cell carcinoma, 285, 286
Koebner phenomenon, 36, 347
KP. *See* keratosis pilaris

lactate dehydrogenase (LDH) level, 292
lamivudine, 237
Langerhans cells, 16
larger-vessel vasculitis, 328
laser therapy, 276, 282, 342
latency
   HSV-1, 170
   HSV-2, 173

LCV. *See* leukocytoclastic vasculitis
LDH level. *See* lactate dehydrogenase level
lentigo
   clinical presentation, 214–215
   differential diagnosis, 215
   epidemiology, 213
   overview, 213
   pathology/histology, 213–214
   patient education, 216
   special considerations, 215
   treatment/management, 215
lentigo maligna melanoma, 290
leptomeninges, 181
lesions, 19
   cauterization of, 46
   HSV-1 and HSV-2, 173
leukocytoclastic vasculitis (LCV)
   clinical presentation, 328–329
   differential diagnosis, 329
   epidemiology, 328
   overview, 327
   pathology/histology, 328
   patient education, 330
   special considerations, 330
   treatment/management, 329–340
leukotrichia, 346
lice
   clinical presentation, 205
   differential diagnosis, 206
   epidemiology, 204
   overview, 204
   pathology/histology, 205
   special considerations, 207
   treatment/management, 206–207
lichenification, 20
lichen planus (LP)
   clinical presentation, 224–225
   differential diagnosis, 225
   epidemiology, 224
   overview, 223
   pathology/histology, 224
   patient education, 226
   special considerations, 226
   treatment/management, 225
lichen simplex chronicus (LSC)
   causes of, 141
   clinical presentation, 140
   differential diagnosis, 140–141
   epidemiology, 139
   overview, 138
   pathology/histology, 139–140
   patient education, 142
   treatment/management, 141
linear lesions, 21
lingua villosa nigra, 98
livedoreticularis, 329
LM. *See* longitudinal melanonychia
localized granuloma annulare, 165, 166

localized lesions, 22
localized vitiligo, 347
longitudinal melanonychia (LM), 238
LP. *See* lichen planus
LSC. *See* lichen simplex chronicus
lymphohistiocytic infiltrate, 158, 164
lymphoma, 159

macule, 19
magnification, diagnostics, 41
Majocchi granuloma, 308
major histocompatibility complex (MHC) Class II molecules, 250
*Malassezia furfur*, 142, 143, 145, 318
malignancy
  for varicella, 187
  workup for herpes zoster, 183
malignant melanoma
  clinical presentation, 290–291
  differential diagnosis, 292
  epidemiology, 289
  overview, 288
  pathology/histology, 289–290
  patient education, 295
  resources for patients, 295
  risk factors, 293
  special considerations, 293–294
  treatment/management, 292–293
marginal inflammatory vitiligo, 347
MCV. *See* molluscum contagiosum virus
medial knee, abrasion, 62
melanocytes, 16, 289, 346
melanocytic nevi, 217–219
melanoma, 28
melanonychia
  clinical presentation, 239
  differential diagnosis, 239
  epidemiology, 238
  overview, 238
  pathology/histology, 238–239
  patient education, 240–240
  special considerations, 239
  treatment/management, 239
metatypical basal cell carcinoma, 285
methicillin-resistant *Staphylococcus aureus* (MRSA) infection, 112
methotrexate, 269
micronodular basal cell carcinoma, 285, 286
microscopic examination of involved skin, 346
*Microsporum audouinii*, 303
*Microsporum canis*, 303
miescher nevi, 219
milia cyst
  clinical presentation, 126
  differential diagnosis, 126
  epidemiology, 125
  overview, 125

  pathology/histology, 126
  patient education, 127
  special considerations, 126
  treatment/management, 126
  types of, 126
Mohs micrographic surgery, 47
moisturizer, 54–55
molluscum contagiosum virus (MCV)
  characteristics of, 231
  clinical presentation, 230–231
  conditions, 231
  differential diagnosis, 231
  epidemiology, 230
  overview, 229
  pathology/histology, 230
  patient education, 233
  special considerations, 232
  treatment/management, 231–232
morbidity, 236
  in pemphigus vulgaris, 249
morbilliform, 21
morpheaform (sclerosing) basal cell carcinoma, 285, 286
mortality in pemphigus vulgaris, 249
mosaic wart, 340
Moxibustion, cultural practices, 28
MRSA infection. *See* methicillin-resistant *Staphylococcus aureus* infection
mucous membranes, 250
multiform lesions, 21
myrmecia warts, 340

nail conditions
  ingrown nails, 235–238
  melanonychia, 238–240
  onychomycosis, 240–243
  paronychia, 243–246
narrow-band ultraviolet (UV)-B phototherapy, 348
National Alopecia Areata Foundation, 77
necrobiosis lipoidica diabeticorum (NLD), 31
neonatal HSV infection, 174
neonatal pemphigus, 251
neonatal varicella, 186
neonates, abrasions/skin tears, 63
neurodermatitis (ND). *See* lichen simplex chronicus (LSC)
neurogenic factors, seborrheic dermatitis, 143
neurogenic inflammation, 256
neurovirulence
  HSV-1, 170
  HSV-2, 173
nevi
  classification of, 217
  clinical presentation, 218–219
  differential diagnosis, 219
  epidemiology, 217
  overview, 216

nevi (cont.)
  pathology/histology, 217–218
  patient education, 220
  special considerations, 220
  treatment/management, 219–220
Nikolsky sign, 36–37
  for pemphigus vulgaris, 251
NLD. See necrobiosis lipoidica diabeticorum
nodular basal cell carcinoma, 284, 286
nodular lesions, 329
nodular melanoma, 290
nonbullous impetigo, 194
nondermatophytic molds, onychomycosis, 240–241
nongenital warts, 337
nonpustular lesions, 274
nonsteroidal anti-inflammatory drugs (NSAIDs), 92, 93
nummular, 21
nummular eczema, refractory cases of, 56, 57
nutritional counseling, 55–56
nystatin suspension, 103
nystatin troche, 103

ocular manifestations, 274
ocular rosacea, 274, 276
older adult, abrasions/skin tears, 62
OM. See onychomycosis
onychomycosis (OM)
  clinical presentation, 241–242
  differential diagnosis, 242
  epidemiology, 240–241
  overview, 240
  pathology/histology, 241
  patient education, 243
  special considerations, 243
  treatment/management, 242–243
Orabase, 82
oral acyclovir, 177
oral antibiotics, 276
  atopic dermatitis/eczema, 137
oral antifungal treatments, for symptomatic infections, 106
oral azole antifungals, 319
oral candidiasis
  clinical presentation, 102–103
  differential diagnosis, 103
  epidemiology, 102
  overview, 102
  pathology/histology, 102
  patient education, 104
  special considerations, 103
  treatment/management, 103
oral contraceptive therapy, 276
oral itraconazole, 310
oral ketoconazole, 305, 310
oral psoriasis, 268
oral terbinafine, 310

order chest radiographs, 160
owl's eye cells, 339

palmar erythema, in pregnancy, 29
palms and soles, 22
papules, 19, 165
papulopustular lesions, 274
papulopustular rosacea, 274
parakeratosis, 266
paronychia
  clinical presentation, 244–245
  differential diagnosis, 245
  epidemiology, 244
  overview, 243
  pathology/histology, 244
  patient education, 246
  special considerations, 246
  treatment/management, 245–246
pathogenetic mechanisms of granuloma annulare, 164
patient education
  actinic keratosis, 283
  basal cell carcinoma, 288
  black hairy tongue, 99
  diaper dermatitis, 101
  malignant melanoma, 295
  oral candidiasis, 104
  psoriasis, 270
  squamous cell carcinoma, 299
  tinea capitis, 306
  tinea corporis, 310
  tinea faciei, 313
  tinea pedis, 316
  tinea versicolor, 320
  vulvovaginal candidiasis, 107
Payne–Martin Classification System, 61
PCR. See polymerase chain reaction
PDT. See photodynamic therapy
Pediculus humanus capitis, 205
Pediculus humanus corporis, 205
pemphigus vulgaris
  clinical presentation, 250–251
  differential diagnosis, 251
  epidemiology, 249–250
  multidisciplinary approach, 252
  overview, 249
  pathology/histology, 250
  patient education, 252–253
  special considerations, 252
  special considerations, 252
  treatment/management, 251–252
penile lentigo, 214
perforating granuloma annulare, 165
perifollicular lymphocytic infiltrates, 346
perioral dermatitis (POD)
  clinical presentation, 256
  differential diagnosis, 256

epidemiology, 255
overview, 255
pathology/histology, 256
patient education, 257
special considerations, 257
treatment/management, 256–257
persistent EM, 155
petaloid type, 144
petechiae, 20, 21
PHN. *See* postherpetic neuralgia
photodynamic therapy (PDT), 121, 282, 342
*phthiraptera*, 205
phymatous rosacea, 274
pigmented basal cell carcinoma, 285, 286
pimecrolimus cream, 257
  seborrheic dermatitis, 145
pityriasiform type, 144
pityriasis rosea (PR)
  clinical presentation, 260–261
  differential diagnosis, 261
  epidemiology, 259
  overview, 259
  pathology/histology, 260
  patient education, 262
  special considerations, 262
  treatment/management, 261–262
pityriasis rosea-like drug eruptions, 260
*Pityrosporum*, 318
plane warts, 340
plantar warts, 337, 338
plaque, 19
  plaque psoriasis, 267
POD. *See* perioral dermatitis
podophyllotoxin, 341
polycystic lesions, 21
polycystic ovarian syndrome (POS), 66
polymerase chain reaction (PCR), to Tzanck smear, 183
POS. *See* polycystic ovarian syndrome
positive Nikolsky sign, 251
postherpetic neuralgia (PHN), 182, 184
poststreptococcal glomerulonephritis, 203
potassium hydroxide (KOH) examination, 40–41, 309
PR. *See* pityriasis rosea
prednisone, 349
pregnancy, 159
  areolas, 29
  diabetes, 30–31
  hair, 30
  palmar erythema, 29
  striae distensae, 29
  and varicella, 187
  varicose veins and, 333
pregnant women, pemphigus vulgaris, 252
preventive care, 52
primary care providers, 4, 5
  dermatology for, 3
primary skin lesion, 19–20, 36

probiotics, atopic dermatitis/eczema, 137
progressive disorder, vitiligo, 345
prominent mucosal involvement, 152
*Propionibacterium acnes*, 66
propolis, 342
proximal subungualonychomycosis (PSO), 241, 242
pruritic rash, 188
pruritus, 189, 260, 261
psoralen photochemotherapy, 348
psoralen with UV-A (PUVA) therapy, 225, 348
psoriasis
  causes of, 266
  clinical presentation, 267–268
  differential diagnosis, 268
  epidemiology, 265
  overview, 265
  pathology/histology, 265–267
  patient education, 270–271
  special considerations, 270
  treatment/management, 268–270
  types of, 267
psoriatic arthritis, 268
*Pthirus pubis*, 205, 207
  transmission, source of, 200
puberty, 29
pulmonary function tests, vascularitis, 330
punch biopsy, 39
purpura, 20, 21
pustular psoriasis, 267
pustule, 19
PUVA lentigo, 214
PUVA therapy. *See* psoralen with UV-A therapy
pyoderma faciale, 274


quadrichrome vitiligo, 347
quality of life, implications, 5


radiation lentigo, 214
radiotherapy, 121
Ramsay Hunt syndrome (herpes zoster oticus), 185
RAS. *See* recurrent aphthous stomatitis
rash, 19
  documentation of, 19
  of zoster, 181
reactivation
  HSV-1, 170
  HSV-2, 173
receptor-selective acetylenic retinoid tazarotene (Tazorac), 287
recurrent aphthous stomatitis (RAS), 79
  diagnosis of, 80
  goals of therapy for, 82
  predisposing factors of, 81
  treatment for, 81
  ulcer caused, 80

regional lymphadenopathy, 176
retinoids, 121, 276, 342
Rituximab, 252
rosacea
   clinical presentation, 274–275
   differential diagnosis, 275
   epidemiology, 273
   overview, 273
   pathology/histology, 274
   patient education, 277
   special considerations, 276
   treatment/management, 275–276
rosacea fulminans, 274
routine skin care, 51–52

salicylic acid, 67
sarcoidosis, 159
sarcomatoid carcinoma, 297
*Sarcoptes scabiei*, 199
scabies
   clinical presentation, 201–202
   differential diagnosis, 202
   epidemiology, 200
   histologic features, 201
   immunodeficiency disorders, 200
   overview, 199
   pathology/histology, 200–201
   patient education, 204
   special considerations, 203
   treatment/management, 203
scalp psoriasis, 268
scar, 20
SCD. *See* systemic contact dermatitis
scleredema diabeticorum, 31
scraping, 40–41
screening for diabetes, 348
sebaceous cysts. *See* epidermal inclusion cysts
sebaceous glands, 16
seborrheic dermatitis (SD)
   clinical presentation, 143–144
   differential diagnosis, 144
   epidemiology, 143
   medications, 145
   overview, 142
   pathology/histology, 143
   patient education, 146
   special considerations, 145
   strategies, 145
   treatment/management, 144–145
   types of, 144
sebum, 16, 27, 66
secondary skin lesion, 20
   anatomy and physiology, 17
self-examination, of skin, 52–53
sensitivity testing, 39
serologic studies, 329
serpiginous lesions, 21

sexually transmitted diseases, 233
sexually transmitted infection (STI), 204
shampoos, 306
   seborrheic dermatitis, 145
Sha rash, 28
shave biopsy, 39
shingles. *See* herpes zoster
simple lentigo, 213
skin
   anatomy and physiology, 15–18
   diagnostic evaluations, 21
   distribution, type, characteristics, and pattern of lesions, 22
   special distribution category, 22
   terminology, 19–20
   vascular lesions, 21
skin assessment
   dermatologic signs, 36–37
   differential diagnosis, 37–38
   family history, 36
   medical history, 35
   physical, 35–36
   social history, 36
skin biopsy, 39
   basal cell carcinoma, 287
   psoriasis, 268
   specimens, 251
   of tinea corporis, 308
   of tinea pedis, 313
skin cancer
   actinic keratosis, 279–283
   basal cell carcinoma, 283–288
   malignant melanoma, 288–295
   overview, 279
   squamous cell carcinoma, 295–299
skin disorders
   epidemiology and statistics of, 4–5
   total economic burden of, 5
skin lesions, excision of, 47
skin self-examination, 52–53
Skin Tear Audit Research (STAR), 61
skin tears
   abrasions. *See* abrasions/skin tears
   categories, 61
smoking, 270
   creating wrinkles, 51
   psoriasis, 270
social history, skin assessment, 36
solar keratosis. *See* actinic keratosis (AK)
solar lentigo, 213
SPF. *See* sun protective factor
SPF 15 sunscreen, consistent use of, 53
spider veins
   clinical presentation, 332–333
   differential diagnosis, 333
   epidemiology, 332
   overview, 331–332
   pathology/histology, 332

patient education, 334
special considerations, 333–334
treatment/management, 333
spindle cell (sarcomatoid)
  carcinoma, 297
spironolactone (Aldactone), 68
spitz nevi, 218, 219
squamous cell carcinoma (SCC)
  clinical presentation, 297–298
  differential diagnosis, 298
  epidemiology, 295–296
  overview, 295
  pathology/histology, 296–297
  patient education, 299
  special considerations, 299
  treatment/management, 298
SSC in situ (SSCIS), 296, 298
*Staphylococcus aureus*, 136, 148, 193, 203
  infection, 95
STAR. *See* Skin Tear Audit Research
stasis dermatitis
  clinical presentation, 147
  differential diagnosis, 147–148
  epidemiology, 146
  overview, 146
  pathology/histology, 146–147
  patient education, 149
  special considerations, 148
  treatment/management, 148
steroids
  lichen simplex chronicus/neurodermatitis, 141
  for varicella, 187
  for varicella-zoster virus, 184
stings
  clinical presentation, 208–209
  differential diagnosis, 210
  epidemiology, 207–208
  overview, 207
  pathology/histology, 208
  patient education, 211–212
  special considerations, 211
  treatment/management, 210–211
*stratum corneum*, 15
*stratum germinativum*, 15
*Streptococcus aureus*, 148, 185
stress, 81
stretch marks. *See* striae distensae
striae distensae, in pregnancy, 29
subcutaneous granuloma annulare, 165
subungual melanoma, 238, 239
sucking lice. *See* anoplura
sulfapyridine, 179
sunburn, 90
  prevention, 94
sun damage, prevention of, 77
sun exposure, 22, 23, 51, 52
sun protective factor (SPF), 51, 54, 94
sunscreen, 54

preventive care, 52
routine skin care, 51–52
superficial basal cell carcinoma, 285, 286
superficial perivascular, 346
superficial spreading melanoma, 290
superficial veins, 332
suprabasal epidermal cells, 250
surgical treatment, cauterization of lesions, 46
symmetrical lesions, 22
symptomatic infections, topical and oral antifungal
  treatments for, 106
synthetic fibers (polyester), protection from sun, 53
systematic review, 6
systemic agents, for warts, 342
systemic azoles, 310
systemic contact dermatitis (SCD), 131
  elicitation stage, 131
  sensitization stage, 131
systemic evaluation, treatment and, 45
systemic phototherapy, 348
systemic retinoids, 269
systemic steroids (prednisone), 262, 349
systemic therapy
  tinea corporis, 309
  tinea versicolor, 319

tanning-bed lentigines, 214
tar, 269
target lesions, 21
Tazorac, 287
TBSA. *See* total body surface area
T-cell-mediated immunity, 260
telangiectasia, 20
telogen effluvium
  clinical presentation, 73
  pathology/histology, 73
telogen phase, 71
terbinafine, 305, 319
terminal hair follicles, 71
therapeutic interventions, for varicella-zoster
  virus, 184
thrush. *See* oral candidiasis
thyrotropin testing, 348
tinea barbae, 310
tinea capitis
  clinical presentation, 304
  differential diagnosis, 305
  epidemiology, 303
  overview, 303
  pathology/histology, 303–304
  patient education, 306
  special considerations, 306
  treatment/management, 305–306
tinea corporis
  clinical presentation, 308
  differential diagnosis, 308–309
  epidemiology, 307

tinea corporis (cont.)
  overview, 306
  pathology/histology, 307–308
  patient education, 310
  special considerations, 310
  treatment/management, 309–310
tinea corporis gladiatorum, 308
tinea corporis purpurica, 308
tinea faciei
  clinical presentation, 311
  differential diagnosis, 311–312
  epidemiology, 311
  overview, 310
  pathology/histology, 311
  patient education, 313
  special considerations, 312
  treatment/management, 312
tinea imbricata, 308
tinea incognito, 308
tinea pedis
  clinical presentation, 314–315
  differential diagnosis, 315
  epidemiology, 313
  overview, 313
  pathology/histology, 313–314
  patient education, 316
  special considerations, 316
  treatment/management, 315
tinea versicolor
  clinical presentation, 318
  differential diagnosis, 319
  epidemiology, 318
  overview, 316–317
  pathology/histology, 318
  patient education, 320
  special considerations, 319
  treatment/management, 319
  types of, 318
TNF-α. *See* tumor necrosis factor-alpha
TNM classification system. *See* tumor-node-metastasis classification system
tobacco, 81
  atopic dermatitis, 136
topical 5-fluorouracil, 287
topical antiacne medications, 257
topical antibiotics, 67
topical antifungals
  tinea versicolor, 319
  symptomatic infections, treatments for, 106
topical anti-inflammatory agents, 257
topical azoles, 309
topical benzoyl peroxide, 67
topical corticosteroids
  seborrheic dermatitis, 144
  treatment, 44
topical emollients, atopic dermatitis/eczema, 136
topical medication, 43–44
  antibacterial, 45
  antifungals, 45

chemotherapeutics, 45
steroids, 44
topical pimecrolimus (Elidel), atopic dermatitis/eczema, 137
topical retinoids, 269
topical steroids, 44, 269
  atopic dermatitis/eczema, 136
  seborrheic dermatitis, 145
topical tacrolimus (Protopic), atopic dermatitis/eczema, 137
topical therapies, 257, 275
topical vitamin D analogs, 269
total body surface area (TBSA), 91
  erythema multiforme (EM), 151–155
  erythema nodosum, 157–160
  granuloma annulare (GA), 165–166
  pityriasis rosea (PR), 261–262
  POD, 256–257
  rosacea, 275–276
  urticaria 324–325
  verruca vulgaris, 340–343
  vitiligo, 348–349
tretinoin, 342
*Trichophyton* infections, 303
*Trichophyton mentagrophytes*, 241, 304, 307
*Trichophyton rubrum*, 240, 241
*Trichophyton tonsurans*, 303
*Trichophyton verrucosum*, 307
trichrome vitiligo, 346
t-TG. *See* gluten-tissue transglutaminase
tumor necrosis factor-alpha (TNF-α), 80
tumor-node-metastasis (TNM) classification system, 291
Tyndall phenomenon, 219
type I allergic immunoglobulin E (IgE) response, 322
type II allergic response, 322
type III immune complex disease, 322
Tzanck smear, 40, 183, 189

ulcer, 20, 329
ultraviolent protection factor (UPF), 53
ultraviolet (UV)-B phototherapy, 262
ultraviolet (UV) rays, 53, 89
unilateral lesions, 22
unintentional injury, patterns of, 22–25
universal lesions, 22
universal vitiligo, 347
UPF. *See* ultraviolent protection factor
urticaria
  clinical presentation, 322–323
  differential diagnosis, 323–324
  epidemiology, 322
  overview, 321
  pathology/histology, 322
  patient education, 326
  special considerations, 325
  treatment/management, 324–325

urticarial vasculitis lesions, 328
U.S. Centers for Disease Control and Prevention, 207
U.S. Surveillance, Epidemiology, and End Results (SEER) program, 288
UV irradiation, 270
UV radiation, 294
UV rays. *See* ultraviolet rays

vagabond skin, 205
varicella, 186, 188
   clinical presentation, 188–189
   differential diagnosis, 189
   epidemiology, 187
   etiology, 186–187
   malignancy, 187
   overview, 186
   pathology/histology, 188
   patient education, 190–191
   pregnancy, 187
   risk factors for, 187
   special considerations, 190
   steroid therapy, 187
   treatment/management, 189–190
   vaccine, 187
varicella-zoster virus (VZV), 180, 181, 183–184, 186
   antivirals, 183
   gabapentin, 184
   steroids, 184
   therapeutic interventions, 184
   treatment for, 183
varicose veins
   clinical presentation, 332–333
   differential diagnosis, 333
   epidemiology, 332
   overview, 331–332
   pathology/histology, 332
   patient education, 334
   special considerations, 333–334
   treatment/management, 333
vascular lesions, 21
vasculitis
   leukocytoclastic, 327–331
   spider and varicose veins, 331–334
VC. *See* verrucous carcinoma
vellus hair follicles, 71
vemurafenib, 293
venous insufficiency syndrome, 331
venous system, history of, 333
verruca plana, 340
verruca vulgaris
   clinical presentation, 339–340
   differential diagnosis, 340
   epidemiology, 337–339
   overview, 337
   pathology/histology, 339
   patient education, 343

   special considerations, 343
   treatment/management, 340–343
verrucous carcinoma (VC), 297
vesicles, 20, 203
vesiculobullous lesions, 152
viral exanthem, of leg, 38
viral pneumonia, 188
visceral angiography, 330
vitamin A deficiency, skin manifestations, 56
vitamin $B_1$ (thiamine) deficiency, skin manifestations, 55
vitamin D analogs, 349
vitamin D deficiency, 271
vitamin K deficiency, skin manifestations, 56
vitiligo, 31
   clinical presentation, 346–347
   differential diagnosis, 347–348
   epidemiology, 346
   overview, 345
   pathology/histology, 346
   patient education, 350
   special considerations, 349
   treatment/management, 348
vulvar lentigo, 214–215
vulvovaginal candidiasis (VVC)
   clinical presentation, 105
   differential diagnosis, 105
   epidemiology, 104
   overview, 104
   pathology/histology, 105
   patient education, 107
   special considerations, 106
   treatment/management, 105–106
VVC. *See* vulvovaginal candidiasis
VZV. *See* varicella-zoster virus

warts. *See* verruca vulgaris
warty squamous cell carcinoma, 297
water-soluble vitamin deficiencies, skin manifestations, 55
wheal, 20
white superficial onychomycosis (WSO), 241, 242
women, vitiligo affects, 349
Wood's light, 41, 205, 304, 319
WSO. *See* white superficial onychomycosis

xeroderma pigmentosum (XP), 24, 299

yeasts, onychomycosis, 241

Zelboraf, 293
Zilactin-B, 82
zinc salts, 121
Zostavax (herpes zoster vaccine), 186